Biomarkers in Dermatology

Robert Norman
Editor

Biomarkers in Dermatology

Springer

Editor
Robert Norman
Professor of Dermatology
Nova Southeastern University
Tampa, USA

ISBN 978-3-031-66512-7 ISBN 978-3-031-66513-4 (eBook)
https://doi.org/10.1007/978-3-031-66513-4

This Springer imprint is published by the registered company Springer Nature Switzerland AG
The registered company address is: Gewerbestrasse 11, 6330 Cham, Switzerland

In Memoriam

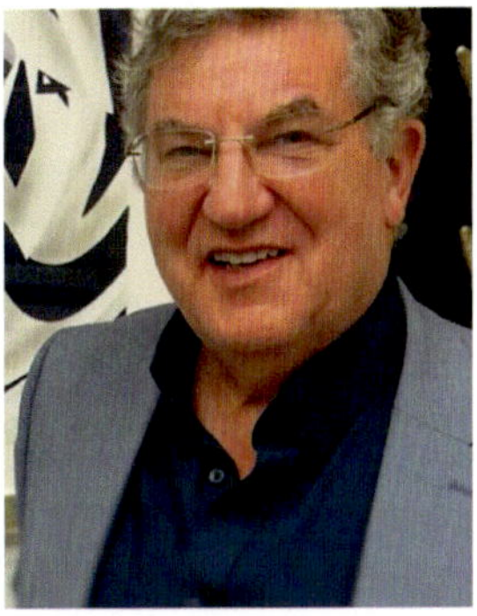

Dr. Rob Norman
1955–2025

Dr. Robert A. Norman, known affectionately as "Rob" or "Zayde" to his family, "Doc Rob" to his friends, and "Doc" to the many patients whose lives he touched, passed away on February 14, 2025, due to complications of pneumonia following a successful stem cell transplant.

His passion for medicine was matched by his love for writing, having authored hundreds of articles and 76 published books. He was passionate about education and, with this title, wanted to communicate the importance of understanding and using biomarkers for early diagnosis and effective treatment of many skin diseases. He had been working on this edition until a few weeks before his death.

Foreword

Dermatologic conditions have a profound impact on physical and social aspects of patients' lives. Although we are in the golden age of treatment modalities, disease monitoring lags. While common conditions such as atopic dermatitis and psoriasis have many treatment options, new treatment options are desperately needed for patients with other chronic skin diseases.

Biomarkers have become an indispensable monitoring and decision-making tool in many non-dermatologic conditions. Since the skin is an open window on its own condition, there has been less pressure to develop biomarkers in dermatology. While skin characteristics may be measured objectively, the patient's subjective experience can complicate management and underlying systemic effects may not be so readily observed. Biomarkers can serve as another objective measure to support drug development, monitor treatment progress, and objectively define disease severity. Biomarkers can support clinical decision-making and relieve stress on the medical system. In patients with recalcitrant disease, frequent visits are necessary to fine-tune medications. Such visits are impractical and costly. Incorporating biomarkers in dermatology may eliminate unnecessary office visits and enhance outpatient monitoring.

The fresh perspective in this book may accelerate the update of biomarkers in dermatology. Dr. Robert Norman has provided that perspective. He was a very active member in the dermatology community and was faculty for several Medical, PA, and ARNP schools. His altruism extended to the international community through medical mission trips to Haiti, Cuba, Jamaica, and Argentina. Dr. Norman has provided his unique perspective and valuable insights in 70 books and now has taken on biomarkers in dermatology.

Dr. Norman's book describes serologic and histologic biomarkers across a wide range of dermatologic conditions and their evolving role in clinical practice. Biomarkers are newcomers in dermatology, and their impact on the field is yet to be realized. This book provides a major step forward in the implementation of biomarkers in dermatology and will help to greatly improve the care of our patients.

Dr. Norman lived his life in service to others, building a brighter future for all. His legacy as mentor, physician, and visionary will leave an everlasting mark on dermatology.

Florida, USA

Chenan Andy Huang

Preface

Biomarkers are exciting new tools granting both physicians and patients the ability to assess patient health status. As a complex, rapidly-emerging medical field, the Food and Drug Administration (FDA) has put in a great deal of effort into formulating and consolidating common definitions to be used in the "Biomarkers, EndpointS, and other Tools," or BEST, resource. Under this system of classification, there are six different subtypes to biomarkers according to their application process: diagnostic, monitoring, pharmacodynamic/response, predictive, prognostic, and safety biomarkers. It is integral to remember that these subtypes have varying degrees of overlap depending on the specific biomarker in question. Utilized together, these different subtypes of biomarkers can paint a comprehensive picture of the patient's current health status, risk of disease development, remission, or progression, and response to various treatments.

Modern technology has made measuring levels of glucose, cytokines, or other markers much easier, to the point that a patient can measure their own levels outside of the clinical setting. Of course, this is a relatively new innovation in medicine that can pair well with the traditional methods involved in hands-on physical diagnosis, medical testing and data collection.

A plethora of benefits exists in utilizing biomarkers for patient health assessment. In certain cases, patients can use a variety of portable and/or wearable devices, ranging from watches to phones to skin-patch monitors, that allow them to measure their biomarker levels from the comfort of their home. Even sweat, saliva, and tears can be collected and processed to measure relevant biomarker data. This saves time for both patients and physicians when it comes to determining the health status of a patient and detect any complications that exist with a particular treatment regimen that a patient is receiving. For instance, diabetic patients are easily able to monitor their glucose levels at home to both assess the minute-to-minute variations in their levels as well as to assess the efficacy of their insulin regimens and adjust accordingly. We know the widespread negative effects of diabetes on the skin and the patient's full health and lifestyle, and every new and effective biomarker can help.

Combined with biomolecular genetic testing and other cutting-edge technology, we will be able to prevent and sometimes eliminate the curse of certain debilitating skin disease such as melanoma and severe bullous disease and lessen the blows of life quality-reducing maladies that inhabit our clinic and hospital patients and waste countless precious hours and dollars.

Another advantage of utilizing biomarkers over traditional methods of data collection is that biomarkers are objective measurements that cannot be readily skewed by observer bias. This ensures more accurate data collection in situations where bias can introduce complications. Most importantly, a combination of traditional medicine and biomarkers can give the physician a more complete picture of the patient's health status, which, as a result, gives them more knowledge on how to proceed. Biomarkers can help identify candidates for medical and/or surgical intervention who are more likely to respond well to treatment, serve as diagnostic tools for even the rarest pathological processes and ensure continuous monitoring of a patient's health status.

We must keep in mind that biomarkers have inherent risks to consider as well as their benefits. We do not yet know enough about the full accuracy of these biomarkers or if they are totally reliable to determine the exact health status of the patient. Biomarkers present complicated issues regarding patient privacy and cybersecurity. These are all questions that need to be answered to ensure that no harm befalls patients who are treated on the basis of biomarker analysis. Enormous research efforts are underway to compare the benefits to the risks.

Much of my interest and research over the last decade has been on the connection between the skin and the brain, including searching for skin biomarkers to detect Alzheimer's disease (AD) and the connection between Parkinson's disease (PD) and melanoma.

Neurodegenerative diseases are characterized by the presence of abnormal aggregates of proteins in brain tissue. Among them, the presence of aggregates of phosphorylated Tau protein (p-Tau) is the hallmark of Alzheimer's disease (AD) and other major neurodegenerative disorders such as corticobasal degeneration and frontotemporal dementia and implicated in Parkinson's disease (PD) among others.

What is Tau? Traditionally, it was considered a cytoplasmic protein whose major biological function would be to stabilize microtubules and facilitate axonal transport. According to this view, in AD there is a hyperphosphorylation of tau that leads to the intracellular accumulation of tau in the form of neurofibrillary tangles. Now we know that Tau protects the nuclear and chromatin organization for proper gene expression throughout neuronal life. Tau protein transfer to the cytoplasm results in loss of the protector role of nuclear Tau and the subsequent global chromatin disorganization. Therefore, the cytoplasmic Tau protein accumulations that characterize AD have been completely reinterpreted, as it is the search for new therapeutic solutions.

PD is a neurodegenerative disorder that triggers death of dopaminergic neurons within the brain's substantia nigra. This disorder is characterized by intracellular inclusions primarily composed of proteinaceous α-synuclein amyloid fibrils. Interestingly, there is a significant coincidence of PD and melanoma that may suggest a shared pathophysiology. Melanocytes are the pigmented cells that give rise to skin, hair and eye color, and melanoma is a potentially deadly cancer arising from melanocytes. Recently, we reported that PD and melanoma patients have increased staining for α-synuclein in their skin. We think that neurons and melanocytes, both derived from neuroectodermal cells, may share protein synthesis and regulation pathways that become dysfunctional in PD and melanoma. Therefore, uncovering the behavior of α-synuclein in melanoma could both provide novel approaches for treating melanoma and insights into the role of α-syn in PD. As Dean and Lee [1] noted, we should investigate how α-synuclein influences melanoma cell survival, because this may reveal new insights into α-synuclein function that may be used to prevent dopaminergic cell death and subsequently PD.

Identifying PD has been limited by inadequate sensitivity and specificity. Various diagnostic tests have been utilized, including olfactory function testing, cardiovascular autonomic testing, biological fluids (including CSF and blood) testing and PET or SPECT imaging. According to Rodríguez-Leyva [2, 3] and Wang and collaborators [4] skin deposition of misfolded α-synuclein is a potential biomarker for PD. For Donadio (2019) "the autonomic skin innervation is a useful site for the search of abnormal α-syn aggregates since peripheral sympathetic nerves could be the earliest affected neural region and autonomic symptoms may precede the classical symptoms of synucleinopathy, such as motor dysfunction in PD [5]."

Although Tau protein has previously been assumed to be exclusive to the central nervous system, it is also found in peripheral tissues. My colleagues Maria E. Jimenez-Capdeville, Ildefonso Rodríguez-Leyva, William Eng and others and I reported our research in 2017 on whether there is a differential Tau expression in oral mucosa cells according to cognitive impairment.

Immunocytochemistry and immunofluorescence revealed the presence of Tau and four p-Tau forms in the cytoplasm and nucleus of oral mucosa cells. More positivity was present in subjects with cognitive impairment than in control subjects, both in the nucleus and cytoplasm, in a speckle pattern. The mRNA expression of Tau by quantitative real-time polymerase chain reaction was higher in SCI as compared with the control group.

Our findings demonstrated the higher presence of p-Tau and Tau transcript in the oral mucosa of cognitively impaired subjects when compared with healthy subjects. The feasibility of p-Tau quantification by flow cytometry supported the prospective analysis of oral mucosa as a support tool for screening of proteinopathies in cognitively impaired patients. Utilizing oral swabs to gather our specimens and detecting biomarkers for dementia hopefully opens pathways for future researchers and patients themselves to assay these crucial markers and make key health decisions [6, 7].

As a clinician and researcher, I truly enjoy working with my colleagues who have inquisitive minds and are searching to unlock the mysteries of human life. Collaboration is a key to our progress and by sharing our important research and clinical findings, we can move ahead at a more effective and rapid pace. Dr. Steve Feldman swept into the scene with his outstanding students and contributed key chapters to our text. Some of my students added their magic and new and old colleagues filled the pages with amazing new insights and research.

Included in this book are a number of fascinating research and clinical approaches to diagnosing and treating various diseases with the use of biomarkers. I hope this book will be read and utilized by those thirsty for knowledge about the future of medicine and looking for ways to help their patients. Delayed by COVID-19, the book is finally seeing the light of day.

Dementia, skin cancer and many of the other issues addressed in this book are among the most important public health issues of our time. The sooner we can create new preventions and treatments based on the successful results of our collective hard work, the quicker we can alleviate the suffering of millions of diseased and debilitated co-inhabitants of our world.

Dr. Robert Norman has died before the publication of this book.

Tampa, USA Dr. Robert Norman

References

1. Dean DN, Lee JC. Linking Parkinson's disease and melanoma: interplay between α-synuclein and Pmel17 amyloid formation. 2021.
2. Rodríguez-Leyva I, Calderón-Garcidueñas AL, Jiménez-Capdeville ME, Rentería-Palomo AA, Hernandez-Rodriguez HG, Valdés-Rodríguez R, Fuentes-Ahumada C, Torres-Álvarez B, Sepúlveda-Saavedra J, Soto-Domínguez A, Santoyo ME, Rodriguez-Moreno JI, Castanedo-Cázares JP. α-Synuclein inclusions in the skin of Parkinson's disease and parkinsonism. Ann Clin Transl Neurol. 2014;1(7):471–8. https://doi.org/10.1002/acn3.78. Epub 2014 Jul 1. PMID: 25356418; PMCID: PMC4184776.
3. Rodríguez-Leyva I, Chi-Ahumada EG, Carrizales J, Rodríguez-Violante M, Velázquez-Osuna S, Medina-Mier V, Martel-Gallegos MG, Zarazúa S, Enríquez-Macías L, Castro A, Calderón-Garcidueñas AL, Jiménez-Capdeville ME. Parkinson disease and progressive supranuclear palsy: protein expression in skin. Ann Clin Transl Neurol. 2016;3(3):191–9. https://doi.org/10.1002/acn3.285. PMID: 27042679; PMCID: PMC4774258.
4. Wang Z, Becker K, Donadio V, Siedlak S, Yuan J, Rezaee M, Incensi A, Kuzkina A, Orrú CD, Tatsuoka C, Liguori R, Gunzler SA, Caughey B, Jimenez-Capdeville ME, Zhu X, Doppler K, Cui L, Chen SG, Ma J, Zou WQ. Skin α-synuclein aggregation seeding activity as a novel biomarker for Parkinson disease. JAMA Neurol. 2020;78(1):1–11. https://doi.org/10.1001/jamaneurol.2020.3311. Epub ahead of print. Erratum in: JAMA Neurol. 2021;78(1):120. PMID: 32986090; PMCID: PMC7522783.
5. Donadio V, Skin nerve α-synuclein deposits in Parkinson's disease and other synucleinopathies: a review. Clin Auton Res. 2019;29(6):577–85.
6. Arredondo LF, Aranda-Romo S, Rodríguez-Leyva I, Chi-Ahumada E, Saikaly SK, Portales-Pérez DP, González-Amaro R, Salgado Bustamante M, Enriquez-Macias L, Eng W, Norman RA, Jimenez Capdeville ME. Tau protein in oral mucosa and cognitive state: a cross-sectional study. Front Neurol. 2017;8:554.
7. Rodríguez-Leyva I, Chi-Ahumada E, Mejía M, Castanedo-Cazares JP, Eng W, Saikaly SK, Carrizales J, Levine TD, Norman RA, Jimenez-Capdeville ME. The presence of alpha-synuclein in skin from melanoma and patients with Parkinson's disease. Mov Disord Clin Pract. 2017;4(5):724–32. https://doi.org/10.1002/mdc3.12494. PMID: 30363411; PMCID: PMC6174388.

Contents

Chapter 1
Mitochondrial DNA Biomarkers in Skin Disease Featuring Skin Aging

Jessica A. Moor, Elizabeth Ruddy, Olusola C. Idowu, and Mark A. Birch-Machin

Abstract The skin is the largest organ of the human body and provides a barrier between the internal environment and stressors from the external environment, including ultraviolet radiation (UVR), pollution and harmful microorganisms. Mitochondria are known as the powerhouse of the cell due to their role in cellular energy production through the generation of adenosine triphosphate (ATP). They possess their own maternally inherited genome (mtDNA) which encodes 37 genes and is considered vulnerable to damage and mutations due to its close proximity to the site of energy production and therefore reactive oxygen species (ROS). Mitochondria have vital roles within the skin including energy generation, maintaining homeostasis and growth. Research suggests that mitochondrial dysfunction through mtDNA damage is associated with skin disorders such as skin aging, skin cancer and other diseases, and studies have identified mtDNA biomarkers in such skin disorders.

Keywords Mitochondria · Mitochondrial DNA · Skin · Skin disease · Skin aging · Reactive oxygen species · Mutations · Biomarkers

---

J. A. Moor · E. Ruddy · M. A. Birch-Machin (✉)
Dermatological Sciences, Translational and Clinical Research Institute, Medical School, Newcastle University, Newcastle upon Tyne NE2 4HH, UK
e-mail: mark.birch-machin@ncl.ac.uk

M. A. Birch-Machin
UK National Innovation Centre for Ageing, The Catalyst, 3 Science Square, Newcastle Helix, Newcastle upon Tyne NE4 5TG, UK

O. C. Idowu
HexisLab Ltd, The Catalyst, Newcastle Helix, Newcastle upon Tyne NE4 5TG, UK

R. Norman (ed.), *Biomarkers in Dermatology*,
https://doi.org/10.1007/978-3-031-66513-4_1

1.1 Introduction

1.1.1 The Skin

1.1.1.1 Skin Structure

The skin is the largest organ of the human body, accounting for 15% of total body weight with an average surface area of 2 m^2, and provides a barrier between the body and the external environment [1]. It is divided into three layers: epidermis, dermis and subcutaneous adipose layer, each containing several sublayers.

The epidermis is the uppermost layer of the skin with a thickness of 0.05–0.1 mm and is subsequently divided into five sublayers: stratum basale, stratum spinosum, stratum granulosum, stratum lucidum and stratum corneum [2, 3]. The most abundant cell type within the epidermis is keratinocytes, accounting for 95% of cells, which are responsible for the production of keratin, a structural protein synthesized for mechanical strength and skin waterproofing [4]. The stratum basale is the deepest layer of the epidermis, containing stem cells which differentiate into keratinocytes and migrate upwards through the layers of the epidermis [4]. Other cells present in this layer are melanocytes and Merkel cells. Melanocytes are responsible for the production of melanin from tyrosine, which offers a degree of protection to keratinocytes against the damaging effects of ultraviolet radiation (UVR). Different skin tones contain varying quantities of melanin in the skin, therefore providing differing levels of natural protection [2, 4]. Merkel cells act as mechanoreceptors for light touch, contributing to the sensory function of the skin [4]. As new keratinocytes are generated within the stratum basale, they migrate into stratum spinosum, contributing to up to 10 cell layers alongside Langerhans cells which are derived from bone barrow and are most prominent within this layer [2]. Langerhans cells interact with lymphocytes to stimulate an immune response, protecting the skin from environmental insults and microbes [4]. The stratum granulosum, also known as the granular layer, is up to 5 cell layers thick. Keratinocytes within this layer become more flattened and produce large quantities of keratin and keratohyalin which accumulate within the cells. The cells also lose their nuclei and begin to die due to increased distance from the blood supply which is located beneath the stratum basale, causing them to be devoid of nutrients and oxygen [3]. The stratum lucidum layer consists of 2–3 cell layers of mainly dead cells; only present in hairless parts of the body, where the skin is thick, such as the palms of hands and feet [5]. In this layer, the keratinocytes contain eleidin protein derived from keratohyalin, which contributes to limiting water loss [2]. The outermost layer of the epidermis is the stratum corneum, the skin layer which can be seen with the naked eye. This layer is hard and protective due to being composed of 15–20 layers of corneocytes which have progressively lost their nuclei and cytoplasmic organelles. Skin cells regenerate and the stratum corneum is replaced approximately every 4 weeks; however, this can differ with various skin conditions [2, 4].

Separating the epidermis from the dermis is the basement membrane, also known as the dermal–epidermal junction. Nutrients and proteins can diffuse from the dermis to the epidermis across this layer, although blood flow does not pass through [3]. The dermis is a connective tissue layer of mesenchymal origin and is divided into two layers: the papillary layer and the deeper reticular layer. The papillary dermis consists of lose connective tissue and vasculature, whereas the reticular dermis is made up of thick elastic fibers and is the principal part of the dermis [4, 6]. Cells present in the dermis are primarily fibroblasts but also include histiocytes, mast cells and adipocytes. Fibroblasts synthesize collagen and elastin contributing to skin elasticity and strength, with collagen types I and III being most predominant [7]. Also present in the dermis are nerve endings, hair follicles and sebaceous glands [5].

The subcutaneous adipose layer is the innermost layer which consists of adipocytes, nerves and blood vessels. This offers a supportive framework and can act as a shock absorber protecting organs, alongside functioning as fat storage and therefore providing thermal insulation [3].

Typically, the skin has an acidic pH ranging between 4.0 and 6.0 with areas of greatest hydration such as skin folds recording the highest pH values. Skin pH may vary depending on hydration of the skin, physical activity levels and external environmental conditions [6]. The maintenance of a healthy skin pH is reliant upon the production of lactic and amino acids, hydrogen and ammonium compounds as well as the composition of the epidermis, with pH having a significant role in limiting transepidermal water loss. Increased pH is associated with increased water loss [6].

1.1.1.2 Skin Function

The skin has many important functions such as acting as a barrier between the body and external environment by providing a degree of protection from the numerous environmental stressors it is regularly exposed to, such as UVR and pollution. Additionally, it possesses roles in immune response, thermoregulation, sensation and metabolism [6].

The barrier function of the skin typically refers to the stratum corneum layer of the epidermis, comprising corneocytes and the intracellular lipid matrix. Ceramides, cholesterol and fatty acids in the stratum corneum are key to the waterproof characteristic of the barrier as they are responsible for making this layer highly hydrophobic. This plays a significant role in preventing transepidermal water loss and the entrance of microorganisms due to being highly impermeable [8, 9].

The skin is the first line of defense from invading pathogens, with infections most likely to occur when the skin is broken such as through a wound. Present in the stratum spinosum and stratum granulosum are anti-microbial peptides, including defensins and cathelicidin, which are transported to the stratum corneum [8]. They possess the ability to kill microorganisms including bacteria, fungi and some viruses [8]. Langerhans cells are antigen presenting cells and also play a role in the protection against microorganisms through entering the dermal lymphatic system in response to epidermal injury in order to activate T-cells [10].

With repeated exposure to harmful external stressors, with UVR from the sun being one of the greatest insults, the skin is the first line of protection to defend against and reduce consequent damage such as photodamage, erythema and skin cancer. The amount of skin damage caused by UVR varies between people due to factors such as skin type, hydration and active usage of photoprotection with sunscreen and clothing. Some of the protective mechanisms of the skin against UVR include epidermal thickening, DNA repair, antioxidant enzymes and skin pigmentation caused by melanin production [11]. As a result of sunlight exposure, melanin is synthesized by melanosomes, produced by melanocytes in the stratum basale of the epidermis, in response to oxidation reactions [12]. The melanin is delivered to keratinocytes, with each melanocyte communicating with up to 40 keratinocytes, acting as a physical barrier through the scattering of UVR and as an absorbent barrier by reducing the amount of UVR able to penetrate through the epidermis [3, 11, 13]. Darker skin types have increased protection from UVR in comparison to lighter skin types due to increased melanin quantities and more efficient distribution, hence why individuals with darker skin types exhibit the clinical skins of photoaging at much later stages in comparison to those with fair skin. On the other hand, melanin has also been identified as a photosensitizer molecule by generating ROS upon UV irradiation [11, 14].

The skin has a significant role in thermoregulation via various mechanisms including secretion and evaporation. As body temperature rises, the skin excretes sweat from glands within the skin, releasing water, salt and urea from the body [6]. Sweat evaporates from the skin, cooling the body and therefore regulating body temperature. Additionally, skin contributes to thermoregulation via radiation and insulation of heat using blood vessels. Vasodilation is the expansion of blood vessels which reach the skin's surface to radiate heat in order to cool the body. The blood vessels can also undergo vasoconstriction to narrow the vessels to prevent heat loss from the skin, retaining body temperature [13].

Finally, sensory function is another vital role of the skin to aid survival, with many sensory receptors and free nerve endings distributed throughout the skin. This allows transmission of environmental information to the body which can lead to a cascade of changes in response to various stimuli [13]. There are many types of mechanoreceptors in the skin which respond to sensory changes including Merkel cells in the stratum basale of the epidermis which detect light touch and texture, Meissner corpuscles in the papillary dermis which detect moving touch, Pacinian corpuscles which detect vibration, located in the deeper dermis, and Ruffini corpuscles which detect stretch [13, 15]. In summary, the skin has a range of functions to execute and the maintenance of skin health is pivotal for the overall health of the internal body.

1.1.2 Mitochondria

Mitochondria are organelles known as the 'powerhouse of the cell' due to their significant role in producing 90% of cellular energy in the form of adenosine triphosphate (ATP). They also have a substantial role in maintaining homeostasis and tissue health.

Mitochondria are located in the cytoplasm of eukaryotic cells at a quantity of 100–1000 mitochondrion per cell which is dependent on energy demand; for example, more mitochondria are present in skeletal muscle in comparison to the skin due to a larger energy demand [16]. They are a double membraned organelle, usually 1–2 μM in length and 0.5–1 μM in diameter, consisting of an outer membrane and an inner membrane. The inner membrane is folded to form cristae, separated by an intermembrane space. Mitochondria contain a maternally inherited genome of 16.569 kilobases which is located in the matrix of the inner mitochondrial membrane [16]. It encodes 37 genes including 13 oxidative phosphorylation (OXPHOS) proteins, 22 tRNAs and 2 rRNAs. The mitochondrial genome is considered to be highly vulnerable due to its close proximity to the electron transport chain (ETC) and lack of protective histones and limited repair mechanisms.

Subsequently, mitochondrial DNA (mtDNA) has a rate of mutation 10–17 times higher than that of nuclear DNA, and these mutations remain within the cell for longer which can lead to various diseases [17, 18]. Current research has identified 27 mitochondrial haplotypes from mtDNA or single nucleotide polymorphisms (SNPs) within a population which have been correlated with several diseases including cancer and skin disorders [19].

Mitochondria have vital functions within the skin, divided into categories of energy, homeostasis and growth [12]. These functions include providing energy to power the regeneration of the epidermis with differentiation and migration of keratinocytes through the epidermis, alongside wound healing, cell signaling, hair growth and skin pigmentation [12]. Mitochondria have been shown to play an important role in defending the skin from microbes with research providing evidence of increased glycolysis and ATP production in response to hypoxia induced metabolic stress, caused by infection of the skin [12]. Therefore, mitochondria are vital in skin health and could be used as a target for treatment for various skin disorders.

1.1.2.1 Electron Transport Chain

As previously mentioned, mtDNA accumulates damage intrinsically due to its close proximity to the ETC within the mitochondrial matrix. The ETC is responsible for producing cellular energy through the generation of ATP, via respiration [16].

Cellular respiration is composed of three pathways: glycolysis, the tricarboxylic acid (TCA) cycle; also known as the Krebs cycle, and OXPHOS. OXPHOS is responsible for generating the main source of cellular ATP [20]. Glycolysis (Fig. 1.1) occurs within the cytoplasm and involves the oxidation of glucose. Glucose is initially converted to fructose-1,6-bisphosphate and requires two molecules of ATP. Fructose-1,6-bisphosphate is then split into dihydroxyacetone phosphate and glyceraldehyde-3-phosphate, with the latter being converted into two molecules of pyruvate. Along with the generation of two molecules of pyruvate, two molecules of nicotinamide adenine dinucleotide (NADH) and four molecules of ATP are also produced during this process. NADH is known as an electron donor and is responsible for transporting electrons into the ETC for the production of ATP through OXPHOS. Each molecule of pyruvate is then decarboxylated to acetyl-CoA by pyruvate dehydrogenase, producing 2 molecules of NADH and 2 molecules of carbon dioxide (CO_2) per molecule of glucose. Acetyl-CoA then feeds into the TCA cycle within the mitochondrial matrix (Fig. 1.1). The generation of pyruvate from glyceraldehyde-3-phosphate is able to occur twice as dihydroxyacetone phosphate can be converted to glyceraldehyde-3-phosphate for subsequent decarboxylation [16, 21].

The TCA cycle was proposed by Hans Adolf Krebs in 1937 and is central to oxidative metabolism [22]. It consists of eight enzymatic reactions that oxidize acetyl-CoA,

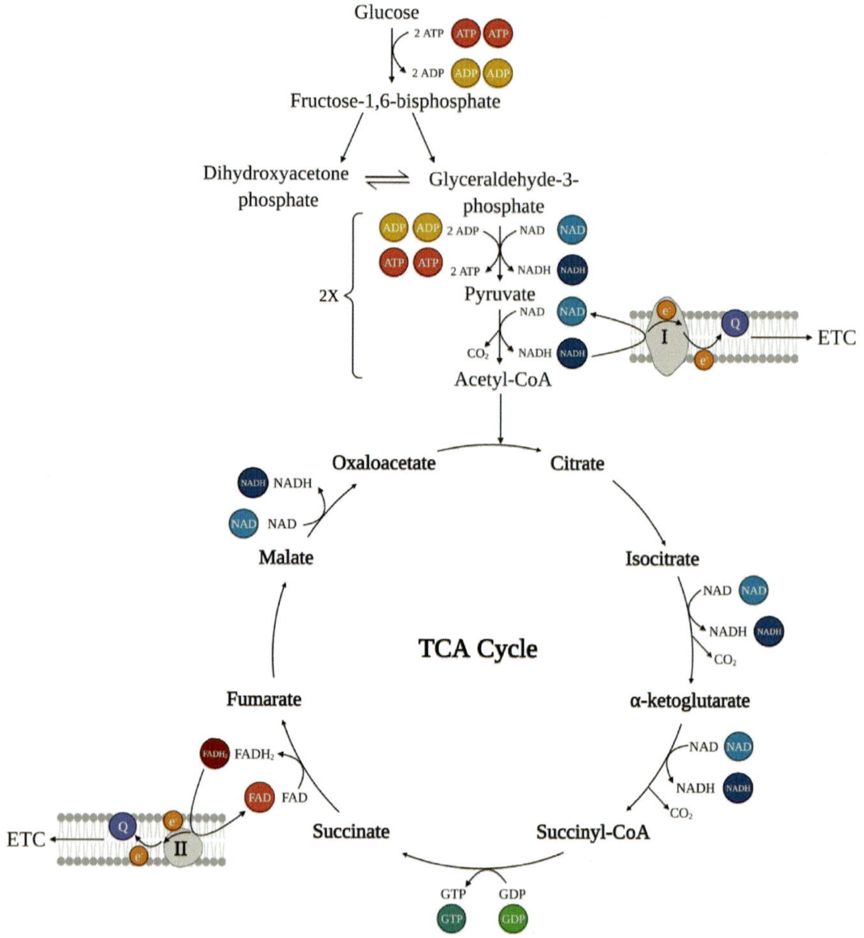

Fig. 1.1 Glycolysis and the tricarboxylic acid (TCA) cycle. Glucose is converted into two molecules of pyruvate which are subsequently converted to Acetyl-CoA by pyruvate decarboxylase. Acetyl-CoA enters the TCA cycle where it is combined with citrate and undergoes multiple enzymatic reactions in order to produce electron donors. Electron donors then provide electrons to complexes within the ETC in order to generate ATP. Created with Biorender.com

resulting in the formation of 2 molecules of CO_2, 1 molecule guanosine triphosphate (GTP), 3 molecules of NADH and 1 molecule of flavin adenine dinucleotide ($FADH_2$), also an electron donor, per cycle. The process is as follows: Acetyl-CoA and oxaloacetate are combined to generate citrate, catalyzed by citrate synthase. Citrate is then converted to cis-aconitase and subsequently isocitrate by aconitase. Isocitrate dehydrogenase converts isocitrate to α-ketoglutarate, producing 1 molecule of NADH and CO_2. This is then converted to succinyl-CoA by αketoglutarate dehydrogenase, similarly, producing 1 molecule of NADH and CO_2. Succinate is generated by succinyl-CoA synthase, generating 1 molecule of GTP from guanosine diphosphate (GDP). Succinate dehydrogenase converts succinate to fumarate, producing 1 molecule of $FADH_2$, followed by the generation of malate from fumarate by fumarase. Finally, malate dehydrogenase converts malate to oxaloacetate, which is able to react with acetyl-CoA in another round of the TCA cycle and generates the final molecule of NADH. Electron donors NADH and $FADH_2$ generated by the TCA cycle feed into the ETC, resulting in the production of large amounts of ATP through OXPHOS [22, 23]. Although there is no direct participation of oxygen in the TCA cycle, it only operates under aerobic conditions [22].

OXPHOS (Fig. 1.2) occurs at the inner mitochondrial membrane. The ETC is responsible for this process and consists of complexes I-V, ubiquinone, also known as coenzyme Q, and cytochrome C. Overall, electrons from NADH and $FADH_2$ are combined with O_2, along with the transfer of H+ across the membrane [16]. The movement of protons through complex V, also known as ATP synthase, down the electrochemical proton gradient, drives the phosphorylation of adenosine diphosphate (ADP) to produce ATP [24]. Transferring electrons from donors to O_2 requires energy, which is generated by the passage of electrons through the complexes of the ETC. Electrons from NADH enter the ETC at complex I, where they are transferred to flavin mononucleotide and then ubiquinone. They are then transferred to complex III, to cytochrome b and finally to cytochrome c. Cytochrome c transfers the electrons to ATP synthase where they are transferred to molecular O_2. In contrast, complex II receives electrons from succinate, part of the TCA cycle, and transfers them to $FADH_2$, then to ubiquinone and subsequently the rest of the ETC. The energy formed by the passage of electrons through the ETC is coupled to the synthesis of ATP from ADP [16].

Approximately 90% of oxygen consumed within eukaryotes is used in oxidative phosphorylation [17]. Under normal physiological conditions, up to 5% of oxygen consumed is converted to reactive oxygen species (ROS), highly reactive oxygen containing species with an unpaired electron. Studies have shown that electrons leak from complexes I and III within the ETC and react with molecules of oxygen (O_2) which are present in high abundance in the mitochondria, resulting in the formation of ROS. Highly reactive superoxide ($O_2^{-\cdot}$) is a major mitochondrial ROS, generated from the interaction between electrons and O_2. Superoxide dismutase (SOD) converts $O_2^{-\cdot}$ to hydrogen peroxide (H_2O_2), a less damaging molecule, which can then be converted to water (H_2O) by catalase and glutathione peroxidase (GPX). Although it is less damaging, H_2O_2 has the ability to cross-membranes easily and in conjugation with transitional Fe(II) drives the generation of the hydroxyl radical ($OH^{\cdot}$) which is

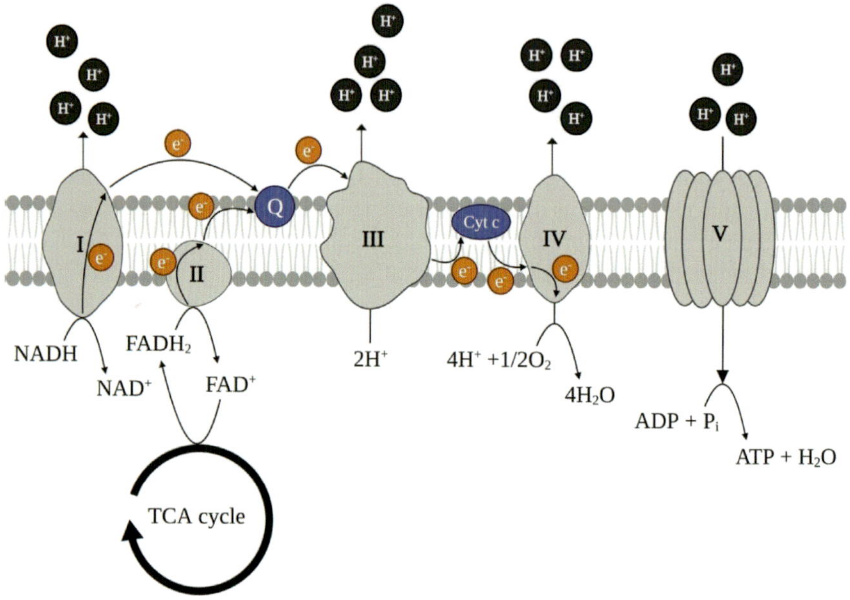

Fig. 1.2 Generation of ATP by the electron transport chain (ETC). Electron donors generated within the TCA cycle provide electrons which move along the ETC. The movement of electrons is coupled with the pumping of H^+ into the intermembrane space in order to generate a proton gradient. At complex IV, H_2O is generated from O_2 and ATP is generated at complex V from ADP and P_i, as well as the movement of H^+ down its proton gradient through the complex. Created with Biorender.com

highly reactive and damaging to cells, resulting in cellular damage including lipid peroxidation. These oxygen radicals can then result in further generation of ROS, ultimately causing cellular oxidative stress if antioxidant defense mechanisms are overwhelmed [18, 24–26]. Studies have also linked bioenergy and oxidative stress with pigment production [26]. Antioxidants within cells offer protection against ROS by providing an electron without becoming unstable, therefore, allowing free radicals to gain an electron, harboring them unreactive. SOD is an example of an antioxidant, in particular an enzymatic scavenger, removing $O_2^{-\cdot}$ from the cell, by converting it to H_2O_2 [16, 18]. ROS is known to damage proteins, membranes and DNA by oxidation, and as mtDNA is situated in close proximity to the site of ROS generation, it is highly susceptible to damage by these species. Oxidative damage to nucleic acids includes adducts of base and sugar groups, single and double-stranded breaks in the DNA backbone and cross-links to other molecules [18]. As we age chronologically, ROS contributes toward structural changes in the skin which affect its ability to function correctly [16]. Respiratory chain complexes I, III and IV are encoded by both mitochondrial and nuclear DNA; however, complex II is encoded by nuclear DNA (nDNA) only. Damaged mtDNA results in the generation of faulty respiratory chain complexes and increased electron leak and genetic damage, and instability outside the nuclear genome has been suggested to contribute to aging. This theory proposed by Harman is termed the 'vicious cycle of ageing', and albeit ROS can be extremely damaging to cells, low levels are continually produced in vivo and are involved in multiple important cellular pathways such as autophagy; however, it is crucial that levels are controlled [25, 27]. Studies have examined the influence of mitochondrial complex II on ROS production in human skin. Research by the Birch-Machin laboratory investigated the relationship between complex II and aging using human skin, showing that the rate of complex II activity significantly decreased with age in fibroblasts which was associated with a significant decline in transcript expression and protein levels. In addition, there was a significant decrease in complex II activity with age that was specific to senescent cells, this being the first study to investigate these differences with senescence and skin aging [26, 28, 29]. Studies also show that mitochondrial ROS generation plays a key regulatory role in the differentiation of various cell lineages via several downstream transcription factors such as C/EBP, Notch and ß-catenin [30].

1.1.2.2 Mitochondrial Deletions in Skin Aging and Disease

Mitochondrial deletions and mutations have been widely linked to both skin aging and skin disease. They have been shown to occur intrinsically due to the high abundance of ROS within the mitochondria and increase with age, such as the 4977 bp 'common deletion', due to accumulation as a result of limited repair mechanisms. It is therefore suggested that the accumulation of mutations within mtDNA is molecular events associated with the human skin aging process. Areas exposed to high levels of environmental stressors such as UVR have also been shown to accumulate mutations more quickly than non-exposed areas; therefore, the skin is vulnerable to damage as a result of both intrinsic and extrinsic stressors, particularly the face and hands [31]. During aging, the level of ROS increases, but the ability of the skin cells to repair this damage declines [32]. Signs of skin aging include reduced elasticity, the appearance of fine lines, deep wrinkles and increased surface roughness, which result from both intrinsic and extrinsic agings [33]. Skin disease also results from mutations within the mitochondrial genome. Studies have highlighted the role of the mitochondria in maintaining skin homeostasis and pigmentation, as well as in disorders such as cancer, inflammatory conditions and rare inherited diseases which are affected when essential mitochondrial functions are impaired [30].

1.2 Biomarkers in Skin Disease

The skin has a high turnover rate and depends on the rapid proliferation of its progenitor cells. The epidermis is a self-renewing layer that depends on the differentiation and migration of the proliferative basal keratinocytes to cornified keratinocytes in the outermost squamous later. This relies on energy generated by mitochondrial respiration in the form of ATP through OXPHOS. As previously discussed, ROS is produced in high amounts during OXPHOS which results in damage to cellular structures if levels are not controlled by antioxidant defense mechanisms. Oxidative damage caused by ROS has been shown to be the molecular basis of multiple pathophysiological conditions, including aging and cancer. The mitochondria are the primary organelle affected during chronological and photoaging, resulting in mitochondrial dysfunction [30].

In addition to skin aging and cancer, mitochondrial dysfunction has also been associated with various common and rare skin disorders. Ten % of patients with primary mitochondrial disorders present skin manifestations that can be categorized into hair abnormalities, pigmentation abnormalities and acrocyanosis (i.e., blueness of extremities) [34]. The underlying molecular mechanisms have been identified for most and mainly involve dysfunctional OXPHOS and high ROS generation, mutations in mtDNA, an imbalance between mitochondrial biogenesis and mitophagy and aberrant expression levels of nuclear-encoded mitochondrial proteins [30].

1.2.1 Cancer

Studies indicate that genetic changes in mtDNA result in a variety of diseases including cancer.

A non-coding mtDNA control region contains three hypervariable regions and a displacement (D-loop) region. Mutations in complexes I, III, IV and V, encoded by mtDNA, as well as mutations in the hypervariable regions constitute some of the mtDNA aberrations found in cancer tissue. Somatic mutations identified in human carcinomas have also been found within the D-loop of mtDNA. Although the D-loop is a non-coding region, it is essential for transcription and replication, with mutations in this region potentially resulting in dysfunctional mitochondria or mtDNA replication errors. Due to the absence of introns in mtDNA, most mtDNA mutations occur in coding sequences [35, 36]. The mitochondrial genome has an accelerated mutation rate in comparison to nDNA and somatic mutations arise in tumor tissue. The high mtDNA copy number within cells enables the detection of important biomarkers, even at low levels. It can also be heteroplasmic; therefore, wild-type and mutant molecules coexist within cells, and the proportion of mutant molecules can vary between tissues and with age. The presence of heteroplasmy is an indication of disease and is found in many human tumors [37, 38].

The incidence of skin cancer is steadily increasing, and it is the most common malignancy affecting humans, accounting for 40% of all cancer cases worldwide. It is classified into non-melanoma skin cancer (NMSC), responsible for approximately 90% of skin cancers including basal-cell carcinoma (BCC) and squamous cell carcinoma (SCC), and the melanocyte-derived melanomas [30, 37]. Although the latter doesn't make up a large proportion of skin cancer cases, melanoma is associated with a significant mortality rate of approximately 25%, as well as metastatic risk [30]. BCCs are the most common form of NMSC and predominantly arise from the basal keratinocytes of the epidermis, as well as from cells in hair follicles and sebaceous glands. They are locally invasive but rarely metastasise, unlike SCCs which may metastasise, although they are also derived from basal keratinocytes. Cutaneous malignant melanoma is a malignant tumor of the melanocytes, usually arising in the epidermis, and is the most lethal of the skin cancers [37]. The risk of developing skin cancer is higher in the Caucasian population due to the low melanin content within the skin. As previously discussed, melanin provides natural protection against UVR which is the cause of the majority of skin cancers [30, 37]. Mitochondria have been implicated in almost all human cancers, primarily due to their role in ROS generation and apoptosis, and congenital and somatic mutations in mtDNA have been detected in most tumors, including those affecting the skin [30].

Durham et al. presented the first detailed study of the distribution of multiple forms of mtDNA damage in NMSC, compared to histologically normal perilesional dermis and epidermis. The results show 20 different deletion species in the major deletion arc, and 4 species in the minor deletion arc [39]. Studies have also shown that the development of malignant melanoma may frequently have mutations in the D-loop region of the mitochondrial genome [34, 35]. Mitochondrial deletions such as the 3895 bp deletion have also been shown to be higher in NMSC samples [40].

1.2.2 Dupuytren Disease

Dupuytren disease is considered as one of the most common hereditary disorders of connective tissue in the Caucasian population [41]. It is a progressive fibroproliferative disorder affecting the palms of the hands with abnormal skin thickening, benign nodules and a cord formation of collagen which pulls the fingers toward the palm of the hand [42]. The disease involves hyperproliferation of type III collagen, forming abnormal myofibroblastic growth with cytokine involvement. The overall prevalence is 4% within the UK and rises to 20% in individuals over the age of 65 years, with the disease being 6 times more common in men than women [43]. In the most severe cases of the disease, the fingers cannot be straightened, negatively impacting the patient's quality of life by restricting everyday movements such as grasping objects. Currently, there is no complete cure available for the disease although treatment options include fasciectomy surgery to remove the affected palmar fascia or dermofasciectomy where the affected skin and palmar fascia are removed. Additionally, corticosteroid injections can be considered for those with nodules [42].

Dupuytren disease is maternally inherited and is a heterogeneous autosomal dominant disease. Research has revealed that the disease may be associated with many genes, suggesting abnormalities in chromosomes 6, 11 and 16 [42]. Although the genetic basis of the disease is complex and still not fully understood, it has been revealed that a mutation in mtDNA may be involved in the disease. Results from a study revealed that 90% of patients that they enrolled had a heteroplasmic C2839A mutation in a gene coding for 16s rRNA [44]. Additionally, it has been established that patients with Dupuytren disease have a large number of mitochondria in their myofibroblasts, which therefore leads to increased ROS and mutations in a vicious cycle [44]. Due to the presence of the mtDNA mutation, the mitochondrial genome may be used as a biomarker in this skin disease.

1.2.3 Non-epidermolytic Palmoplantar Keratoderma

Non-epidermolytic palmoplantar keratoderma (NEPPK) is a disease which causes hyperkeratosis across the palms of the hands and soles of the feet which clinically presents as thickened skin with peripheral erythema and no intraepidermal blistering [45]. There are several types of NEPPK, each of which differ regarding modes of inheritance, age of onset and biochemical compositions. These include diffuse keratodermas affecting the palms of the hands and soles of the feet, focal keratodermas affecting pressure areas and punctate-type keratoderma which presents as small lumps on the palms of the hands and soles of the feet. The most accurate way to differentiate between the types of NEPPK is to identify the genetic defect present [45]. NEPPK can be inherited with symptoms presenting at a very young age as well as being acquired at an older age [45].

Research into NEPPK with hearing loss has been associated with a homoplasmic point mutation (A7445G) in the heavy strand of mtDNA with an adenine to guanine transition, affecting the ETC complex IV subunit I, resulting in a decrease in cellular respiration [46]. This type of NEPPK is currently the only type to be associated with a mutation in mtDNA and has only been demonstrated in 5 families, with penetrance and expression varying between families [47]. This suggests that the disease is not solely caused by a genetic disorder, and other environmental factors may also have an influence [47]. This provides evidence that mtDNA could be utilized as a biomarker for this disease; however, there are limited studies which have investigated the prevalence of this mutation in patients and further research into the function of this mutation is required.

1.2.4 Bullous Pemphigoid

Bullous pemphigoid (BP) is a skin disorder associated with autoimmune subepidermal tense blistering and typically affects individuals over the age of 75 years, with equal incidence in males and females [48]. The incidence of BP in the UK is reported as 42.8 cases per year per 1 million people [49]. Patients present with fluid-filled lesions and generalized itching, and symptoms can be treated with topical or systemic immunosuppressants depending on the severity of the disease [48]. The blisters are caused by immunoglobulin G (IgG) autoantibodies against the hemidesmosome proteins BP180 and BP230 in the dermal–epidermal junction and the extracellular matrix [50]. Studies have identified multiple gene polymorphisms associated with the disease including those in the human leukocyte antigen (HLA) region and cytokine genes, with research supporting a genetic predisposition [51].

The mitochondrial genome has been found to be involved in the pathogenesis of BP. A study has recently shown the relationship between BP IgG cell dysfunction and mitochondrial dysfunction, with increased ROS production [52]. Additionally, a polymorphism in the ATP synthase 8 gene (MT-ATP8), encoded my mtDNA, has been previously associated with BP. Further mitochondrial single nucleotide polymorphisms (mtSNP) have recently been identified, including m.16051A > G, m.16162A > G and m.16263 T > C of the non-coding D-loop region and a mtSNP m11914 in MT-ND4 gene [51]. The MT-ATP8 polymorphism can increase keratinocyte susceptibility to apoptosis and reduce epidermal integrity, leading to the blistering in BP [53]. This offers insight for mtDNA to be used as a biomarker for BP and also offers a potential target for therapeutic interventions.

1.2.5 Pemphigus Vulgaris

Similar to BP, pemphigus vulgaris (PV) is an IgG autoantibody disease which causes blistering of the skin, but also affects oral surfaces which can lead to difficulties eating, drinking and talking. PV affects the epidermal layer of the skin with blistering being caused by a suprabasal split in the epithelium, whereas BP is associated with the dermal–epidermal junction [54]. Detachment of keratinocytes, termed acantholysis, is a major mechanism in the disease which is thought to be caused by IgG antibodies binding to the desmoglein 3 protein in keratinocytes, resulting in blistering [54]. The age of onset ranges from between 30 and 60 years and can be treated with steroids in conjunction with immunosuppressives in severe cases, although the disease can be life-threatening with a mortality rate of 12% [54, 55].

Research has found that patients with PV produce pathogenic antibodies against mitochondria in keratinocytes which are significant in disease pathology. The IgGs produced in PV enter keratinocytes and bind to mitochondrial self-antigens, causing keratinocyte detachment and affects many mitochondrial functions, including decline in ATP production, increased ROS production, increased lipid peroxidation and alterations to the mitochondrial membrane [56]. The pathogenic antibodies can bind to target proteins in the mitochondrial matrix as well as the mitochondrial inner and outer membranes and can therefore disrupt a range of mitochondrial functions and processes, making mitochondrial dysfunction a key factor in PV [54]. Recent developments have shown that mitochondrial protecting drugs such as nicotinamide are a substantial therapeutic agent in PV patients; therefore, future work could investigate other effective treatments and therapies that restore mitochondrial function [54].

1.3 Mitochondrial DNA Biomarkers in Skin Aging

Aging is the progressive loss of structural integrity and physiological function and can be both extrinsic and intrinsic (Fig. 1.3). Intrinsic aging, also known as chronological aging, occurs at a genetically determined rate and cannot be controlled. In contrast, extrinsic aging occurs as a result of extrinsic factors such as UVR, pollution, smoking, diet and physical activity levels, and exposure can be controlled [57, 58]. Both intrinsic and extrinsic agings occur as a result of the accumulation of oxidative stress due to the imbalance between ROS generation and antioxidant defense mechanisms, termed the 'vicious cycle of ageing'. This results in the loss of cells, as well as extracellular matrix, which is the network of extracellular macromolecules including collagen, enzymes and glycoproteins [18]. UVR exposure has been shown to result in damage to the mitochondrial genome in the form of the 4799 bp deletion, known as the 'common deletion', 3895 bp deletion and T414G mutation, which have been proposed as an underlying cause of the aging process [14, 40, 59]. Mitochondrial DNA is commonly used as a biomarker of UVR-induced DNA damage, with multiple studies highlighting the presence of mitochondrial DNA lesions in UV-exposed skin [17, 40, 60, 61].

1.3.1 Ultraviolet Radiation

Human skin is frequently exposed to UVR which is known to be damaging and result in photoaging, characterized by deep wrinkles, laxity and a leathery appearance [25, 62]. UVR is composed of UVA, UVB and UVC, classified by their wavelength. UVR exposure from the sun reaching the earth's surface is composed of approximately 95% UVA (320–400 nm) and the remainder is UVB (280--320 nm), each having different effects on the skin in terms of penetration. UVC does not reach the earth's surface due to being blocked by the ozone layer and therefore does not contribute to photodamage of the skin [63]. UVB has a shorter wavelength and is mainly absorbed by the epidermis, predominantly keratinocytes. As UVA has a longer wavelength, it is able to penetrate deeper into the skin to the dermis and interact with both epidermal keratinocytes and dermal fibroblasts [14]. The half-life of collagen, the major structural protein in skin, has been calculated to be 15 years and is reduced further in skin that is severely sun damaged due to the presence of ROS, which are responsible for collagen oxidation and degradation. ROS also interferes directly with signal transduction pathways involved in the expression of genes which are important in the regulation of collagen metabolism [25]. Research shows collagen degradation results from matrix metalloproteinases (MMP) that are released from keratinocytes and fibroblasts. MMP levels in the skin increase with age as well as following UV exposure. Naturally aged skin also shows a decrease in the synthesis of procollagen in comparison to young skin. A transient reduction is also seen following UV exposure,

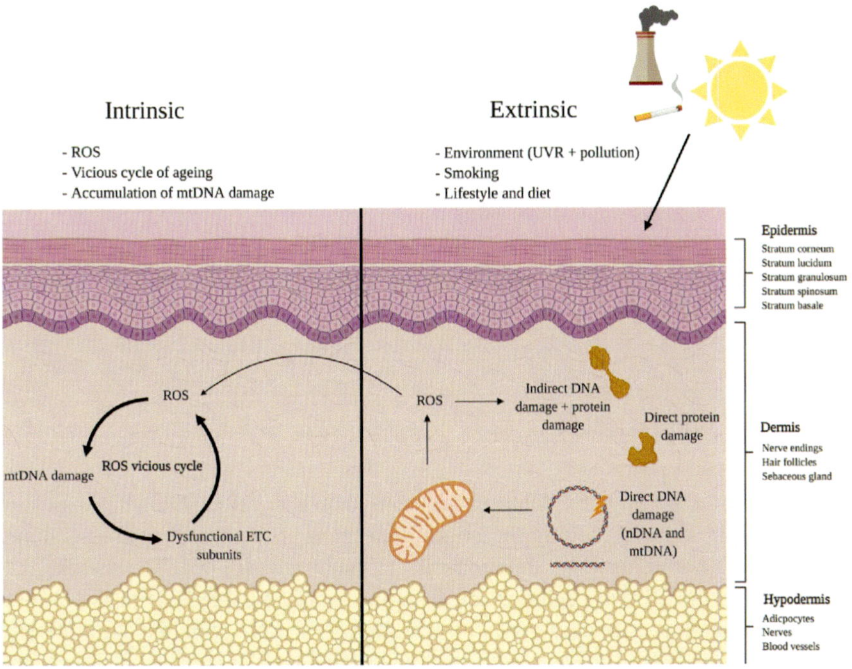

Fig. 1.3 Effects of both intrinsic and extrinsic agings on the mitochondria. Intrinsic aging occurs naturally with age, resulting from a build-up of ROS and subsequently oxidative stress due to the vicious cycles of aging theory. Extrinsic aging results from extrinsic factors such as UVR and can result in direct and indirect damage. UVR damages both proteins and DNA directly. Damaged mitochondrial DNA results in the production of faulty mitochondrial subunits and therefore increased ROS production; once again, resulting in the vicious cycle of aging theory

with a sustained reduction in old photodamaged skin, in comparison to photoprotected skin [64]. Studies provide evidence for the damaging effects of ROS produced following irradiation of the skin with UVA and UVB to mtDNA [25]. UVA and UVB have the ability to generate mtDNA damage, both directly and indirectly. The DNA directly absorbs UVB photons which results in subsequent structural changes such as DNA photoproducts, including cyclobutene pyrimidine dimers (CPDs) and pyrimidine [64] pyrimidone photoproducts, which cannot be repaired [63]. UVA is thought to damage mtDNA through the generation of ROS, including superoxide ($O_2^{-\cdot}$), singlet oxygen ($^1O_2$), hydrogen peroxide (H_2O_2) and the hydroxyl radical ($OH^\cdot$). ROS is generated by the absorption of photons by endogenous photosensitizer molecules, which then react with oxygen (O_2). A number of photosensitizers in human skin have been identified, including porphyrins, flavins, pterins and melanin. Oxidative stress as a result of high levels of ROS generation can subsequently result in lipid and protein peroxidation, generation of DNA strand breaks and activation of transcription factors. UVB is also able to generate ROS, but to a much lesser extent than UVA. Although UVA is poorly absorbed by DNA, like UVB, it has been shown to induce CPDs in both human skin and mice, but to a much lower level than UVB. UVA-generated $^1O_2$ has been identified to cause the mitochondrial common deletion, which has also been shown to occur at higher rates in photoaged skin [14, 25, 63, 65]. Evidence highlights base excision repair of oxidative damage; however, there is no evidence of nuclear excision repair for the repair of DNA photoproducts (e.g., CPDs) in mtDNA. Each cell can contain up to several thousand copies of the mitochondrial genome; therefore, mitochondria can tolerate up to 90% of damaged mtDNA through complementation of the remaining wildtype. These factors lead to the accumulation of photodamage in mtDNA without compromising cell function, hence making it an effective biomarker for UV damage [40, 66].

1.3.2 3895 bp Deletion

The presence of the 3895 bp deletion has been shown increase following exposure to UVR and it is present within the minor arc region of the mitochondrial genome which doesn't harbor as many deletions as the major arc [40, 66]. The regions that are deleted in the 3895 bp deletion are from the mtTF1 binding site in the D-loop to tRNA methionine. Deleted genes also include 12s rRNA, 16s rRNA, ND1 and also the promoters for the transcription of both the H and L strands. Research has shown a significantly greater deletion frequency in 'usually' sun exposed compared with 'occasionally' sun-exposed body sites in both the dermis and epidermis in human skin samples. In vitro work has also linked the 3895 bp deletion to the UVR component of sunlight by inducing the deletion with repetitive sublethal doses of UVA and UVB. The frequency of the deletion was also shown to be higher in NMSC samples [40]. Studies have also shown that the dermis harbors a higher level of the 3895 bp deletion than the epidermis, in both occasionally sun-exposed and usually sun-exposed samples. This links to previous reports that show more mtDNA damage in tissues that turn over more slowly. The high turnover of keratinocytes in the epidermis may give little time for the accumulation of mtDNA damage in comparison to the low proliferative rate of the fibroblasts in the dermis [66, 67]. A skin swab technique was used by Harbottle et al. to obtain mtDNA and determine the level of the 3895 bp deletion in different body sites. Results showed the highest level of the 3895 bp deletion in the nose, followed by the arm and then the heel, with each body site being exposed to a lower level of UVR. Due to the fact that the epithelial swab can detect the 3895 bp deletion in the epidermis despite the increased cell turnover in the epidermis in comparison to the dermis, the results suggest that the age of the individual has no significant effect on the damage present. This therefore suggests that epidermal skin swabs are measuring recent UVR exposure rather than long-term chronic damage [68].

1.3.3 4977 bp Deletion

The 4977 bp deletion is considered the 'common deletion' due to substantial levels of investigation revealing that the deletion is present in several mitochondrial diseases and it has been shown to arise more frequently in sun-exposed skin. The deletion is attributed to 12 mitochondrial genes, encoding several units of the electron transport chain. This includes four genes associated with complex I, one gene associated with complex IV, two associated with ATP synthase and five tRNA genes [31]. The deletion has been found to be present in different proportions depending on the tissue type, with a greater presence of the deletion in tissues such as the brain and muscles which are of low mitotic activity and a high metabolic rate [69]. The deletion has been found in sun-protected skin although is of a higher of heteroplasmy in skin exposed to UVR; therefore, the mutation is used as a biomarker for photoaged skin and is detected through the use of quantitative polymerase chain reaction (qPCR) methodology [70]. Research has found high levels of this deletion in the dermis in comparison to the epidermis which is thoughts to be due to the lower turnover rate of the dermis, hence the accumulation [69]. Additionally, no relationship was discovered between age and quantity of the 4977 bp deletion, suggesting that it is an effective biomarker for photoaging of the skin as opposed to chronological aging [39].

1.3.4 T414G Mutation

A T414G transversion mutation has been identified as a mtDNA biomarker for skin aging. The mutation is considered the most prevalent control region mutation in fibroblasts, occurring in mtDNA promoter regions for RNA primer synthesis of mtDNA heavy-strand synthesis and for light-strand transcription [59]. The mutation has been correlated with intrinsic skin aging but is also found in Alzheimer's disease and other age-related diseases [12]. Research has shown that the mutation is exacerbated in dermal fibroblasts with exposure to UVR, uncovering a direct link between oxidative stress and the mutation [12]. The presence of the T414G mutation in photoaged skin has also been found to have a genetic linkage with the 3895 bp deletion with a study reporting a break-point of the 3895 bp deletion lies close to the T414G mutation [59]. It was also suggested that a common stress mechanism may result in both mutations to be common together in photoaged skin with the potential for one mutation to predispose the other [59].

1.3.5 Tandem Duplications

The D-loop is a key regulatory site of the mitochondrial genome and any type of mutation in the regulatory elements in the D-loop can cause alterations in mtDNA replication and/or transcription [65, 71]. A 260 bp tandem duplication (TD) has previously been reported in the D-loop and was proposed to be associated with large-scale deletions such as the common deletion. TDs of 150 bp and 200 bp in size, and the previously reported 260 bp TD, have been found to occur in an age-dependent manner in tissues such as muscle, testis and skin. They have also been reported to occur at a higher frequency in sun-exposed skin, in comparison to non-exposed skin, with TDs being present in 25% of usually sun-exposed samples, in comparison to 9% of occasionally sun-exposed samples [65, 71]. A higher frequency was also seen in the dermis in comparison to the epidermis, thought to be due to the higher activity of antioxidant enzymes in the epidermis which keep levels of ROS controlled. Antioxidants' superoxide dismutase, glutathione peroxidase and glutathione reductase have been shown to be higher in the epidermis compared to the dermis by 126%, 61% and 215%, respectively [65, 72].

Acknowledgements We would like to thank ERDF IIIP for funding support.

References

1. Slominski AT, Zmijewski MA, Semak I, Kim T-K, Janjetovic Z, Slominski RM, et al. Melatonin, mitochondria, and the skin. Cell Mol Life Sci. 2017;74(21):3913–25.
2. Yousef H, Alhajj M, Sharma S, editors. Anatomy, skin (integument), epidermis. 2019.
3. Venus M, Waterman J, McNab I. Basic physiology of the skin. Surgery. 2011;29:471–4.
4. Lai-cheong JE, McGrath JA. Structure and function of skin, hair and nails. Medicine (Abingdon 1995, UK ed Print). 2013;41(6):317–20.
5. Agarwal S, Krishnamurthy K. Histology, skin. StatPearls. Treasure Island (FL): StatPearls Publishing Copyright © 2020. StatPearls Publishing LLC; 2020.
6. Boer M, Duchnik E, Maleszka R, Marchlewicz M. Structural and biophysical characteristics of human skin in maintaining proper epidermal barrier function. Postepy Dermatol Alergol. 2016;33(1):1–5.
7. Brown TM, Krishnamurthy K. Histology, dermis. StatPearls. Treasure Island (FL): StatPearls Publishing Copyright © 2020. StatPearls Publishing LLC; 2020.
8. Lee SH, Jeong SK, Ahn SK. An update of the defensive barrier function of skin. Yonsei Med J. 2006;47(3):293–306.
9. Elias PM. Skin barrier function. Curr Allergy Asthma Rep. 2008;8(4):299–305.
10. Kusuma S, Vuthoori R, Piliang M, Zins J. Skin anatomy and physiology. 2010. pp. 161–71.
11. Brenner M, Hearing VJ. The protective role of melanin against UV damage in human skin. Photochem Photobiol. 2008;84(3):539–49.
12. Stout R, Birch-Machin M. Mitochondria's role in skin ageing. Biology (Basel). 2019;8(2).
13. Abdo JM, Sopko NA, Milner SM. The applied anatomy of human skin: a model for regeneration. Wound Med. 2020;28:100179.
14. Berneburg M, Plettenberg H, Krutmann J. Photoaging of human skin. Photodermatol Photoimmunol Photomed. 2000;16(6):239–44.

15. Marzvanyan A, Alhawaj AF. Physiology, sensory receptors. StatPearls. Treasure Island (FL): StatPearls Publishing Copyright © 2020. StatPearls Publishing LLC; 2020.
16. Tulah AS, Birch-Machin MA. Stressed out mitochondria: the role of mitochondria in ageing and cancer focussing on strategies and opportunities in human skin. Mitochondrion. 2013;13(5):44453.
17. Birch-Machin MA, Swalwell H. How mitochondria record the effects of UV exposure and oxidative stress using human skin as a model tissue. Mutagenesis. 2009;25(2):101–7.
18. Beckman KB, Ames BN. The free radical theory of aging matures. Physiol Rev. 1998;78(2):547–81.
19. Bussard KM, Siracusa LD. Understanding mitochondrial polymorphisms in cancer. Cancer Res. 2017;77(22):6051–9.
20. Wilson DF, Erecińska M, Drown C, Silver IA. The oxygen dependence of cellular energy metabolism. Arch Biochem Biophys. 1979;195(2):485–93.
21. Fernie AR, Carrari F, Sweetlove LJ. Respiratory metabolism: glycolysis, the TCA cycle and mitochondrial electron transport. Curr Opin Plant Biol. 2004;7(3):254–61.
22. Akram M. Citric acid cycle and role of its intermediates in metabolism. Cell Biochem Biophys. 2013;68(3):475–8.
23. Bowtell JL, Marwood S, Bruce M, Constantin-Teodosiu D, Greenhaff PL. Tricarboxylic acid cycle intermediate pool size: functional importance for oxidative metabolism in exercising human skeletal muscle. Sports Med. 2007;37(12):1071–88.
24. Cogliati S, Lorenzi I, Rigoni G, Caicci F, Soriano ME. Regulation of mitochondrial electron transport chain assembly. J Mol Biol. 2018;430(24):4849–73.
25. Wlaschek M, Tantcheva-Poór I, Naderi L, Ma W, Schneider LA, Razi-Wolf Z, et al. Solar UV irradiation and dermal photoaging. J Photochem Photobiol B. 2001;63(1–3):41–51.
26. Birch-Machin MA, Bowman A. Oxidative stress and ageing. Br J Dermatol (1951). 2016;175(S2):26–9.
27. Sena Laura A, Chandel NS. Physiological roles of mitochondrial reactive oxygen species. Mol Cell. 2012;48(2):158–67.
28. Bowman A, Birch-Machin MA. Age-dependent decrease of mitochondrial complex II activity in human skin fibroblasts. J Investig Dermatol. 2016;136(5):912–9.
29. Anderson A, Bowman A, Boulton SJ, Manning P, Birch-Machin MA. A role for human mitochondrial complex II in the production of reactive oxygen species in human skin. Redox Biol. 2014;2(C):1016–22.
30. Sreedhar A, Aguilera-Aguirre L, Singh KK. Mitochondria in skin health, aging, and disease. Cell Death Dis. 2020;11(6):444.
31. Yang JH, Lee HC, Lin KJ, Wei YH. A specific 4977-bp deletion of mitochondrial DNA in human ageing skin. Arch Dermatol Res. 1994;286(7):386–90.
32. Tahara S, Matsuo M, Kaneko T. Age-related changes in oxidative damage to lipids and DNA in rat skin. Mech Ageing Dev. 2001;122(4):415–26.
33. Trojahn C, Dobos G, Lichterfeld A, Blume-Peytavi U, Kottner J. Characterizing facial skin ageing in humans: disentangling extrinsic from intrinsic biological phenomena. Biomed Res Int. 2015;2015:1–9.
34. Feichtinger RG, Sperl W, Bauer JW, Kofler B. Mitochondrial dysfunction: a neglected component of skin diseases. Exp Dermatol. 2014;23(9):607–14.
35. Takeuchi H, Fujimoto A, Hoon DSB. Detection of mitochondrial DNA alterations in plasma of malignant melanoma patients. Ann N Y Acad Sci. 2004;1022(1):50–4.
36. Penta JS, Johnson FM, Wachsman JT, Copeland WC. Mitochondrial DNA in human malignancy. Mutat Res Rev Mutat Res. 2001;488(2):119–33.
37. Parr RL, Dakubo GD, Thayer RE, McKenney K, Birch-Machin MA. Mitochondrial DNA as a potential tool for early cancer detection. Hum Genomics. 2006;2(4):252–7.
38. Legros F. Organization and dynamics of human mitochondrial DNA. J Cell Sci. 2004;117(13):2653–62.
39. Durham SE, Krishnan KJ, Betts J, Birch-Machin MA. Mitochondrial DNA damage in nonmelanoma skin cancer. Br J Cancer. 2003;88(1):90–5.

40. Krishnan KJ, Harbottle A, Birch-Machin MA. The use of a 3895 bp mitochondrial DNA deletion as a marker for sunlight exposure in human skin. J Investig Dermatol. 2004;123(6):1020–4.
41. Michou L, Lermusiaux J-L, Teyssedou J-P, Bardin T, Beaudreuil J, Petit-Teixeira E. Genetics of Dupuytren's disease. Joint Bone Spine. 2012;79(1):7–12.
42. Anderson ER, Burmester JK, Caldwell MD. Evaluation of a mitochondrial DNA mutation in maternally inherited and sporadic cases of Dupuytren disease. Clin Med Res. 2012;10(3):122–6.
43. Hindocha S, McGrouther DA, Bayat A. Epidemiological evaluation of Dupuytren's disease incidence and prevalence rates in relation to etiology. Hand (NY). 2009;4(3):256–69.
44. Bayat A, Walter J, Lambe H, Watson JS, Stanley JK, Marino M, et al. Identification of a novel mitochondrial mutation in Dupuytren's disease using multiplex DHPLC. Plast Reconstr Surg. 2005;115(1):134–41.
45. Martin L, Toutain A, Guillen C, Haftek M, Machet MC, Toledano C, et al. Inherited palmoplantar keratoderma and sensorineural deafness associated with A7445G point mutation in the mitochondrial genome. Br J Dermatol. 2000;143(4):876–83.
46. Maász A, Komlósi K, Hadzsiev K, Szabó Z, Willems PJ, Gerlinger I, et al. Phenotypic variants of the deafness-associated mitochondrial DNA A7445G mutation. Curr Med Chem. 2008;15(13): 125762.
47. Caria H, Morim de Matos T, Oliveira-Soares R, Santos A, Galhardo I, Soares-de-Almeida L, et al. A7445G mtDNA mutation present in a Portuguese family exhibiting hereditary deafness and palmoplantar keratoderma. J Eur Acad Dermatol Venereol JEADV. 2005;19:455–8.
48. Baigrie D, Nookala V. Bullous pemphigoid. StatPearls. Treasure Island (FL): StatPearls Publishing Copyright © 2020. StatPearls Publishing LLC; 2020.
49. Langan SM, Smeeth L, Hubbard R, Fleming KM, Smith CJP, West J. Bullous pemphigoid and pemphigus vulgaris—incidence and mortality in the UK: population based cohort study. BMJ. 2008;337: a180.
50. Genovese G, Di Zenzo G, Cozzani E, Berti E, Cugno M, Marzano AV. New insights into the pathogenesis of bullous pemphigoid: 2019 update. Front Immunol. 2019;10(1506).
51. Russlies J, Fähnrich A, Witte M, Yin J, Benoit S, Gläser R, et al. Polymorphisms in the mitochondrial genome are associated with bullous pemphigoid in Germans. Front Immunol. 2019;10:2200.
52. Tie D, Da X, Natsuga K, Yamada N, Yamamoto O, Morita E. Bullous pemphigoid IgG induces cell dysfunction and enhances the motility of epidermal keratinocytes via Rac1/proteasome activation. Front Immunol. 2019;10:200.
53. Grando SA. The mitochondrion is a common target of disease pathophysiology in pemphigus and pemphigoid. Exp Dermatol. 2015;24(9):655–6.
54. Kalantari-Dehaghi M, Chen Y, Deng W, Chernyavsky A, Marchenko S, Wang PH, et al. Mechanisms of mitochondrial damage in keratinocytes by pemphigus vulgaris antibodies. J Biol Chem. 2013;288(23):16916–25.
55. Kridin K. Emerging treatment options for the management of pemphigus vulgaris. Ther Clin Risk Manag. 2018;14:757–78.
56. Chernyavsky A, Chen Y, Wang PH, Grando SA. Pemphigus vulgaris antibodies target the mitochondrial nicotinic acetylcholine receptors that protect keratinocytes from apoptolysis. Int Immunopharmacol. 2015;29(1):76–80.
57. Farage MA, Miller KW, Elsner P, Maibach HI. Intrinsic and extrinsic factors in skin ageing: a review. Int J Cosmet Sci. 2008;30(2):87–95.
58. Hudson L, Bowman A, Rashdan E, Birch-Machin MA. Mitochondrial damage and ageing using skin as a model organ. Maturitas. 2016;93:34–40.
59. Birket MJ, Birch-Machin MA. Ultraviolet radiation exposure accelerates the accumulation of the aging-dependent T414G mitochondrial DNA mutation in human skin. Aging Cell. 2007;6(4):55764.
60. Bowman A, Martinez-Levasseur LM, Acevedo-Whitehouse K, Gendron D, Birch-Machin MA. The simultaneous detection of mitochondrial DNA damage from sun-exposed skin of three whale species and its association with UV-induced microscopic lesions and apoptosis. Mitochondrion. 2013;13(4):342–9.

61. Boulton SJ, Bowman A, Koohgoli R, Birch-Machin MA. Skin manifestations of mitochondrial dysfunction: more important than previously thought. Exp Dermatol. 2015;24(1):12–3.
62. Kang S, Chung JH, Lee JH, Fisher GJ, Wan YS, Duell EA, et al. Topical N-acetyl cysteine and genistein prevent ultraviolet-light-induced signaling that leads to photoaging in human skin in vivo. J Investig Dermatol. 2003;120(5):835–41.
63. Swalwell H, Latimer J, Haywood RM, Birch-Machin MA. Investigating the role of melanin in UVA/UVB- and hydrogen peroxide-induced cellular and mitochondrial ROS production and mitochondrial DNA damage in human melanoma cells. Free Radical Biol Med. 2012;52(3):626–34.
64. Fligiel SEG, Varani J, Datta SC, Kang S, Fisher GJ, Voorhees JJ. Collagen degradation in aged/photodamaged skin in vivo and after exposure to matrix metalloproteinase-1 in vitro. J Investig Dermatol. 2003;120(5):842–8.
65. Krishnan KJ, Birch-Machin MA. The incidence of both tandem duplications and the common deletion in mtDNA from three distinct categories of sun-exposed human skin and in prolonged culture of fibroblasts. J Investig Dermatol. 2006;126(2):408–15.
66. Harbottle A, Birch-Machin MA. Real-time PCR analysis of a 3895 bp mitochondrial DNA deletion in nonmelanoma skin cancer and its use as a quantitative marker for sunlight exposure in human skin. Br J Cancer. 2006;94(12):1887–93.
67. Cortopassi GA, Shibata D, Soong NW, Arnheim N. A pattern of accumulation of a somatic deletion of mitochondrial DNA in aging human tissues. Proc Nat Acad Sci PNAS. 1992;89(16):7370–4.
68. Harbottle A, Maki J, Reguly B, Wittock R, Robinson K, Parr R, et al. Real-time polymerase chain reaction analysis of a 3895-bp mitochondrial DNA deletion in epithelial swabs and its use as a quantitative marker for sunlight exposure in human skin. Br J Dermatol. 2010;163(6):1291–5.
69. Cortopassi GA, Shibata D, Soong NW, Arnheim N. A pattern of accumulation of a somatic deletion of mitochondrial DNA in aging human tissues. Proc Natl Acad Sci USA. 1992;89(16):7370–4.
70. Eshaghian A, Vleugels RA, Canter JA, McDonald MA, Stasko T, Sligh JE. Mitochondrial DNA deletions serve as biomarkers of aging in the skin, but are typically absent in nonmelanoma skin cancers. J Invest Dermatol. 2006;126(2):336–44.
71. Lee H-C, Pang C-Y, Hsu H-S, Weia Y-H. Ageing-associated tandem duplications in the D-loop of mitochondrial DNA of human muscle. FEBS Lett. 1994;354(1):79–83.
72. Shindo Y, Witt E, Han D, Epstein W, Packer L. Enzymic and non-enzymic antioxidants in epidermis and dermis of human skin. J Investig Dermatol. 1994;102(1):122–4.

Chapter 2
Serological Biomarkers

Jalal Ibrahim, Torrin Jacobsen, Adina Boulos, and Robert Norman

Abstract In medicine, obtaining reliable and precise information is fundamental in diagnosing conditions. Given this, the introduction and relative rise in the use of measured biomarkers have given physicians a more efficient way to diagnose conditions. The method of measuring these serum biomarkers is minimally invasive and cost-effective for the clinicians and patients involved. Serum biomarkers range from specific cytokines, immunoglobulins, and interleukins to other more specific nucleic acid measurements. These quantifications might soon be commonly used by dermatologists and others to confirm the skin-based diseases that were previously in question. These biomarkers can help diagnose conditions such as atopic dermatitis, autoimmune bullous skin diseases, psoriasis, cutaneous malignancies, and other chronic inflammatory skin diseases via an efficient and less invasive manner. However, further clinical trials are needed to develop significant evidence that will enable development in biomarker technology.

Keywords Serum biomarkers · Minimally invasive · Cytokines · Interleukins · Autoantibodies · IgA · IgG · Circulating tumor cells (CTCs) · Atopic dermatitis · Psoriasis · Autoimmune bullous skin diseases · Cutaneous malignancies · Chronic inflammatory skin diseases · Hidradenitis suppurativa · Inflammatory bowel disease (IBD)

J. Ibrahim · T. Jacobsen · A. Boulos
Lake Erie College of Osteopathic Medicine, Bradenton, FL, USA

R. Norman (Deceased) (✉)
Nova Southeastern University, Tampa, USA
e-mail: skindrrob@aol.com

R. Norman (ed.), *Biomarkers in Dermatology*,
https://doi.org/10.1007/978-3-031-66513-4_2

2.1 Introduction

2.1.1 Serum Biomarkers

Dermatological disorders consist of a large range of pathologies, each determinable by histologic, genetic and serum-based informatics. Recent worldwide research has been increasingly centered on unveiling potential biomarkers in hopes to predict treatment efficacy and further innovate new biologic treatments [1]. Serum biomarkers are defined as indicators of normal or pathogenic responses shown in the blood. These markers could include small proteins or chemical compositions that are commonly released into circulating serum as a result of normal or pathologic processes. Proteins such as cytokines, gaseous compositions, and chemokines serve as commonplace biomarkers and are especially present in literature researching allergic diseases [2]. Although dermatological disorders do include allergic processes (and these too will be highlighted), many other dermatologic disorders follow an alternate pathologic process. In addition to proteins and chemical compositions, circulating nucleic acids (ctDNA, mRNA, microRNA) and tumor cells (CTCs) are equally important and most prominent in the understanding of oncologic disease processes [3]. This chapter aims to collect worldwide research and highlight the important biomarkers across the dermatologic spectrum.

2.1.2 Role of Serum Biomarkers in Medicine

Medicine has been progressively advancing toward patient-specific treatment and testing. Dubbed "precision medicine", this patient-oriented arm of medicine aims to utilize genetic and epigenetic makeups, quantitative biomarker profiles and molecular phenotypes. These tools help predict a more efficacious treatment, monitor disease progression, predict future prognosis, and better understand disease recurrence risk [4]. As the community of medicine and informatics continues to intertwine, more advanced technologies will allow for more cost-effective and efficient techniques. From its inception, precision medicine has been geared toward revealing insights into oncological disease processes. However, as research innovates, equipment advances, and accessibility increases, we have started seeing more specialty-focused usage of these tools. In 2019, the Joint American Academy of Dermatology and National Psoriasis Foundation guidelines recognized the necessity to understand biomarkers involved in dermatological pathologies more extensively, with that understanding leading the way to creating a patient centered approach for these conditions [5]. In this chapter, we will explore the novel identifications of biomarkers and how the dermatological understanding has evolved recently to include the concepts of precision medicine.

2.2 Serum Biomarkers in Dermatologic Conditions

Serum biomarkers exist within the blood and flow through all organs, including the skin. This serum gives an unique window of insight into what is going on within our body. Given this understanding, it is imperative that we reaffirm and expand on these serum biomarkers and their relationship to dermatologic conditions. Within dermatological conditions, a few key players measurable in the blood rise to the top, such as: cytokines (immunoresponse molecules), immunoglobulins, miRNA (lysed cell nucleic acid material), and ctDNA (lysed *tumor* cell nucleic acid material). In addition, there are lipid infused vesicles in the blood (EV) that can be found using liquid biopsy, as well as circulating tumor cells (CTC) which are found using RT-PCR, liquid biopsy, and techniques like ISET [6–8]. EVs can contain clues such as protein, lipids, and nucleic acids from an origin cell [7]. CTCs are various forms of tumor cells that shed from a cancer lesion into circulation; thus, these are important considerations for oncogenic processes [6].

Many more examples can be given; however, we need to further explore our understanding of the role of biomarkers in autoimmune bullous skin diseases, cutaneous malignancies, atopic dermatitis, hidradenitis suppurativa, psoriasis, and chronic inflammatory skin diseases. Serum biomarkers can help paint a comprehensive picture of the patient's current health status, risk of disease development, remission, progression, and treatment response [9]. This can give dermatologists a faster and clearer idea on how to address the specific condition. Measuring a specific biomarker shown in the serum of a patient can give invaluable insight to a dermatologist, providing the capability to quickly provide treatment, with a more directed diagnosis.

2.2.1 Serum Biomarkers in Autoimmune Bullous Skin Diseases

Serological biomarkers can diagnose based off unique autoantibodies, associated with specific disease groups. These serum biomarkers have been shown to detect autoimmune bullous skin diseases (AIBDs). A group of skin disorders that damage structural components that help maintain cell–cell adhesion, such as desmosomes and hemidesmosomes. Key AIBDs include pemphigus related diseases, acquired epidermolysis bullosa (EBA), and dermatitis herpetiformis [10]. Pemphigus diseases produce autoantibodies against the cell adhesion desmosome proteins desmoglein (Dsg)3 and desmoglein (Dsg)1. Dysfunction of these two main proteins results in loss of epidermal cell–cell adhesion with blisters as the outcome [10]. The severity of skin lesions and blisters is variable among patients, so being able to assess such serum biomarkers gives dermatologists a faster ability treating this disease before it worsens. To dive more into this, it is important to analyze how similar pemphigus foliaceus and pemphigus vulgaris are, yet how their markers and pathologies differ.

In pemphigus foliaceus, IgG antibodies are only directed against Dsg1, resulting in blistering being confined to the skin surface. With pemphigus vulgaris, autoantibodies are against both Dsg1 and Dsg3 and the blistering may be more severe and involve the mucous membrane. The difference between the two diseases and being able to measure the specific biomarkers has made diagnosing more accurate and faster. In addition, the combination of these membrane biomarkers and salivary biomarkers can create more valuable combination diagnostics for assessing mucous membrane specific pemphigus diseases [11].

The next AIBD to review is acquired epidermolysis bullosa. This condition is a severe blistering dermatosis with autoantibodies against type VII collagen, a key component for our connective and structural tissues [10]. This is the key serum biomarker that would be shown with this condition. The manifestation of acquired epidermolysis bullosa is subepidermal blisters that causes erosions in response to irritation of the skin, but ultimately affects both the skin and mucous membranes. The next AIBD to cover is dermatitis herpetiformis, an itchy dermatosis that majorly affects patients with celiac disease, and manifests as blisters in the sub-epidermis of the elbows, knees or buttocks [10]. The primary serum biomarker expressed with dermatitis herpetiformis is IgA autoantibodies against endomysium tissue/epidermal transglutaminase (anti-tTG/-eTG) or deamidated gliadin (IgA/IgG) [10].

AIBDs are quite rare and potentially fatal disorders of the skin and mucous membranes which can be associated with IgA or IgG autoantibodies that disrupt the homeostasis of adhesion molecules of the epidermis and dermis [12]. The common types of AIBDs have been covered here with their respective serum biomarkers; however, the diagnostic approach of these biomarkers is necessary to understand. Simply put, it's the quantification of immunoglobulins in circulation (serum biomarkers). Serological testing for detecting these biomarkers is the best in regards to being minimally invasive and overall more suitable for simple diagnostic purposes [10].

2.2.2 *Serum Biomarkers of Cutaneous Malignancies*

From 2001 to 2010, the third most common referral and visit diagnosis to dermatologists was non-melanoma skin cancer (NMSC) [13]. NMSC consists of squamous cell carcinoma, basal cell carcinoma, and other rare skin disorders. Other cutaneous malignancies, such as malignant melanoma, although not as common, can be fatal and it is extremely important to be able to recognize and treat quickly and effectively. Research on serum biomarkers for cutaneous malignancies such as those mentioned is a high priority for the future of dermatology. For a high-yield analysis, we will focus on metastatic melanoma, squamous cell carcinoma, and basal cell carcinoma.

Older research recognized three important serum biomarkers for melanoma: lactase dehydrogenase (LDH) and melanocyte lineage antigens S100-beta and melanoma inhibitory activity (MIA). LDH is shown to be the strongest prognostic indicator of disseminated stage IV melanoma. S100-beta and MIA are also good correlative indicators of tumor load in later stage, with S100-beta having the advantage over MIA at better predicting tumor progression, relapse, and metastasis [14]. As time has progressed, simple quantification of serum protein biomarkers S100-beta and LDH remains confined to only a *minimal* clinical value [15].

In addition to protein analysis, earlier research searching biomarkers of melanoma employed RT-PCR to find circulating tumor cells (CTC). CTCs can be found using short-lived mRNAs in the circulating blood that can be linked back to its "origin" tumor cell using RT-PCR. Using this method, biomarkers such as tyrosinase, Melan-A/Mart-1, gp100, and MAGE have been found [8]. Previous research from Voit et al. showed CTCs to correlate with disease progression in Stage II-III melanoma. This research also showed patients that were repetitively negative for RT-PCR tyrosinase testing had greater survival rates than those who tested positive [16]. More recently however, advancements in this space such as the CellSearch® Circulating Tumor Cell Kit have allowed for simple and quick blood testing analysis of CTCs, thus allowing prompt quantification of CTC type counts. A recent study found that patients with greater than 1 type of CTC (vs. zero) found via the simple blood assay were at risk for relapse of stage III node-positive melanoma [17].

In addition to CTC analysis, development in precision medicine has unveiled nucleic acid biomarkers such as ctDNA and microRNA. These novel avenues in biomarker science show possible applications within the understanding of melanoma. ctDNA has been shown correlate with tumor burden and detect recurrence [18–20]. It also has been shown to identify patients at high risk for relapse of Stage III melanoma [20–22]. A 2023 meta-analysis covering 648 melanoma and 578 control patients showed that circulating lysed tumor cell microRNA (miRNA) could be used as a diagnostic biomarker for melanoma. Examples of miRNA in the study included miR-320a-5p, miR-21-5p, miR-210-3p, miR-185-5p, miR-221-3p, and miR-1246d and combinations of miR-149-3p, miR-150-5p, and miR-193a-3p. Interestingly, the analysis showed miRNA biomarkers as a better diagnostic for patients of European descent compared to other subgroups [23]. Overall, pooled sensitivity was 0.87 and specificity was 0.81, meaning that in theory 87% of melanoma patients *should* test positive for their melanoma using a form of miRNA assay testing [23]. Studies like these show the future possibilities of highly individualized medicine, as increased data is narrowing down the best possible form of testing.

Squamous cell carcinoma and basal cell carcinoma are not nearly as extensively researched as melanoma. However, they are equally important to understand as they impact a significant portion of the dermatological visits. Because of their often-localized nature, many of the biomarkers are within the lesion and found through immunohistochemical techniques (biopsy). For example, from older literature on SCC, p-STAT3, a transcription factor, was found to be increased in more poorly differentiated lesions. E-Cadherin, an intracellular adhesion molecule, was found to be inversely correlated to increased metastasis and better differentiated lesions [14]. However, through novel methods, serum biomarkers have been found. Liquid biopsy of extracellular vesicles (EV) in the blood (lipid "capsules" of cell parts), SCC has been found to be associated with upregulated Ct-SLCO1B3 (a gene from an EV) in patients with RDEB. A circular RNA circ-CYP24A1 was also found to be upregulated to the greatest extent in serum RNA analyzed from patients with SCC [24]. Cañueto et al. in 2017 found that miRNA-203 and 205 were associated with prognosis of SCC. Expression of miRNA-203 was found to be an indicator of a more favorable outlook, while expression of miRNA-205 was an indicator of a poor outlook [25, 26]. This shows a trend of transition from lesion specific to disseminated biomarkers of clinical prognostic and diagnostic value. In addition, BCC has important serologic biomarkers to understand and utilize. From Hu et al. in 2019, a poor BCC prognosis was found to be associated with low levels of miRNA-34a [26, 27]. Through many years and a variety of evolving methods, the biomarkers found for cutaneous malignancies have allowed medicine to shift from relying solely on biopsies to having reliable information in the blood. These findings shape the outlook for cutaneous malignancy treatments and offer insight into the possibilities of precision medicine in the future.

2.2.3 Serum Biomarkers in Patients with Atopic Dermatitis

Atopic dermatitis (AD), commonly referred to as eczema, is a well-known dermatologic condition that is relatively common among patients. AD is not contagious nor fatal, with usual onset at childhood. However, it can occur at any age. AD is a chronic disease that causes redness, inflammation, and irritation of the skin [28]. For AD, there are a multitude of serum biomarkers that are elevated when measured. To begin with, relatively known inflammatory biomarkers such as IL-5, IL-1b, IL-7, IL-1R1, and IL-15 were all elevated in the serum of patients with AD [28]. Not only is AD a dermatologic condition, but with the measurements of serum biomarkers being elevated, it gives us an idea that it can also be a systemic disease. Being able to recognize these inflammatory biomarkers in the serum of patients gives us a faster and more reliable way to fully confirm a diagnosis, but of course, there are many more biomarkers out there.

In another study, researchers measured the immunoinflammatory biomarkers in serum in relation to disease severity. Patients with different severities of atopic dermatitis, ranging from mild to severe [29]. Researchers correlated serum biomarkers with the "SCORAD" scale, which determines the severeness of AD. Abnormal measurements of serum biomarkers CCL17, CCL26, total IgE, IL-33, and IL-5 correlated with higher levels of SCORAD for AD patients [29]. The data concluded elevated serum biomarkers in more severe disease was related to the Th2 pathway. These findings equip dermatologists to better understand the specific condition a patient might have.

Expanding on this relationship between AD and the T helper cell responses, it was also shown that Th1, Th17, and Th22 cell-based responses play a role in atopic dermatitis pathogenesis [30]. The clinical severity of AD also correlates strongly with serum levels of TARC (thymus activated-regulated chemokine), S100 proteins, CCL22, eosinophil count, IL-22, IL-4, IL-13, and more [30, 31], giving more insight into the biomarkers associated with AD.

2.2.4 Serum Biomarkers in Patients with Hidradenitis Suppurativa

Hidradenitis suppurativa (HS) is a devastating chronic inflammatory disease that takes the form of deep-seated nodules and abscesses, draining tracts, and ultimately leads to fibrotic scars [32]. Novel biomarkers relating to collagen catabolism and anabolism have been found. These include metabolite biomarkers for collagen type I, III, IV, VII degradation (C1M, C3M, C4M, C7M) and peptide biomarkers for type III, IV, VI formation (PRO-C3, PRO-C4, PRO-C6). Biomarkers for citrullinated vimentin (modified protein that anchors organelles in the cytosol) and calprotectin (protein complex secreted during inflammation by neutrophils) degradation (VICM, CPa9-HNE) were also found to be associated [33–35]. In addition, C1M, C3M, C4M, C7M, VICM, CPa9-HNE have also been found to be increased in higher severity patients. With C1M and C4M showing strong and moderate correlations respectively with inflammatory protein CRP [35]. These biomarkers could conceivably indicate the prognosis of in HS in patients.

In addition to these, non-specific IgG quantification has been found to be a possible prognostic biomarker in HS. Patients with high severity showed increased amounts of IgG compared to lesser severities. IgG also showed to be a better prognostic indicator than NLC and SII (inflammatory indicators) [36]. Although non-specific, this provides a possible option to be used as an adjunct biomarker in diagnostics. Similar research found that specific B-cells whose receptors (BCR's) favored activation signaling via Bruton's tyrosine kinase (BTK) and spleen tyrosine kinase (SYK) pathways were most heavily involved "players" in HS patients [37]. B-cells and BCRs can be analyzed through blood draw. Although this is not a specific dermatological diagnostic yet by any measure, future clinical trials may reveal its association and allow for a diagnostic significance.

2.2.5 Serum Biomarkers Found in Inflammatory Bowel Disorders and Chronic Inflammatory Skin Diseases

Among chronic dermatological diseases, inflammatory pathologies represent the largest proportion [38]. Inflammation is linked to many pathological disorders across the spectrum of medicine and manifests often as chronic symptoms on the skin. Within all medical specialties, there may be room to draw associations between varying pathologies and the inflammatory mechanisms that overlap them. Inflammatory bowel disorders (IBD) may affect approximately 1% of the US populations, a significant number [39]. Chronic inflammatory skin diseases (CISDs) consist of diseases such as atopic dermatitis (AD). AD ranks 15th most common among non-fatal diseases and has the highest burden on life for patients with skin diseases [40, 41]. Given the sheer quantity of patients affected, it is imperative to understand the associations between IBD and CISD.

From a longitudinal study observing patients from 2004 to 2020, Schneeweiss et al. found that the presence of IBD was a 100% increase for patients with hidradenitis suppurativa, 30% increase in psoriasis, and a 12% increase in atopic dermatitis [42]. Given the marked association, understanding overlapping biomarkers present among these diseases is crucial. Tumor necrosis factor-alpha (TNF-α), IL-17, and IL-23 are overlapping cytokine biomarkers found in IBD, psoriasis, and hidradenitis suppurativa [42]. IL-17 and IL-23 induce a proinflammatory state and promote release of molecules TNF-α, IFN-γ, IL-22, lymphotoxin, IL-1b, and lipopolysaccharide (LPS). IL-17 and IL-23 and TNF-α are especially important in the pathology of Crohn's disease, with TNF-α inhibitors (such as ustekinumab) being used to treat patients. This treatment was found to help Crohn's symptoms and simultaneously reduce psoriasiform lesions [43]. Evidence like this indicates that these three cytokines are reliable biomarkers.

In other current research, the trend certainly reaffirms the serum-based approach. Biasci et al. have found an optimal 17-gene sequence in blood using qPCR that predicts the prognosis and thus can direct treatment in Crohn's disease and ulcerative colitis patients [44]. Similar research has been done that focused not on the genes themselves, but on miRNA which influences genes. Five miRNAs (2355–3p, 4264, 2355–5p, 29c-5p, and 361–3p) were found to be significantly increased in Chronic Spontaneous Urticaria. The miRNA targets genes surrounding none other than, genes regulating inflammation [45]. Unfortunately, there is not much research intending to quantify IBD and CISD biomarkers and their relationship. However, seeing the similarities among these newfound biomarkers is a hopeful outlook that we will be able to better diagnose, associate, and predict the interaction of these inflammatory pathologies in the future, being possible through a simple blood test.

2.2.6 Serum Biomarkers in Psoriasis

The last condition to be reviewed here is psoriasis. Psoriasis is a chronic skin disease caused by multiple inflammatory pathways and produces a scaly red plaque, specifically on the extensor sites of the extremities [46]. Patients with psoriasis experience a Th17 dominant immune response, which increases the inflammatory cytokines: IL-17, IL-22, and IL-23. Along with elevated levels of thymus activation-regulated chemokine (TARC) and many others [46]. Given this information, a dermatologist suspecting psoriasis in a patient will be able to measure the serum biomarkers and fully determine if the diagnosis is likely psoriasis and if so, how severe it is. All this may be possible from simple diagnostic information such as Th17-related cytokines and interleukins obtained from blood. This is an enormous advantage that can ensure that a patient is treated with the correct medication.

Another study conducted by Ramessur et al., showed genomic biomarkers in patients with psoriasis. Given this information, they concluded that the biomarkers obtained, such as HLA-C*06:02, LCE3D, IL-23R, NFKBIL1, and IL-23A, were all good diagnostic biomarkers for psoriasis [47]. This is a promising study, as they were able to assess the likeliness of getting psoriasis based on these specific biomarkers. Although this was a meta-analysis analyzing genomic information from various studies, genomic data can be obtained through the blood. Moving forward, this shows the possibility that these diagnostics could be simplified and offered routinely, ultimately enabling physicians to treat the condition earlier, alter the prognosis, and grant the patient a better quality of life.

2.3 Summary Key Points

- Serum biomarkers allow for a minimally invasive diagnostic tool that gives insight into the prognosis of many dermatological diseases.
- Autoimmune skin blistering diseases (AIBDs) demonstrate marked serum changes in immunoglobulins or autoantibodies specific to collagen and other cell membrane-based structures.
- Important proteins, CTCs, and nucleic acid-based biomarkers have been found to be associated with melanoma, SCC, and BCC. These serum biomarkers can give insight into disease severity, prognosis, and possible relapse risk.
- Atopic dermatitis patients express a dominant Th2 response with abnormal levels of related inflammatory markers in serum. Th1, Th17, and Th22 also showed correlations with atopic dermatitis. This assists with ruling in or out other conditions not involving these immune pathways.
- Collagen anabolism and catabolism serum biomarkers, as well as simple immunoglobulin techniques, can be used to determine prognosis in patients with Hidradenitis Suppurativa. Hidradenitis suppurativa may also soon be diagnosed using unique B-cells.
- Inflammatory-based diseases of the skin and the digestive system show serum biomarkers that control similar inflammatory-related functions. These diseases have overlapping qualities and incidences, prompting further necessity for research involving the specific profiles shared among them.
- Psoriasis diagnosis and prognosis can be determined based off serum biomarkers such as inflammatory cytokines, interleukins, and certain gene products.
- Reliable serum biomarkers in most dermatological diseases require more research. Concrete data from clinical trials need to be collected in order to further develop reliable technology and diagnostic criterion.

References

1. Wu Y, Gu C, Wang S, et al. Serum biomarker-based endotypes of atopic dermatitis in China and prediction for efficacy of dupilumab. Br J Dermatol. 2023;188(5):649–60. https://doi.org/10.1093/bjd/ljad032.

2. Ogulur I, Pat Y, Ardicli O, et al. Advances and highlights in biomarkers of allergic diseases. Allergy. 2021;76(12):3659–86. https://doi.org/10.1111/all.15089.
3. Gahan PB. Circulating nucleic acids in plasma and serum: diagnosis and prognosis in cancer. EPMA J. 2010;1(3):503–12. https://doi.org/10.1007/s13167-010-0021-6.
4. Olivier M, Asmis R, Hawkins GA, Howard TD, Cox LA. The need for multi-omics biomarker signatures in precision medicine. Int J Mol Sci. 2019;20(19). https://doi.org/10.3390/ijms20194781.
5. Zakria D, Brownstone N, Armstrong AW, et al. Integrating precision medicine into medical dermatology clinical practice: an expert consensus panel. J Drugs Dermatol. 2023;22(6):588–93. https://doi.org/10.36849/JDD.7432.
6. Zhu Z, Hu E, Shen H, Tan J, Zeng S. The functional and clinical roles of liquid biopsy in patient-derived models. J Hematol Oncol. 2023;16(1):36. https://doi.org/10.1186/s13045-023-01433-5.
7. Liu J, Chen Y, Pei F, et al. Extracellular vesicles in liquid biopsies: potential for disease diagnosis. Biomed Res Int. 2021;2021:6611244. https://doi.org/10.1155/2021/6611244.
8. Khoja L, Lorigan P, Dive C, Keilholz U, Fusi A. Circulating tumour cells as tumour biomarkers in melanoma: detection methods and clinical relevance. Ann Oncol. 2015;26(1):33–9. https://doi.org/10.1093/annonc/mdu207.
9. Califf RM. Biomarker definitions and their applications. Exp Biol Med (Maywood). 2018;243(3):213–21. https://doi.org/10.1177/1535370217750088.
10. Heckler I, Hong M, Amart Sinha A, Venkataraman I. Serological biomarkers and their detection in autoimmune bullous skin diseases. Dermatol Pract Concept. 2022;12(2): e2022116. https://doi.org/10.5826/dpc.1202a116.
11. Carey B, Setterfield J. Mucous membrane pemphigoid and oral blistering diseases. Clin Exp Dermatol. 2019;44(7):732–9. https://doi.org/10.1111/ced.13996.
12. Hertl M, Niedermeier A, Borradori L. Autoimmune bullous skin disorders. Ther Umsch. 2010;67(9):465–82. https://doi.org/10.1024/0040-5930/a000080.
13. Wilmer EN, Gustafson CJ, Ahn CS, Davis SA, Feldman SR, Huang WW. Most common dermatologic conditions encountered by dermatologists and nondermatologists. Cutis. 2014;94(6):285–92.
14. Utikal J, Schadendorf D, Ugurel S. Serologic and immunohistochemical prognostic biomarkers of cutaneous malignancies. Arch Dermatol Res. 2007;298(10):469–77. https://doi.org/10.1007/s00403-006-0726-5.
15. Huang N, Lee KJ, Stark MS. Current trends in circulating biomarkers for melanoma detection. Front Med (Lausanne). 2022;9: 873728. https://doi.org/10.3389/fmed.2022.873728.
16. Voit C, Kron M, Rademaker J, et al. Molecular staging in stage II and III melanoma patients and its effect on long-term survival. J Clin Oncol. 2005;23(6):1218–27. https://doi.org/10.1200/JCO.2005.04.098.
17. Lucci A, Hall CS, Patel SP, et al. Circulating tumor cells and early relapse in node-positive melanoma. Clin Cancer Res. 2020;26(8):1886–95. https://doi.org/10.1158/1078-0432.CCR-19-2670.
18. McEvoy AC, Warburton L, Al-Ogaili Z, et al. Correlation between circulating tumour DNA and metabolic tumour burden in metastatic melanoma patients. BMC Cancer 2018;18(1):726. https://doi.org/10.1186/s12885-018-4637-6.
19. McEvoy AC, Pereira MR, Reid A, et al. Monitoring melanoma recurrence with circulating tumor DNA: a proof of concept from three case studies. Oncotarget. 2019;10(2):113–22. https://doi.org/10.18632/oncotarget.26451.
20. Beasley AB, Chen FK, Isaacs TW, Gray ES. Future perspectives of uveal melanoma blood based biomarkers. Br J Cancer. 2022;126(11):1511–28. https://doi.org/10.1038/s41416-022-01723-8.
21. Lee JH, Saw RP, Thompson JF, et al. Pre-operative ctDNA predicts survival in high-risk stage III cutaneous melanoma patients. Ann Oncol. 2019;30(5):815–22. https://doi.org/10.1093/annonc/mdz075.

22. Tan L, Sandhu S, Lee RJ, et al. Prediction and monitoring of relapse in stage III melanoma using circulating tumor DNA. Ann Oncol. 2019;30(5):804–14. https://doi.org/10.1093/annonc/mdz048.
23. Wu N, Sun H, Sun Q, et al. Circulating microRNAs as diagnostic biomarkers for melanoma: a systematic review and meta-analysis. BMC Cancer. 2023;23(1):414. https://doi.org/10.1186/s12885-023-10891-6.
24. Lee IT, Shen CH, Tsai FC, Chen CB, Ma KS. Cancer-derived extracellular vesicles as biomarkers for cutaneous squamous cell carcinoma: a systematic review. Cancers (Basel). 2022;14(20). https://doi.org/10.3390/cancers14205098.
25. Cañueto J, Cardeñoso-Álvarez E, García-Hernández JL, et al. MicroRNA (miR)-203 and miR-205 expression patterns identify subgroups of prognosis in cutaneous squamous cell carcinoma. Br J Dermatol. 2017;177(1):168–78. https://doi.org/10.1111/bjd.15236.
26. Dobre EG, Constantin C, Neagu M, Skin cancer research goes digital: looking for biomarkers within the droplets. J Pers Med. 2022;12(7). https://doi.org/10.3390/jpm12071136.
27. Hu P, Ma L, Wu Z, Zheng G, Li J. Expression of miR-34a in basal cell carcinoma patients and its relationship with prognosis. J BUON. 2019;24(3):1283–8.
28. Yu L, Li L. Potential biomarkers of atopic dermatitis. Front Med (Lausanne). 2022;9:1028694. https://doi.org/10.3389/fmed.2022.1028694.
29. Holm JG, Hurault G, Agner T, et al. Immunoinflammatory biomarkers in serum are associated with disease severity in atopic dermatitis. Dermatology. 2021;237(4):513–20. https://doi.org/10.1159/000514503.
30. Brunner PM, Guttman-Yassky E, Leung DY. The immunology of atopic dermatitis and its reversibility with broad-spectrum and targeted therapies. J Allergy Clin Immunol. 2017;139(4S):S65–76. https://doi.org/10.1016/j.jaci.2017.01.011.
31. Renert-Yuval Y, Thyssen JP, Bissonnette R, et al. Biomarkers in atopic dermatitis-a review on behalf of the International Eczema Council. J Allergy Clin Immunol. 2021;147(4):1174-1190.e1. https://doi.org/10.1016/j.jaci.2021.01.013.
32. StatPearls. 2023.
33. Stríz I, Trebichavský I. Calprotectin—a pleiotropic molecule in acute and chronic inflammation. Physiol Res. 2004;53(3):245–53.
34. Katsumoto T, Mitsushima A, Kurimura T. The role of the vimentin intermediate filaments in rat 3Y1 cells elucidated by immunoelectron microscopy and computer-graphic reconstruction. Biol Cell. 1990;68(2):139–46. https://doi.org/10.1016/0248-4900(90)90299-i.
35. Groen SS, Nielsen VW, Ravn Jørgensen A-H. 33530 Novel serological biomarkers are associated with disease severity and systemic inflammation in patients with hidradenitis suppurativa. J Am Acad Dermatol. 2022;87(3, Supplement):AB86. https://doi.org/10.1016/j.jaad.2022.06.376.
36. Mintoff D, Borg I, Pace NP. Serum immunoglobulin G is a marker of hidradenitis suppurativa disease severity. Int J Mol Sci. 2022;23(22). https://doi.org/10.3390/ijms232213800.
37. Gudjonsson JE, Tsoi LC, Ma F, et al. Contribution of plasma cells and B cells to hidradenitis suppurativa pathogenesis. JCI Insight. 2020;5(19). https://doi.org/10.1172/jci.insight.139930.
38. Liu Y, Wang H, Taylor M, et al. Classification of human chronic inflammatory skin disease based on single-cell immune profiling. Sci Immunol. 2022;7(70):eabl9165. https://doi.org/10.1126/sciimmunol.abl9165.
39. Weisman MH, Oleg Stens, Seok Kim H, Hou JK, Miller FW, Dillon CF. Inflammatory bowel disease prevalence: surveillance data from the U.S. National Health and Nutrition Examination Survey. Prev Med Rep. 2023;33:102173. https://doi.org/10.1016/j.pmedr.2023.102173.
40. Flohr C, Hay R. Putting the burden of skin diseases on the global map. Br J Dermatol. 2021;184(2):189–90. https://doi.org/10.1111/bjd.19704.
41. Laughter MR, Maymone MBC, Mashayekhi S, et al. The global burden of atopic dermatitis: lessons from the Global Burden of Disease Study 1990–2017. Br J Dermatol. 2021;184(2):304–9. https://doi.org/10.1111/bjd.19580.
42. Schneeweiss MC, Kirchgesner J, Wyss R, et al. Occurrence of inflammatory bowel disease in patients with chronic inflammatory skin diseases: a cohort study: classification: epidemiology. Br J Dermatol. 2022;187(5):692–703. https://doi.org/10.1111/bjd.21704.

43. Schmitt H, Neurath MF, Atreya R. Role of the IL23/IL17 pathway in crohn's disease. Front Immunol. 2021;12: 622934. https://doi.org/10.3389/fimmu.2021.622934.
44. Biasci D, Lee JC, Noor NM, et al. A blood-based prognostic biomarker in IBD. Gut. 2019;68(8):1386–95. https://doi.org/10.1136/gutjnl-2019-318343.
45. Lin CE, Kaptein JS, Sheikh J. Differential expression of microRNAs and their possible roles in patients with chronic idiopathic urticaria and active hives. Allergy Rhinol (Providence). 2017;8(2):67–80. https://doi.org/10.2500/ar.2017.8.0199.
46. Honma M, Nozaki H. Molecular pathogenesis of psoriasis and biomarkers reflecting disease activity. J Clin Med. 2021;10(15). https://doi.org/10.3390/jcm10153199.
47. Ramessur R, Corbett M, Marshall D, et al. Biomarkers of disease progression in people with psoriasis: a scoping review. Br J Dermatol. 2022;187(4):481–93. https://doi.org/10.1111/bjd.21627.

Chapter 3
Biomarkers in Psoriasis

Ananya Koripella, Esther Balogh, and Steven Feldman

Abstract Psoriasis is an inflammatory skin condition involving the overactivation of the innate and adaptive immune responses. Its dermatological manifestations greatly reduce patients' health and quality of life. While there may be no cure for psoriasis yet, many biomarkers have been identified in the blood and tissue of psoriasis patients, the levels of which may be informative about diagnosis, prognosis, treatment efficacy, and monitoring comorbidities in this condition. These biomarkers include keratin proteins, apoptotic proteins, and several inflammatory mediators like cytokines and TNF-α. Many genetic biomarkers for psoriasis that may inform susceptibility to the condition have also been researched and discovered. These genetic markers play a role in the pathogenesis and maintenance of psoriasis. While no gene therapy has been developed to reduce the expression of these genes, these biomarkers serve as important indicators of disease progression and response to treatment. The chapter will further expand on the role of biomarkers in psoriasis and its pathogenesis as well as its possible role in the future development of drug therapy.

Keywords Apoptosis · Biologics · Blood · Genetic · HLA-Cw6 · IL-17 · IL-23 · Keratin · Th17 · Tissue · TNF-alpha

---

A. Koripella (✉)
322 Glenolden Ct, Cary, NC 27513, USA
e-mail: ebalogh@wakehealth.edu

E. Balogh
Wake Forest School of Medicine, 4618 Country Club Road, Winston-Salem, NC 27104, USA

S. Feldman
Professor of Dermatology, Pathology and Social Sciences & Health Policy, Wake Forest School of Medicine, 4618 Country Club Road, Winston-Salem, NC 27104, USA
e-mail: sfeldman@wakehealth.edu

R. Norman (ed.), *Biomarkers in Dermatology*,
https://doi.org/10.1007/978-3-031-66513-4_3

3.1 Introduction

Psoriasis is an immune-mediated inflammatory skin disease which affects two percent of patients worldwide [1, 2]. Its systemic manifestations include erythema, scaly skin lesions, papules, plaques, and the involvement of nails and joints. The skin lesions typically become pruritic and a source of pain [2]. Although psoriasis is a genetically pre-determined skin condition, its onset and exacerbation are usually associated with a variety of stressful environmental and immunological risk factors [2, 3]. As a multifactorial disease, its complete immunopathogenesis has not yet been completely understood, making treatment of psoriasis difficult and the course of the disease unpredictable [4]. Because psoriasis is a visually apparent skin condition, the severity of which can most often be determined clinically without the need for laboratory tests, the clinical utility of biomarkers in psoriasis may not be as profound as in conditions with little to no visually apparent manifestations, such as diabetes mellitus. Because of this, choice of treatment in psoriasis is usually based upon visual manifestations of skin lesions, comorbidities, and access to care [4, 5].

However, biomarkers may provide an additional tool to assess disease severity and to monitor the appearance or progression of psoriasis comorbidities that may not have a visually apparent manifestation, such as cardiovascular disease. They are important characteristics that are evaluated and measured to identify deviations from normal biological functions [4]. According to the World Health Organization, they are 'any substance, structure, or process that can be measured in the body or its products and influence or predict the incidence of outcome or disease' [6]. In addition to locating pathogenic processes and monitoring disease progression, they can also be used to evaluate pharmacological response in various diseases [4]. Different classes of biomarkers include screening biomarkers that identify risk of disease development, diagnostic biomarkers for disease identification, prognostic biomarkers for disease progression and response to therapy, as well as biomarkers for comorbidities to identify associated health issues [6].

As an immune disease, the pathogenesis of psoriasis involves the interaction of inflammatory mediators and immune cells, as well as genes that control their expression. These substances and structures may potentially serve as important biomarkers to better classify disease severity in some patients, as well as track disease progression and the development of certain comorbidities which are not easily visualized clinically [4]. In addition, identifying biomarkers for psoriasis has also led to the development of new biologics, such as IL-17 inhibitors, that have drastically improved the quality of life of psoriatic patients [7]. This chapter will discuss specific biomarkers found in the DNA, blood, and tissue of psoriasis patients as well as their implications on disease susceptibility, diagnosis, prognosis, and risk for comorbidities.

3.2 Methods

A literature search was conducted using the PubMed search engine. Keywords used included psoriasis, risk factors of psoriasis, psoriasis biomarkers, biomarkers for psoriasis, HLA psoriasis, pathogenesis psoriasis, IL-17 psoriasis, psoriasis biologics, tumor necrosis factor-alpha psoriasis, keratin in psoriasis, psoriasis apoptosis, psoriasis pharmacogenomics, and GlycA psoriasis cardio biomarker. One article discussing the World Health Organization's definition of biomarkers was also reviewed and included in the final bibliography.

The articles perused for this chapter were limited to publications since 2010 written in English. Search results were prescreened by reviewing abstracts and conclusions. Additional articles were found by utilizing the 'similar results' feature on PubMed. The results include 20 articles total on biomarkers in psoriasis.

Data collected on biomarkers in psoriasis were categorized into blood biomarkers, tissue biomarkers, and genetic biomarkers. Blood biomarkers were further categorized by biomarkers aiding in diagnosis, those aiding in determining prognosis of disease, and biomarkers tracking development and progression of comorbidities. Our information on tissue biomarkers focused on biomarkers aiding in diagnosis, while our discussion of genetic biomarkers focused on biomarkers potentially aiding in determining susceptibility to disease.

3.3 Pathogenesis of Psoriasis

All the biomarkers discussed in this chapter play a role in the onset and maintenance of psoriasis. To understand their importance, the pathogenesis of psoriasis must first be understood. Under normal conditions, when the skin faces any form of stress such as trauma or infection, signal transductions that mediate an immune response are controlled to maintain homeostasis. However, in psoriasis, the signal transduction pathways are amplified. External stimuli that serve as triggers for psoriatic lesions cause the release of antimicrobial peptides and self-nucleic acids from keratinocytes and dying epidermal cells, respectively [3]. These autoantigens activate the plasmacytoid dendritic cells and macrophages in the dermis through different toll-like receptors [3, 8]. Once activated, plasmacytoid dendritic cells and macrophages secrete type 1 interferon (IFN) and tissue necrosis factor-alpha (TNF-α) which activate the classical dendritic cells. The classical dendritic cells will then produce IL-23, a cytokine which plays a role in skewing the education of naïve T cells and differentiating them into Th1, Th17, and Th22 subsets [3, 8]. The now differentiated T cells react to autoantigens such as antimicrobial peptide LL-37 and the disintegrin-like and metalloprotease domain containing thrombospondin type 1 motif-like 5 (ADAMSTL5) [3].

Once the T cells have been activated through the innate immune response, they mediate a prolonged adaptive immune response. This response consists of reorganized dermal T cell infiltration as well as formation of dendritic cell and T cell clusters in the inflammatory lesions [3, 5]. The dermal dendritic cells and recruited macrophages continue to produce IL-23 which, in turn, stabilizes and stimulates the T cells in the psoriatic lesions to also continue producing IL-17. The cytokines associated with the Th1 (IL-17, 21, and 22) and Th17 (TNF-α and IFN-γ) subsets cause the proliferation of keratinocytes in the epidermis leading to hyperkeratosis [3, 8]. The keratinocytes can be triggered in the same manner as before and continue to drive and maintain the psoriatic inflammatory loop [3, 5].

Psoriasis is mainly a dermatological disease; it also affects the joints and is associated with multiple other diseases. The inflammation that is seen on the skin in psoriasis is not limited to the skin but, rather, is systemic. When compared to individuals without psoriasis, patients with psoriasis have higher rates of hyperlipidemia, hypertension, coronary artery disease, type 2 diabetes, and obesity [5].

3.4 Blood Biomarkers

Since psoriasis is an autoimmune disease, early studies have shown that patients have increased serum levels of non-specific inflammatory markers such as C-reactive protein (CRP), haptoglobin, and platelet P-selectin. There is also a marked increase in pro-inflammatory cytokine levels such as TNF-α, IFN-γ, IL-6, IL-8, IL-12, and IL-18 [4]. High circulating levels of Th1, Th17, and Th22 cells are also seen in patients with psoriasis. In line with the significance of the IL-23/17 axis in the pathogenesis of psoriasis, there is also an increase in the expression of IL-23R on the circulating T cells [4]. There is also evidence of increased production of IL-17A in cells and an upregulation of IL-17A related genes in the skin of psoriasis patients [9].

As important biomarkers of psoriasis, many medications now target several of these pro-inflammatory mediators. Therapeutic benefits have been noted with administering anti-TNF therapy, using an IL-17 blockade, and targeting IL-12/23. There is decreased infiltration of Th1 and Th17 cells after anti-TNF therapy [4]. Targeting the IL-23/IL-17A axis has also significantly improved skin and joint symptoms in mild-to-severe psoriasis cases [9].

3.4.1 Diagnostic Biomarkers

3.4.1.1 TNF-α

Early studies on TNF-α led to the understanding of its role in innate inflammatory pathways for diseases such as psoriasis, rheumatoid arthritis, and inflammatory bowel disease [9]. Many of its roles in inducing inflammation in psoriasis overlap with those of IL-17. TNF-α mostly activates keratinocytes to produce inflammatory mediators through the NF-κB pathway [10]. Through this pathway, TNF-α promotes the transcription of multiple genes that code for pro-inflammatory mediators and cytokines including inducible Nitric Oxide Synthase (iNOS), cyclooxygenase-2 (COX-2), IL-1β, IL-8, IL-12, IL-23, and more TNF-α [3]. The serum and plasma levels as well as the skin lesions of patients with psoriasis exhibit increased levels of TNF-α. In a study of 79 patients with psoriasis vulgaris and 29 patients with psoriatic arthritis, psoriasis patients had higher circulating levels of TNF-α DNA levels than patients without psoriasis. This indicates that this serum marker may have utility in confirming diagnosis of psoriasis, although the actual clinical utility of this may be limited as visible skin lesions offer a convenient and noninvasive avenue through which to evaluate the psoriasis patient [11].

3.4.1.2 IL-23/IL-17

The onset and maintenance of psoriasis, however, are mainly promoted by the IL-23/IL-17 axis. They are the key inflammatory mediators in psoriasis. IL-23 stimulates the differentiation, activation, and proliferation of T cells into the Th1 and Th17 subsets. These subsets secrete effector cytokines like IL-17. IL-17 then promotes inflammation, coagulation, and bone/joint damage that is seen in patients with psoriasis. IL-23 is more 'upstream' in its effects on the pathogenic process of psoriasis, while IL-17 is more 'downstream' in its effects and directly impacts tissue [9].

IL-17A is one of the main cytokine effectors in psoriatic lesions. Its transcriptional activation is proportionally higher in the cells of psoriatic patients than that of IL-22 or IFN-γ. IL-17 also increases the expression of the autoantigens LL-37 and ADAMTSL5. The IL-17 family consists of six members in total: 17A-17F. Within the family, IL-17A, 17C, and 17F are thought to be a part of psoriatic pathogenesis since their expression is approximately eight times higher in psoriatic lesions than that of their other family members. When compared to each other, the levels of IL-17C and 17F are far higher than the level of 17A. However, 17A is more biologically active in stimulating keratinocytes to secrete more cytokines and chemokines. Given the increased expression of these markers in psoriasis patients, it is possible that serum levels of these cytokines may aid in the diagnosis of psoriasis in cases where additional information is needed besides the clinical picture of skin lesions.

For many years, it was thought that IL-17 is only secreted from Th17 cells. However, recent data also suggest that there are other sources of IL-17 including innate lymphoid cells, extracellular neutrophil traps, and mast cells. The mast cell extracellular trap formation, induced by IL-23 and IL-1β, is also associated with the secretion of IL-17. When triggered, mast cells degranulate and release many cytokines and chemokines such as IL-17, TNF-α, and C-X-C Chemokine Ligand 2 (CXCL2). They can capture, store, and release IL-17A when needed and prompt its secretion from Th1 and Th17 cells as well. Innate lymphoid cells that express IL-17A and chemokine receptor type 6 (CCR6) are seen in high levels in the blood and tissue of patients with psoriasis. Their levels decrease with anti-TNF therapy. CCR6 serves as a cell surface marker for T cells expressing IL-17A. When IL-17A is in the epidermis, it increases keratinocyte expression of chemokine ligand 20 (CCL20). This chemokine, in turn, recruits CD8+ T cells and CCR6+ CD4+ T cells into the skin. CCR6 and CCL20 are involved in the interaction of dendritic cells with T cells, and ultimately, with the activation of T cells [9]. Because blood and tissue levels of CCR6 are increased in patients with psoriasis, like TNFα and IL-23/IL-17, this biomarker may be useful in aiding or confirming a diagnosis of psoriasis as well.

3.4.2 Prognostic Biomarkers

3.4.2.1 TNF-α

While TNF-α has been known as one of the first biomarkers of psoriasis, new studies are now also exploring circulating cell-free DNA of TNF-α as another possible biomarker. Circulating cell-free DNA (cfDNA) is released from apoptotic or necrotic cells. It serves as an indicator of cell damage. The gene encoding for TNF-α is in the cfDNA in increased levels in patients with psoriasis and is positively correlated with the severity of symptoms. The cfDNA of TNF-α has a longer half-life than the TNF-α protein itself. With further studies, it is possible that, in the future, the TNF-α cfDNA can serve as a better biomarker for psoriasis severity than the TNF-α protein [11]. In the study of psoriasis patients mentioned in Sect. 4.1.1, levels of TNF-α DNA copies in cfDNA correlated positively with the Psoriasis Area and Severity Index (PASI) score in patients with scores of 10 or higher, which corresponds to severe psoriasis. Consequently, levels of TNF-α DNA copies in cfDNA may have utility as a biomarker for disease severity and disease progression in psoriasis patients when a quantitative objective marker is needed to complement the BSA or PASI score.

3.4.2.2 IL-23/IL-17

In addition to serving as diagnostic biomarkers, many of the same inflammatory mediators also serve as prognostic biomarkers to understand a patient's response to therapy. Before IL-23/IL-17 inhibitors were developed, anti-TNF-α therapy was initially used to treat psoriasis [9]. TNF-α blockers are first-generation biologics for psoriasis and include etanercept, infliximab, adalimumab, and certolizumab pegol [3]. However, their therapeutic benefits do not only arise from the sole inhibition of TNF-α but also from the indirect inhibition of the IL-23/IL-17A axis. This was evident in the clinical trials of etanercept, an anti-TNF-α medication, where a downregulation of IL-17A signaling was also noticed. When IL-17A blockade alone is administered, however, it is highly effective in alleviating psoriasis symptoms by itself. This led to the conclusion that while both IL-17 and TNF-α function to stimulate keratinocytes, the IL-23/IL-17A axis is the key mediator in psoriatic pathogenesis and TNF-α plays a more supporting role in promoting inflammation [9]. Because inhibiting the IL-23/IL-17A axis has been such an effective therapeutic target in psoriasis, it follows that measuring levels of these cytokines may provide clinical utility in determining disease severity. However, because psoriasis is a visually apparent and usually clinically diagnosed condition, measuring levels of these biomarkers may not be as clinically useful in psoriasis as in other conditions wherein the pathology is not easily visualized clinically.

There is also evidence that biologic therapy that solely targets IL-17A decreases the gene expression of multiple cytokines and chemokines. For example, two weeks of IL-17A blockade normalized 765 genes in comparison to TNF-α inhibition that has normalized less than 200 genes. Therapy with IL-17 blockade has also cleared psoriatic skin lesions more effectively than TNF-α inhibition has [9]. Monitoring TNFα levels to determine potential response to treatment may have had more clinical utility when TNFα inhibition was one of the only therapeutic options and only a smaller percentage of patients showed clinical response to it. However, given that a much higher percentage of patients show clinical response to inhibitors of the IL-17/IL-23 axis, measuring serum levels of these cytokines may have less clinical utility in determining drug choice since the majority of patients respond well to these agents. The biologic therapies that are currently being used and developed to target the IL-23/IL-17 axis differ based on their mechanism of actions. IL-23 inhibitors include guselkumab, risankizumab, tildrakizumab, and mirikizumab. Ustekinumab is an IL-23/IL-12 inhibitor. Bimekizumab is an IL-17A inhibitor. Brodalumab is an IL-17A receptor antagonist [12].

3.4.2.3 Th17 Cells

The Th1, 17, and 22 subsets of CD4+ T helper cells are important in the pathogenesis of psoriasis. The pro-inflammatory mediators such as IL-23, drive their differentiation and maintain their increased levels in blood and psoriatic skin plaques [3]. Th17 cells are more largely implicated since they secrete IL-17. Biologics such as secukinumab, bimekizumab, and ixekizumab that block IL-17 show a significant alleviation in psoriasis symptoms [3, 13]. IL-36, a cytokine that is a part of the IL-1 cytokine family that stimulates the proliferation of Th17 cells, is also a target for biologics. These include IL-36R blockers such as spesolimab and imsidolimab. Anakinra, on the other hand, is an IL-1R antagonist that also inhibits the proliferation of Th17 cells downstream [3]. While measuring serum levels of biomarkers secreted by these Th cells such as IL-23, IL-17, and IL-36 could potentially be useful in monitoring progression of psoriatic disease severity and response to treatment, psoriasis is an overwhelmingly clinical diagnosis. Skin lesions and corresponding disease severity are readily visible clinically, and therefore, measuring levels of these biomarkers may not have as much clinical utility in psoriasis as in other conditions without cutaneous manifestations.

3.4.3 *Biomarkers of Comorbidities*

3.4.3.1 GlycA

Evidence shows that psoriasis as an independent factor increases a patient's risk for myocardial infarction, stroke, and death due to cardiovascular disease. The chronic low-grade inflammation in psoriasis increases the rate of vascular disease development [5]. A new biomarker found in the blood and serum of psoriasis patients has been associated with atherosclerotic cardiovascular disease [5, 14]. Using nuclear magnetic resonance (NMR) spectroscopy, GlycA, a glycan N-acetylglucosamine residue, was identified [5]. During systemic inflammation, acute phase proteins undergo many cycles of changes in concentrations and glycosylation patterns. These changes are seen in the NMR signals of GlycA since the proteins circulating throughout the body are at high concentrations to contribute to the signal. Since it is a composite marker rather than a single glycoprotein component, its signaling stays stable over time and eliminates any possible individual variability [14].

GlycA is not only a biomarker for comorbidities such as cardiovascular disease and systemic inflammation but is also a biomarker for disease prognosis. GlycA shows a positive correlation with ongoing disease severity and inflammation. With both pharmaceutical therapy and nonpharmaceutical therapy like exercise and weight loss, a decrease in GlycA concentrations is seen [5, 14]. Clinical measurement of GlycA may have utility in monitoring the status and avoiding the progression of conditions that occur comorbidly in patients with psoriasis and could potentially inform the necessity of treatment of these comorbidities. Biomarkers to assess hidden comorbidity risks of psoriasis may have more utility than biomarkers of psoriasis severity, since psoriasis severity can easily be measured directly.

3.5 Tissue Biomarkers

With skin manifestations being the main concern in psoriasis, tissue provides easy access to identifying biomarkers. Most of the associated biomarkers are related to abnormalities in keratinocyte differentiation and proliferation [4].

3.5.1 *Diagnostic Biomarkers*

3.5.1.1 Keratin

When the skin faces trauma, keratinocytes react and secrete alarming molecules that trigger an innate immune response [15]. In psoriasis, this immune response is dysregulated and leads to uncontrolled inflammation and, later on, an abnormal keratinocyte response that drives the maintenance of the skin plaques and lesions [5, 15]. Keratins are important structural proteins in keratinocytes. Depending upon the stage of differentiation of keratinocytes, different keratins are secreted [15].

Keratinocytes in psoriasis downregulate the expression of keratin (K)1 and (K)10 and upregulate K6, 16, and 17. These three proteins are involved in the hyperproliferation, inflammation, and innate immune activation of keratinocytes [4, 15]. Normally, these proteins help the keratinocytes protect themselves against injury and with the regulation of immune system homeostasis. Genome-wide studies have recently identified mutations in these three proteins that are associated with psoriasis. These mutations are clustered together in the rod domain of the keratin proteins resulting in detrimental effects to their stability and expression. Unfortunately, their implications in the pathogenesis of psoriasis are not yet completely understood [15].

Though the measurement of the levels of K proteins could theoretically be useful in confirming a diagnosis of psoriasis, clinically, this may have limited utility as psoriasis lesions have a characteristic morphology and the disease state is usually easy to identify from the clinical picture alone. Therefore, further tissue examination and testing may not be necessary in most cases and may even lead to unnecessary intervention and risk. In a patient with a family history of psoriasis, it is possible that genetic testing to identify potentially mutated K proteins could possibly serve to highlight increased propensity for the development of psoriasis; however, the clinical usefulness of discovering increased propensity for a condition which has not yet clinically manifested and which does not have a cure is uncertain.

3.5.1.2 Apoptotic Proteins

Not only is there hyperproliferation of keratinocytes in psoriasis, but there is also an abnormality in the cells' apoptotic processes [4, 16]. In psoriasis, the epidermis contains significantly less apoptotic cells than the epidermis of a healthy individual without dermatological issues. The keratinocytes also are resistant to the pro-apoptotic signals that induce cell death. The weakening of the mechanisms of apoptosis leads to an increase in the number of autoimmune cells recruited to the area of tissue in question, thus leading to the tissue inflammation seen in psoriasis [16].

Apoptosis is regulated by pro-apoptotic and anti-apoptotic proteins. The pro-apoptotic proteins include Bax, Bak, and Bad; the anti-apoptotic proteins include Bcl-2 and Bcl-xL [16]. In the epidermis of psoriasis patients, there are higher levels of the anti-apoptotic protein Bcl-xL due to the increased expression of the gene that codes for this protein. This leads to epidermal acanthosis [16]. One of the reasons for the increased expression of Bcl-xL is due to the high secretion of TNF-α: TNF-α not only increases the expression of the gene for Bcl-xL but also for the anti-apoptotic protein Bcl-2 and the pro-apoptotic protein Bax [16]. Although expression for the pro-apoptotic proteins also increased, the expression for the anti-apoptotic proteins is much higher. Ratio wise, if the expression of Bax is increased six times, the expression of Bcl-xL is increased 22 times [17].

The mechanism of effect of TNF-α is not yet completely understood, but its role as an inducer in the hyperexpression of certain genes in psoriasis led to the use of TNA-α inhibitors as a first-generation treatment for the condition [16]. The Fas receptor, a transmembrane protein, is a part of the TNF family as well. It is expressed in high levels in the serum and keratinocytes of psoriasis patients [16]. As a result, measurement of anti-apoptotic protein and Fas receptor levels could theoretically aid in diagnosing psoriasis and determining response to therapy; however, because of the visually apparent nature of psoriasis pathology and the extent to which the condition is an overwhelmingly clinical diagnosis, the actual clinical utility of measuring these markers is not apparent.

3.6 Genetic Biomarkers

It has been well documented that psoriasis can be inherited. Recently, with genome-wide association studies, more than 60 psoriasis susceptibility loci have been identified that increase one's susceptibility for psoriasis [1, 18]. Genome-wide association studies investigated an excess of a single nucleotide polymorphism (SNP) allele in cases of psoriasis when compared with matched controls. The genes identified in these regions have various functions in antigen presentation, the IL-23 axis, T cell development and polarization, negative regulation, and innate immunity. Through these studies, the Human Leukocyte Antigen (HLA)-Cw6 was found to have the most risk for psoriasis. Other genes that were identified include ERAP1, TYK2, STAT3, and CARD14 [13].

These genome-wide association studies are helpful in the identification of genes that serve as genetic biomarkers which increase susceptibility to developing psoriasis [1]. While the many biologics that have been developed are effective in treating psoriasis, their efficacy is variable from one patient to another. Identifying the biomarkers that a patient expresses may help physicians to not only identify patients who are potentially at risk for developing psoriasis, but also to predict responses to treatments in existing psoriasis patients and create a more effective, personalized therapeutic regimen [19]. For example, a patient with an SNP in TNF-related genes such as TNFAIP3 will have a better response to anti-TNF therapy [13]. Additionally, if a patient was to express the HLA-Cw6 allele, they are less likely to respond to adalimumab, etanercept, or infliximab [20].

3.6.1 Susceptibility Biomarkers

3.6.1.1 Antigen Presentation

Psoriasis has its greatest association with nine loci identified as PROS1-9. Out of the nine loci, PROS1 has the strongest link to psoriasis susceptibility. This is because it is in the major histocompatibility region and is therefore associated with 35–50% heritability of psoriasis [3]. Within the MHC region, the allele that is known as the psoriasis susceptibility allele of PSORS1 is HLA-Cw6 [1]. HLA-C's general role is presenting antigens to and activating the CD8+ T cells. One of its serotypes, HLA-Cw6, serves as a biomarker for psoriasis due to its higher affinity for certain psoriatic autoantigens such as the antimicrobial peptide LL-37 [3]. HLA-Cw6 is linked to type 1 early-onset psoriasis, guttate psoriasis, and the Koebner phenomenon. Patients who are HLA-Cw6 positive have a better response to drugs such as methotrexate and interleukin (IL)-12/23, 17, and 23 targeting agents and a decreased response to anti-tumor necrosis factor drugs [18], making HLA-Cw6 positivity a potentially useful biomarker in choosing targeted therapy for individual psoriasis patients.

While HLA-Cw6 is prevalent in most populations, its prevalence is lower in Asian populations. For many patients with psoriasis that are a part of the Asian population, there is a stronger association with HLA-Cw1 than with HLA-Cw6. HLA-Cw1 is associated with erythrodermic and pustular psoriasis as well as an axial form of psoriatic arthritis. HLA-Cw1 is also linked to cases in which patients' symptoms are not responsive to conventional treatment; therefore, identification of HLA-Cw1 in a psoriasis patient, along with a corresponding clinical picture, may point toward susceptibility to refractory disease and the need for more aggressive treatment and thus influence management decisions. There are currently no known triggers or autoantigens that are associated with HLA-Cw1 [18].

Different alleles in another class of HLA also play a role in psoriasis. HLA-B27 is specific for psoriatic arthritis. HLA-B22, on the other hand, is a protective allele against psoriasis [4]. Two other genes that are postulated to be associated with psoriasis are ERAP1 and ERAP2. ERAP1 and 2, also known as endoplasmic reticulum aminopeptidases, are involved in the processing of peptides that are loaded onto MHC class 1 presenting cells. ERAP1 and 2 are thought to increase the efficacy of HLA-Cw6. If the autoantigens of psoriasis can be more easily processed by ERAP1 and 2, they can be more quickly presented by HLA-Cw6 and therefore trigger a stronger T cell-mediated reaction. However, more research must be conducted to understand this process and identify the specific autoantigens that would be involved in the ERAP processing [13].

3.6.1.2 IL-23

IL-23 is very important in the pathogenesis of psoriasis as a Th17 polarizing cytokine. IL-23 consists of p40 and p19 subunits. Expression of both subunit levels and IL-23 levels is increased in psoriatic lesions. Several single nucleotide polymorphisms that indicate susceptibility to psoriasis are seen in two genes associated with the subunits of IL-23. Those genes are ILI12Bp40 and IL23Ap19. Several others are seen in IL-23R which is the gene for the IL-23 receptor. The IL-23 receptor does not have intrinsic signaling activity and, therefore, relies on downstream signaling molecules. Genome-wide association studies have found connections between psoriasis and TYK2, JAK2, and STAT3. These genes encode for a tyrosine kinase protein, a Janus kinase 2 (JAK2) protein, and a signal transducer/activator of transcription 3, respectively. All these proteins are involved in the downstream signaling of IL-23 [13]. Genetic identification of polymorphisms related to IL-23 subunits may serve as useful biomarkers of susceptibility to development of clinical psoriasis in patients with a family history of the condition. Furthermore, because IL-23 levels are increased in psoriatic lesions, measurement of this biomarker has the potential to be used as a gauge of treatment efficacy, although this is typically clinically determined in psoriasis through the status of visible lesions making the practical utility of such tissue testing questionable.

3.6.1.3 T Cell Polarization and Development

T helper cell subsets are widely known blood and tissue biomarkers for psoriasis [4]. Some of the genes that code for them can also be used as biomarkers for susceptibility to clinical development of psoriasis. RUNX3 encodes a transcription factor necessary for CD8+ T cell development and the polarization of Th1 and Th17 cells. RUNX1, another gene in the Runt-domain family, also has psoriasis-associated mutations. However, the manner in which these genes' mutations contribute to psoriasis has still not been ascertained. STAT3 is a genetic biomarker for IL-23 but can also be considered a biomarker for psoriatic T cells since the downstream signaling of IL-23 is one of the main mediators of T cell polarization. Other genes like TAGAP, the T cell activation RhoGTPase activating protein, are also implicated in their contribution to the onset of psoriasis. More research is needed to understand their functions and associations to psoriasis; however, these biomarkers may in the future serve to detect susceptibility to developing clinically apparent psoriasis and thus encourage early detection and management in high-risk individuals, such as those with a family history of the condition [13].

3.6.1.4 Negative Regulation

While the human body has mechanisms to induce an immune response, there are also pathways to suppress immune responses to maintain homeostasis. There are a few mutations associated with psoriasis susceptibility in genes involved in the downregulation of the NF-κB pathway. Two of these genes are TNFAIP3 for tumor necrosis factor-alpha-induced protein 3 and TNIP1 that codes for TNFAIP3 interacting protein 1, annexin A6. These two genes work together to inhibit NF-κB signaling through the degradation of IκB, the inhibitor for NF-κB. However, mutations result in a reduced ability to suppress signaling, leading to a more flagrant inflammatory reaction in those with psoriasis [13]. As with other previously mentioned biomarkers which can identify increased susceptibility to psoriasis development, identifying genetic mutations in the NF-κB pathway may also potentially serve to detect disease susceptibility in higher risk patients.

3.6.1.5 Innate Immunity

An initial activation of the innate immune system is seen at the beginning of the pathogenesis of psoriasis. Some of the genes involved in the innate immune system have associations with psoriasis. These associations indicate a susceptibility to psoriasis and a decreased threshold for the adaptive immune response to begin and continue the pathologic inflammatory response [13].

TNF-α is one of the inflammatory cytokines that activates the NF-κB pathway. NF-κB is an important transcription factor for the induction of inflammatory gene expression in immune responses. Out of its multiple subunits, c-Rel has increased susceptibility in psoriasis and regulates keratinocyte growth. There is also an SNP in TRAF3IP2 gene that codes for the TRAF3 interacting protein 2. This SNP also increases susceptibility to psoriasis. The SNP results in an increased activation of the NF-κB pathway, leading to the overproduction of more pro-inflammatory mediators that can trigger the adaptive immune response [13].

CARD14 is located on the PSORS2 loci [3]. CARD-proteins are involved in the activation of the signaling pathway of NF-κB [13]. This pathway stimulates the production of pro-inflammatory cytokine mediators. CARD14, also known as caspase recruitment domain family member 14, is produced in high levels in keratinocytes [3]. Mutations in this gene lead to the increased activation of the NF-κB pathways leading to the increased recruitment and activation of immune cells. Therapy with a TNF-α blockade helps decrease the expression of the NF-κB protein in the psoriatic skin lesions and decrease the activation of its pathway [13]. Thus, it is possible that patients with this particular mutation in CARD14 may have a superior response to TNF-α as compared to patients without this mutation, a consideration that may impact treatment decisions in this subset of patients.

In genome-wide studies, psoriasis susceptibility is associated with increased expression of interferon and anti-viral response genes. These genes, RIG-1 and MDA5, function to recognize nucleic acid sequences of pathogens. Mutations in these genes cause them to bind to self-identifying molecules, which is a key step in initiating lesion development. Treatment of the skin lesions with phototherapy drastically reduces their expression [13]. Because of this, it is possible that patients with these particular mutations may be especially good candidates for phototherapy.

3.7 Discussion

Research over the years has been able to identify many biomarkers for psoriasis. Those identified in the DNA, blood and tissue are involved in the pathogenesis of psoriasis and their levels can be measured to provide information on susceptibility to disease, diagnosis, disease status, progression, and prognosis, as well as information on development and status of certain comorbidities in psoriasis which cannot be easily visualized, such as cardiovascular disease [4].

Early research quickly identified TNF-α as a diagnostic and prognostic biomarker of psoriasis. As a result, anti-TNF therapy became the first line of treatment in psoriasis [3]. As more research was conducted and the importance of IL-23 and IL-17's roles in the pathogenesis of psoriasis became more evident, development of biologics turned toward antagonizing these inflammatory mediators. These medications provided more relief for patients and drastically improved their quality of life [9].

Because serum levels of these biomarkers are elevated in psoriasis patients as opposed to controls without psoriasis, it is possible that clinical measurement of these biomarkers could provide some useful information regarding solidifying a clinical diagnosis or efficacy of a patient's treatment regimen. High levels of tissue biomarkers like keratin and apoptotic proteins that are not a part of the inflammatory and immune processes have also been identified [15, 16]. Further research may delve into understanding how these biomarkers play a role in directly manifesting the psoriasis plaques and lesions and how their levels could be clinically useful in determining disease severity and response to treatment. However, because psoriasis is a visible cutaneous condition which is almost exclusively clinically diagnosed, and the disease progression can be monitored clinically through the utilization of skin lesion scoring systems such as the PASI, the clinical utility of the measurement of such markers remains uncertain and may be more useful in conditions such as diabetes mellitus wherein the pathology is not easily visualized.

Identification of biomarkers consistent with comorbidities prevalent in psoriasis patients, such as GlycA levels in psoriasis patients with cardiovascular comorbidities, has helped to identify the presence and progression of psoriasis-associated diseases that patients may suffer from that may not be as visually and clinically apparent as cutaneous lesions, and the status and progression of which cannot be easily determined from the clinical picture alone.

In addition to being pathognomonic for psoriasis, genetic biomarkers also serve as indicators of increased susceptibility to this condition. Genome-wide association studies have identified many loci, genes, and SNPs that play a factor in the onset and maintenance of psoriasis [1]. However, while we understand the implications of most of these genetic biomarkers on psoriasis, for many of them, the mechanisms of effects are still not clear. For example, T cell polarization and proliferation are integral to the pathogenesis of psoriasis. However, the roles of the mutated genes RUNX1, RUNX3, and TAGAP that have known associations with psoriasis are still unknown [13]. While substantial research has been conducted to identify genetic biomarkers, more research should now be tailored to understand their mechanisms of effects and what can be done to address the pathology they cause.

Another way that the genetic biomarkers prove to be useful is in identifying effective therapeutic regimens for patients who express certain SNPs or alleles [13]. While psoriasis symptoms in patients are similar, the triggers of onset can be different because of genetic code. Therefore, treatment to address the underlying pathology could potentially be different from person to person [13]. With more knowledge of how these biomarkers work, it may be possible that treatment, in the future, could be tailored to address specific genetic markers.

However, certain limitations to the utility of biomarkers in psoriasis also do exist. While it would be beneficial to tailor therapy to each patient depending on their expressed genetic biomarkers, it would be expensive and potentially inefficient to test each patient's genetic makeup, especially considering that certain biologic drugs, such as those targeting the IL-17/IL-23 axis, are remarkably effective in a very large percentage of psoriasis patients, therefore leaving this kind of genetic testing potentially clinically unimportant. There is also currently no development of new therapeutics that take the susceptibility biomarkers into consideration that specifically target the prevention of psoriasis. The treatments, including current biologic therapy, that are offered solely focus on alleviating the dermatologic manifestations that are seen in psoriasis. For biomarkers to be completely utilized in addressing psoriasis, new methods of management and innovative methods of prevention must be developed that are efficient, cheap, and easily duplicated from patient to patient.

3.8 Conclusion

As a multifactorial disease, it is difficult to find one main cause that triggers the onset of psoriasis in a patient. Likewise, it is difficult to find one sole target for curative treatment. The identification of various biomarkers that are expressed in psoriasis allow for a better understanding of its pathogenesis, maintenance, and response to therapy. Multiple biomarkers for psoriasis can be found in patients' genetic code, blood, and tissue. Enhanced knowledge of these biomarkers and the role they play in psoriasis can potentially aid in assessing susceptibility to the condition, diagnosis, treatment efficacy, and the status of common comorbidities which occur in psoriasis patients. However, psoriasis is and will probably remain a condition which is primarily assessed through examination of skin lesions, through which disease severity and response to treatment can be very easily assessed. Therefore, while blood, tissue, and genetic biomarkers may play some small role in aiding the evaluation of susceptibility, diagnosis, evaluation of treatment efficacy and comorbidities in psoriasis, as a visually apparent disease, the primary evaluation of psoriasis will most likely remain clinical.

References

1. Ogawa K, Okada Y. The current landscape of psoriasis genetics in 2020. J Dermatol Sci. 2020;99(1):2–8.
2. Weigle N, McBane S. Psoriasis. Am Fam Physician. 2013;87(9):626–33.
3. Tseng JC, Chang YC, Huang CM, Hsu LC, Chuang TH. Therapeutic Development based on the immunopathogenic mechanisms of psoriasis. Pharmaceutics. 2021;13(7).
4. Villanova F, Di Meglio P, Nestle FO. Biomarkers in psoriasis and psoriatic arthritis. Ann Rheum Dis. 2013;72 Suppl 2:ii104–10.
5. Rendon A, Schakel K. Psoriasis pathogenesis and treatment. Int J Mol Sci. 2019;20(6).

6. Thijs JL, van Seggelen W, Bruijnzeel-Koomen C, de Bruin-Weller M, Hijnen D. New developments in biomarkers for atopic dermatitis. J Clin Med. 2015;4(3):479–87.
7. Kamiya K, Kishimoto M, Sugai J, Komine M, Ohtsuki M. Risk factors for the development of psoriasis. Int J Mol Sci. 2019;20(18).
8. Bugaut H, Aractingi S. Major role of the IL17/23 axis in psoriasis supports the development of new targeted therapies. Front Immunol. 2021;12: 621956.
9. Blauvelt A, Chiricozzi A. The immunologic role of IL-17 in psoriasis and psoriatic arthritis pathogenesis. Clin Rev Allergy Immunol. 2018;55(3):379–90.
10. Chiricozzi A, Guttman-Yassky E, Suarez-Farinas M, Nograles KE, Tian S, Cardinale I, et al. Integrative responses to IL-17 and TNF-alpha in human keratinocytes account for key inflammatory pathogenic circuits in psoriasis. J Invest Dermatol. 2011;131(3):677–87.
11. Sakamoto R, Sawamura S, Kajihara I, Miyauchi H, Urata K, Otsuka-Maeda S, et al. Circulating tumor necrosis factor-alpha DNA are elevated in psoriasis. J Dermatol. 2020;47(9):1037–40.
12. Kamata M, Tada Y. Efficacy and safety of biologics for psoriasis and psoriatic arthritis and their impact on comorbidities: a literature review. Int J Mol Sci. 2020;21(5).
13. Harden JL, Krueger JG, Bowcock AM. The immunogenetics of psoriasis: a comprehensive review. J Autoimmun. 2015;64:66–73.
14. Mehta NN, Dey AK, Maddineni R, Kraus WE, Huffman KM. GlycA measured by NMR spectroscopy is associated with disease activity and cardiovascular disease risk in chronic inflammatory diseases. Am J Prev Cardiol. 2020;4: 100120.
15. Zhang X, Yin M, Zhang LJ. Keratin 6, 16 and 17-critical barrier alarmin molecules in skin wounds and psoriasis. Cells. 2019;8(8).
16. Krawczyk A, Miskiewicz J, Strzelec K, Wcislo-Dziadecka D, Strzalka-Mrozik B. Apoptosis in autoimmunological diseases, with particular consideration of molecular aspects of psoriasis. Med Sci Monit. 2020;26: e922035.
17. Wang B, Han D, Li F, Hou W, Wang L, Meng L, et al. Elevated IL-22 in psoriasis plays an anti-apoptotic role in keratinocytes through mediating Bcl-xL/Bax. Apoptosis. 2020;25(9–10):663–73.
18. Huang YW, Tsai TF. HLA-Cw1 and psoriasis. Am J Clin Dermatol. 2021;22(3):339–47.
19. Munoz-Aceituno E, Martos-Cabrera L, Ovejero-Benito MC, Reolid A, Abad-Santos F, Dauden E. Pharmacogenetics update on biologic therapy in psoriasis. Medicina (Kaunas). 2020;56(12).
20. Caputo V, Strafella C, Cosio T, Lanna C, Campione E, Novelli G, et al. Pharmacogenomics: an update on biologics and small-molecule drugs in the treatment of psoriasis. Genes (Basel). 2021;12(9).

Chapter 4
Biomarkers in Atopic Dermatitis

Shirley P. Parraga, Madison K. Cook, and Steven R. Feldman

Abstract Atopic dermatitis (AD) is an inflammatory skin disorder characterized by periods of chronic skin flares. Currently available treatment options include topical therapies, phototherapy, and immunosuppressants, but these therapeutics have undesired side effects and the variability in patient presentation requires individualized treatment plans. Biomarkers have a large role in many fields of medicine and could potentially assess limitations in disease diagnosis, prognosis, and management of AD. This chapter focused on analyzing the biomarkers most closely associated with clinical outcomes in AD patients. We conducted a literature review of twelve biomarkers and used classification standards provided by the World Health Organization. Through our review we found that there are measurable levels of cytokines, antibodies, and proteins that are associated with AD diagnosis, prognosis, and responses to treatment. While there are biomarkers being investigated for their use in AD management, the benefit for such laboratory medicine in a historically clinically diagnosed disease is not known.

Keywords Biomarkers · Atopic dermatitis · IgE · TARC · ECP · MDC · CCL-22 · Filaggrin

S. P. Parraga (✉)
East Carolina University, E 5th St, Greenville, NC 27858, USA
e-mail: parragas20@students.ecu.edu

M. K. Cook
Wake Forest School of Medicine, Winston-Salem, NC, USA
e-mail: madison.kathleen.cook@live.mercer.edu

S. R. Feldman
Professor of Dermatology, Pathology and Social Sciences & Health Policy, Wake Forest School of Medicine, 4618 Country Club Road, Winston-Salem, NC 27104, USA
e-mail: sfeldman@wakehealth.edu

R. Norman (ed.), *Biomarkers in Dermatology*,
https://doi.org/10.1007/978-3-031-66513-4_4

4.1 Introduction

Atopic dermatitis is a skin disorder characterized by periods of chronic, inflammatory skin flareups [1]. The disease progression involves a multifactorial combination of immunological and biological skin barrier dysfunction [1, 2]. Key features of AD include inflammation, immune dysregulation, skin barrier dysfunction, and heightened IgE sensitization to external allergens [3]. Atopy is characterized as the overproduction of IgE antibodies in response to environmental exposures or other triggers. This commonly occurs through the activation of the Th2 signaling pathway responsible for IgE antibody recruitment and subsequent production of memory B cells, plasma cells, and eosinophils [2, 4, 5]. The hallmark symptom of AD is pruritus [1]. Other common symptoms of AD include xerosis, cheilitis, hyperlinear palms and eyelids, ichthyosis, keratosis pilaris, lichenification, papules, and urticaria. Different symptoms may present based on the severity of the disease [1, 6]. AD diagnosis is made based on the clinical presentation of symptoms, making it subject to observer differences [1].

Treatment options for mild to severe cases of AD include topical therapies, phototherapy, immunosuppressants, and targeted biologics. Emollients and low dose topical steroid options typically offer better safety profiles in comparison to systemic immunosuppressants which have higher potential for toxicities and drug-drug interactions [6]. While these therapeutic options offer symptom relief for AD, there currently is no cure. Signs and symptoms of AD vary among patients; treatment plans should be individualized accordingly.

Biomarkers have been utilized in medicine to diagnose diseases, predict disease outcomes, assess the risk of disease, and monitor a patient's response to treatments. While biomarkers have a well-defined role in many fields of medicine, their role in dermatology is less well characterized. Because AD, like many other skin diseases, can be diagnosed and measured by direct inspection, the role of biomarkers may have less clinical applicability compared to conditions like diabetes that is not so easily directly measured. However, because AD relies on clinical diagnosis, diagnosis and severity assessment are subject to inter and intra-observer variability, a limitation biomarkers could address.

According to the World Health Organization, a biomarker is classified as a substance, structure or process in the patient's body that can affect the outcome of their disease [7, 8]. Multiple biomarkers are being investigated for their clinical applicability and potential role in management of AD [8]. Biomarkers are useful in understanding disease pathogenesis in addition to offering support to the clinical diagnosis [8]. The application of biomarkers can involve a relatively noninvasive and inexpensive procedure that might facilitate objective, quantitative monitoring of disease progression. Measuring serum levels of specific biomarkers involved in AD might provide insight regarding the potential efficacy of proposed treatment plans [7, 8].

In this chapter we focused on biomarkers that could potentially assess limitations in the diagnosis, prognosis, and management of AD. The selected AD biomarkers were classified based on characteristics assigned by the World Health Organization. The subtypes assigned to the biomarkers included screening (those that helped identify the population of patients at risk), monitoring (those that correlated with higher disease severity), prognostic (those with indicative serum or tissue levels), pharmacodynamic (those that allowed analysis of specific pharmacologic approaches), and diagnostic (those that facilitated diagnosis of disease) [7].

4.2 Methods

A literature search was performed through PubMed using key words covering the topic of biomarkers in atopic dermatitis. Key words used included; *biomarkers, atopic dermatitis, pathophysiology of atopic dermatitis, and role of biomarkers in atopic dermatitis.* The search resulted in 42 articles which were prescreened by reviewing the abstracts and relevant sections. Articles published between January 2000 and October 2021 written in English were reviewed and included based on relevance to the chapter. Information regarding each biomarker was categorized into one of the five classifications defined by the WHO; screening, prognostic, monitoring, pharmacodynamic, and diagnostic.

4.3 IgE as a Biomarker for Atopic Dermatitis

4.3.1 Role of IgE in Atopic Dermatitis Pathogenesis

AD patients are categorized as either having extrinsic or intrinsic IgE phenotypes. The extrinsic phenotype represents the classic phenotype, corresponding to approximately 80% of AD patients. This phenotype develops high serum IgE levels due to exposure to environmental triggers. In contrast to other phenotypes, extrinsic AD patients have higher disease severity along with complex FLG gene mutations and increased skin barrier dysfunction [9]. The intrinsic phenotype is similar in terms of clinical presentation of AD, but patients have normal serum levels of IgE. In addition, these patients normally display delayed disease onset and uncompromised skin barrier function as determined by trans-epidermal water loss [10].

4.3.2 Biomarker Classification

Monitoring IgE levels in AD patients has potential to be a diagnostic marker for disease phenotype. Patients with allergic conditions typically present with high serum IgE levels. Patients with intrinsic AD normally have normal or lower serum levels of

IgE compared to extrinsic AD patients [8]. The reason for higher serum IgE levels in the extrinsic AD subgroup is due to the sensitization to multiple environmental allergens [8]. In addition, IgE levels are associated with the disease severity of AD patients. Extrinsic AD patients who present with higher serum IgE levels tend to display more severe clinical symptoms [8]. However up to 20% of AD patients do not display elevated IgE levels, which inhibits IgE from serving as a reliable monitoring or diagnostic biomarker for all AD phenotypes [11].

Analysis of serum IgE levels can also potentially assist the long-term management of AD progression. Patients with high IgE levels are associated with more severe forms of childhood AD [7]. Therefore, detecting elevated IgE serum levels can potentially serve as a prognostic biomarker and allow for management in the earlier stages of pathogenesis for these patients. During AD therapy trials, serum IgE levels had predictive capabilities for pharmacological approaches, however there is not much evidence supporting its use a pharmacodynamic biomarker [11].

Two biologics, omalizumab and ligelizumab, target distinct binding epitopes in the FC region of the IgE antibody and prevent IgE from binding to several inflammatory cell types including mast cells, basophils, and eosinophils. For patients with the extrinsic phenotype of AD, these biologics can reduce overall presentation of urticaria and common symptoms of allergic disorders including pruritus [10, 11]. Using IgE as a diagnostic marker to determine whether a patient has the extrinsic or intrinsic AD phenotype can potentially help determine whether or not a patient would respond to certain biologics such as omalizumab and ligelizumab [11]. Omalizumab is currently FDA approved for treatment of severe allergic asthma and chronic urticaria, but results in AD treatment are mixed. For some patients with more complex genetic mutations, targeting IgE did not improve their symptoms. However, IgE is an important mediator of the atopic march responsible for AD development and is a target area of interest [2, 11].

4.4 TARC as a Biomarker in Atopic Dermatitis

4.4.1 Role of TARC in Atopic Dermatitis Pathogenesis

Thymus and activation-regulated chemokine (TARC) is a member of the Th2 cytokine family and is a key player in the AD inflammatory pathway [12]. TARC is produced by dendritic and endothelial cells. Through chemokine receptors 4 and 8 (CCR4 and CCR8, respectively), TARC can recruit other inflammatory cells of the same class [13]. TARC is also expressed in epithelial keratinocytes indicating its importance in inflammatory skin pathology. Elevated levels of TARC are noted in lesional and non-lesional skin samples acquired from AD patients [13].

4.4.2 Classification of Biomarker

TARC is a potential monitoring biomarker for AD. TARC serum levels have higher correlative properties to AD disease severity when compared to other biomarkers. Longitudinal and cross-sectional studies indicate correlation coefficients of approximately 0.60 and 0.64, respectively [7]. Through reliance on TARC serum levels, clinicians can potentially obtain a more specific indicator of disease severity for AD patients [12–14]. There are limitations to the use of TARC as a biomarker for AD severity, including that it is not a skin-specific biomarker and its levels can be affected by the presence of other atopic diseases [15]. We don't know if measuring TARC serum levels has value for diagnostic, prognostic, screening, or pharmacodynamic purposes in AD; although TARC serum levels correlate with disease severity in patients with AD, measuring those levels may not be superior to clinical assessments of disease severity.

4.5 Eosinophilic Cationic Protein (ECP) as a Biomarker in Atopic Dermatitis

4.5.1 Role of ECP in Atopic Dermatitis Pathogenesis

AD is characterized by alterations in regulators of cellular and humoral immunity [16]. Eosinophils are important in AD pathogenesis. Patients with AD frequently have elevated blood eosinophil levels [16, 17]. Eosinophilic granule release in inflammatory pathogenic states such as those observed in AD can be of use clinically. ECP offers the potential for analysis of the eosinophilic influx observed in patch-tests performed on AD patients [16, 17].

4.5.2 Classification of Biomarker

ECP as a monitoring and pharmacodynamic biomarker can potentially offer clinical support to assessment of disease severity and possible clinical improvement [16]. ECP levels correlate with disease severity during acute AD exacerbations. In a study conducted at intervals before and after hospital admission, there was a correlation ($p < 0.001$) between ECP serum levels and disease severity based on clinical severity scoring and symptom analysis [16, 17]. These effects were mainly noted on symptoms of papule formation and lichenification [16]. However, limitations of ECP use must also be considered. Levels of ECP only correlate with AD severity during times of active flares, limiting its use for monitoring disease progression [9]. Future reliance on ECP as a biomarker for AD management requires objective quantification of its benefit over traditional clinical monitoring of symptoms.

4.6 MDC/CCL22 as a Biomarker in Atopic Dermatitis

4.6.1 Role of MDC/CCL22 in Atopic Dermatitis Pathogenesis

Macrophage-Derived Chemoattractant (MDC)/CCL22 is a subset of T-lymphocytes associated with the inflammatory skin presentation of AD [18]. MDC/CCL22 participates in diseases involved with the infiltration of TH2-type cells. MDC/CCL22 is a selective chemoattractant for cells expressing the CC chemokine receptor 4 (CCR4) as well as thymus and activation-regulated chemokine (TARC), two factors that are associated with higher disease severity in AD patients [18]. However, the primary role in dermal immunoreactivity is through MDC/CCL22 association with dendritic cells, resulting in the lesional skin presentation of AD [18].

4.6.2 Classification of Biomarker

MDC/CCL22 is a biomarker with potential to assess disease severity in allergic diseases [7, 18]. Use of this biomarker has previously assisted in management of psoriasis vulgaris [18]. Analysis of MDC serum levels correlate with the Scoring AD (SCORAD) index, a measure of disease severity for AD. The value of serum MDC/CCL22 was higher in AD patients compared to psoriasis vulgaris ($p < 0.001$) [18]. This finding offers insight into the potential use of MDC/CLC22 as a screening biomarker for AD [7, 18]. In addition, MDC/CCL22 may also serve as a pharmacodynamic biomarker [7]. A study found serum MDC/CCL22 levels were decreased after initial treatment of skin eruptions with corticosteroids and antihistamine drugs. There was an improvement in the SCORAD index of 29.6 ± 10 points ($p < 0.001$) [4]. The clinical utility of this biomarker over traditional diagnosis of AD has not been determined.

4.7 CTACK as a Biomarker in Atopic Dermatitis

4.7.1 Role of CTACK in Atopic Dermatitis Pathogenesis

Cutaneous T-cell attracting chemokine (CTACK) serves as a ligand for chemokine receptor 10, a chemokine receptor found on melanocytes and skin-homing T-cells. It chemoattracts cutaneous lymphocyte-associated antigen (CLA) memory T-cells into sites of inflammation and is part of the Th2 response present in AD pathogenesis. CTACK is only found in the skin and is expressed in epidermal keratinocytes [19].

4.7.2 *Classification of Biomarker*

CTACK has the potential to serve as a diagnostic and monitoring biomarker for patients with AD. Serum levels are greater in patients with AD than in healthy controls. CTACK serum levels also are increased in patients with greater AD severity, with levels having a direct correlation to patients' SCORAD score (correlation coefficient 0.70, $p < 0.001$) [19]. Two strengths of the potential use of CTACK as a biomarker is that it is only expressed in the skin and is unaffected by the presence of other atopic diseases. CTACK levels are also greater in patients with psoriasis, however, weakening its use as an AD specific diagnostic biomarker [15]. There is limited evidence supporting the use of CTACK as a pharmacodynamic or prognostic biomarker.

4.8 Filaggrin Gene as a Biomarker for Atopic Dermatitis

4.8.1 *Role of Filaggrin in Atopic Dermatitis Pathogenesis*

The filaggrin (FLG) gene is responsible for the development of the profilaggrin protein which is located within the granular epidermal layer and contributes to the integrity of the epidermis [1]. Approximately 10% of AD patients present with loss of function of the FLG gene, which results in a greater than 50% protein downregulation [1]. FLG gene mutations contribute to the skin barrier dysfunction and increased susceptibility to foreign pathogens experienced by AD patients [1]. FLG is responsible for the regulation of epidermal differentiation [1]. Patients with mutations in this gene present with greater trans-epidermal water loss representing a weakened barrier matrix [1]. The loss of matrix results in greater penetration of the skin by allergens and other AD triggering agents [1]. Current therapies aim toward restoring the skin barrier of AD patients and preventing systemic flare ups [20]. Biotechnological intervention of FLG gene mutations is a future venture for the treatment of AD that could be especially beneficial in patients who have mutations in their filaggrin gene [21].

4.8.2 *Classification of Biomarker*

Filaggrin is a critical component in the development of many of the symptoms associated with AD [7]. Filaggrin serves as a potential screening factor for AD that could help to identify the population of patients at risk for AD. Associations exist with certain mutations in the FLG gene and the development of greater disease severity of AD [7, 22, 23]. These mutations are more frequent with patients that present with early onset AD. In a randomized, double blind multicenter study of patients diagnosed with AD, there was an association ($P < 0.00008$) between loss of function mutations in the filaggrin gene and early age of onset [24]. Through the identification and measurement of FLG gene mutations in patients at risk for AD development (with a positive family history), AD can potentially be detected earlier, which allows for quicker treatment planning in these patients [7]. The filaggrin gene also has predictive biomarker qualities as defects in this gene have also been associated with the development of other conditions including severe ichthyosis, peanut allergy, contact dermatitis, and high-risk skin infections [1]. To know if filaggrin gene mutations would be useful as a pharmacodynamic or prognostic biomarker would require information on specificity and sensitivity that is not yet well characterized.

4.9 IL-4 as a Biomarker in Atopic Dermatitis

4.9.1 Role of IL-4 in Atopic Dermatitis Pathogenesis

The increase in IL-4 cytokines marks a key diagnostic feature of AD [6]. IL-4 is a glycosylated cytokine produced by Th2 cells [25]. It signals through two different receptor complexes. The first is a type one receptor expressed on hematopoietic cells and is composed of an IL-4 alpha chain and common gamma chains. The type one receptor is activated specifically by IL-4 cytokines. The second is a type two receptor expressed on non-hematopoietic cells and consists of IL-4 alpha and IL-13 alpha1 subunits. The type two receptor can be activated by both IL-4 and IL-13 cytokines [25].

The signaling of IL-4 results in the mediation of several pathways [25]. Th2 cytokines, IL-4 and Il-13 have been implicated in the loss of function of the FLG gene experienced by AD patients. These cytokines may achieve this via the inhibition of regulatory mRNAs [2]. Within the scope of T-cells, IL-4 allows for the differentiation of naïve CD4 T-cells into Th2 cells, which play a large role in the pathogenesis of AD [25]. The association of IL-4 with B cells leads to the induction of IgE production [25].

IL-4 is also responsible for the amplification of type two inflammation via modulation of dendritic cell activity and resultant downregulation of IL-12 and MHC class II molecules. This type 2 inflammation pathway leads to the development of skin lesions [25]. The upregulation of IL-4 results in the presentation of lesional and non-lesional skin abnormalities [6]. The overexpression of IL-4 results in AD histopathological features, which include skin inflammation, increased bacterial colonization, and higher levels of pruritus [25]. Dupilumab is a monoclonal antibody against IL-4Ra, which forms part of the IL-4 and IL-13 receptors [2, 6]. It inhibits the signaling pathway of IL-4 and IL-13 [2, 6]. Currently, it is the only FDA-approved biologic for AD [2, 6].

4.9.2 Classification of Biomarker

IL-4 as a biomarker has potential to serve as a diagnostic tool for AD [7]. IL-4 levels correspond to AD symptoms related to skin inflammation, such a pruritus. Based on a histological analysis, acute skin lesions are commonly composed of cells expressing higher levels of Th2 cytokines including IL-4, as opposed to chronic skin lesions which express higher levels of interferon (INF)-gamma [2]. Its use alone as a biomarker to assess treatment response is debatable. AD often involves a polymorphism of cytokine presentation, therefore, interpreting serum IL-4 together with other cytokines involved in the Th2 signaling pathway, such as IL-13, may offer more therapeutic relevance in understanding treatment success or failure in patients, rather than measuring IL-4 levels alone [25]. The prognostic and monitoring qualities of IL-4 as a biomarker are not well defined in literature. Although, IL-4 is associated with symptoms of AD and found in histological tissue samples of skin lesions of patients with AD, a benefit of measuring its levels in serum or tissue over clinical diagnosis has not yet been demonstrated.

4.10 IL-5 as a Biomarker in Atopic Dermatitis

4.10.1 Role of IL-5 in Atopic Dermatitis Pathogenesis

IL-5 mediates the inflammatory cascade in response to environmental or allergen triggers [26]. It achieves this by binding to the alpha chain of the IL-5 receptor and inducing the maturation of eosinophils [26]. Once eosinophils become activated, they lead to the activation of inflammatory cells, which allows for the development of atopic dermatitis. A core component of AD, eosinophilic inflammation, is regulated by cytokines including IL-5 and TNF-alpha. Depending on the cytokine and inflammatory pathway activated, skin lesions may present differently. Due to the role IL-5 has in the acute phase reactant inflammatory cascade, elevated IL-5 levels are associated more with acute AD lesions rather than chronic [6, 26]. Biologic therapies targeting IL-5, such as mepolizumab, aim to reduce overall inflammation caused by hyper-eosinophilic conditions. The clinical applicability of such biologics remains unclear [6].

4.10.2 Classification of Biomarker

IL-5 has some qualities of a monitoring and pharmacodynamic biomarker. IL-5 is an indicator of the activation of the eosinophilic cascade and increased levels of IL-5 correlate with more severe AD symptom presentation [6]. Within this context, decreasing levels of IL-5 indicate improvement after initial clinical treatment [6].

While the clinical efficacy of biologics targeting IL-5 is still unclear, focusing on changes in overall IL-5 concentrations can determine the efficacy of the biologics used [6, 26]. The potential use of IL-5 as a prognostic and diagnostic biomarker is not well known and the advantages of measuring IL-5 levels in serum to monitor disease severity over clinical severity assessment has not been determined.

4.11 IL-13 as a Biomarker in Atopic Dermatitis

4.11.1 Role of IL-13 in Atopic Dermatitis Pathogenesis

IL-13 shares many similarities and functions with IL-4 [27]. They are both encoded by adjacent genes and engage in signaling pathways by binding of a common receptor [27]. IL-13 mediates specific tissue responses, such as eosinophil recruitment during allergic reactions [27]. Signaling of the IL-13-mediated inflammation cascade occurs through a series of receptor binding steps [27]. The receptor is characterized as heterodimeric and is composed of the IL-4R alpha and IL-13R1 alpha subunits [27].

The binding of the IL-4R alpha and IL-13R1 subunits by IL-13 results in the downstream production of inflammatory mediators including Janus kinase 2 (JAK2) and Tyrosine kinase 2 (TYK2), inducing the expression of sensory fibers and activation of itch sensation associated with AD [27]. OVOL-1 is an upstream transcription factor necessary to produce the epidermal barrier formed by keratinocytes. This transcription factor is commonly disrupted during AD pathogenesis [27]. Prior research indicates IL-13 and IL-4 activation inhibit FLG expression via inhibition of OVOL-1 [27]. Tralokinumab and Lebrikizumab are humanized neutralizing antibodies that work by inhibiting the binding of IL-13 to IL-4R alpha and IL-13R alpha1, preventing downstream inflammatory signaling [6, 28]. Clinical trials indicate reduction in inflammatory AD symptoms as observed by the Eczema Area and Severity Index (EASI) compared to placebo interventions [6].

4.11.2 Classification of Biomarker

Based on histological analysis, cells expressing higher levels of Th2 cytokines including IL-13 are more prevalent in acute skin lesions documented, as opposed to chronic skin lesions which express higher levels of IFN-gamma [2]. IL-13 levels are also associated with increases in AD disease severity [29]. Consequently, IL-13 analysis could potentially serve as a monitoring biomarker during AD disease progression [7]. There is no current evidence suggesting the potential use of IL-13 as a prognostic or pharmacodynamic biomarker and while there is a correlation between IL-13 levels and disease severity in patients with AD, the benefit of measuring IL-13 levels to determine the severity state of disease over clinical severity assessment is not known.

4.12 IL-31 as a Biomarker in Atopic Dermatitis

4.12.1 Role of IL-31 in Atopic Dermatitis Pathogenesis

IL-31 is produced by T-cells and is a mediator of the intense pruritus symptoms experienced by AD patients [7]. It is one of the effector cytokines involved in the inflammatory cascade activated by the Th2 signaling pathway [30]. IL-31 signals through the IL-31 alpha receptor and activates inflammatory signal transducers including the Janus kinase (JAK), activator of transcription (STAT), mitogen-activated protein kinase (MAPK), and phosphoinositide-3-kinase (PI3K) [30]. There are two common pathways through which IL-31 is believed to lead to AD development [7]. The first involves binding of the IL-31 alpha receptor, which activates the skin sensory neurons [7]. Subsequent activation of these fibers corresponds to the sensation of itch [30]. The second involves a physical disruption of the skin barrier in patients with AD [7]. Ten percent of AD patients with elevated levels of IL-31 have mutations in the filaggrin gene [30]. Agents acting against IL-31, such as nemolizumab, inhibit moderate to severe atopic itch and inflammation present in many AD patients [7, 30].

4.12.2 Classification of Biomarker

4.12.2.1 Diagnostic Biomarker [7]

Elevated IL-31 serum levels correspond to the itch-associated scratching behavior, which could be useful for clinical diagnosis of AD, however other measures would have to be used to confirm diagnosis, making its use as a diagnostic biomarker weak [30]. IL-31 levels directly correlate with SCORAD scores ($R > 0.35$, $p < 0.001$) in patients with AD. This correlation with disease severity allows IL-31 to potentially serve as a monitoring biomarker for disease progression in patients with AD [7]. There is limited evidence on the potential role of IL-31 as a pharmacodynamic or screening biomarker. Its beneficial use as a monitoring and diagnostic biomarker over clinical assessment and diagnosis has not been determined.

4.13 TSLP as a Biomarker in Atopic Dermatitis

4.13.1 Role of TSLP in Atopic Dermatitis Pathogenesis

TSLP is a keratinocyte-derived cytokine [6]. Keratinocytes in AD have increased expression of TSLP [31]. Activation of TSLP stimulates dendritic cells to activate the Th2 signaling pathway responsible for many of the inflammatory symptoms associated with AD [6]. In addition to its role with the Th2 signaling pathway, TSLP compromises filaggrin-deficient skin by activating Th22 cells [31]. In patients with filaggrin loss-of-function mutations, Th2/Th22 signaling becomes activated [31, 32]. Th22 cytokines correspond with increased immune dysregulation and skin barrier impairment in AD patients [31, 32].

TSLP also facilitates a positive feedback loop of chronic inflammation by activating cutaneous innate lymphoid cells (ILCs), which results in the production of inflammatory cytokines IL-4, IL-5, and IL-13 [31]. Cutaneous ILCS are surrounded by Th2 cells in AD lesions, which suggests a close interaction between the two cell types [31]. Cytokines IL-33 and IL-25 also activate cutaneous ILCs in AD [31]. IL-22 has been implicated in the prolonged production of IL-33 and TSLP [31]. Together, these cytokines and molecular regulators interact in a cycle that promotes the inflammatory conditions of AD [31]. Tezepelumab is an Anti-TSLP antibody that is currently in phase 2b trials. It prevents the interaction of TSLP with its receptor [33].

4.13.2 Classification of Biomarker

Epidermal TSLP protein expression has potential to serve as an early screening biomarker in children at increased risk of AD development [7]. In a cohort study of 70 infants, epidermal TSLP protein expression correlated with the later development of AD in patients as young as 2 months old ($p < 0.1$) [34]. In addition, tracking TSLP levels can potentially help predict which patients would likely respond optimally from biologics optimizing TSLP inhibition [7]. In a study conducted on AD patients, serum TSLP levels were higher compared to healthy controls, but no differences were observed between children and adult AD samples. In the study, there was a correlation between TSLP and IL-31 activation in AD patients ($p < 0.001$), there is a low correlation between TSLP protein levels specifically and disease severity in patients with AD [35]. Therefore, there is no current evidence of its potential use as a monitoring biomarker for AD [36].

4.14 OX40 as a Biomarker in Atopic Dermatitis

4.14.1 Role of OX40 in Atopic Dermatitis Pathogenesis

OX40 is a costimulatory molecule found on effector and regulatory T-cells [6, 37]. It is a subtype of the TNF receptor [6, 37]. The binding of OX40 with the OX40 ligand plays a critical role in autoimmunity, resulting in the amplification of cytokine production and cell proliferation via the development of T-cell tolerance [37]. In addition, this molecular association results in the facilitation of Th1 and Th2 signaling pathways, causing an upregulation of TNF-alpha secretion under chronic inflammatory conditions [37]. Because Ox40 is also present in regulatory T-cells, the OX40-OX40L pathway may represent additional targets for inhibition of immunoinflammatory effects. This can allow for in-depth analysis and determination of clinical improvement during AD treatment.

4.14.2 Classification of Biomarker

Analysis of OX40 in the skin of patients with AD indicates elevated levels of immune modulating cells, specifically, dendritic cells in comparison to normal skin and patients with AD have elevated blood levels of OX40 compared to those without the disease [6, 37, 38]. OX40 therefore has the potential to serve as a diagnostic biomarker for AD. OX40 can allow for a more targeted analysis of specific lesions of AD as sites of inflammation have upregulation of OX40 expression in AD patients [37]. In a study done in pediatric patients with AD, OX40 levels in the serum correlated with SCORAD scores of patients, indicating it could be a potential monitoring biomarker for AD severity ($r = 0.72$, $p < 0.01$) [38]. The use of measuring OX40 serum levels to indicate therapeutic success or to screen for AD development has not been well reported. Additionally, the advantages of monitoring OX40 levels to diagnose and assess AD severity over clinical diagnosis and severity assessment is not known.

4.15 Discussion

Biomarkers play a large role in the diagnosis and management of many chronic diseases such as diabetes, yet their potential for use in evaluating and managing dermatological diseases is less known. Atopic dermatitis is the most common chronic inflammatory skin disease. It typically presents in childhood but can persist into adulthood [39]. Presentation of AD is highly variable and multiple phenotypes exist. As with other skin diseases, AD is primarily diagnosed clinically through direct observation of patients' lesions from a trained physician and severity of disease is assessed using clinician-rated severity scores such as SCORAD and EASI are subject to high inter and intra-observer variability [40]. Biomarkers could potentially address these limitations of clinical variability and serve as a tool for achieving a more precise clinical diagnosis and severity assessment of patients with AD.

In this chapter, twelve biomarkers that are closely associated with clinical outcomes in AD patients were analyzed regarding their potential use in AD screening, monitoring, prognosis, diagnosis, and pharmacodynamic evaluation. Identification of key biomarkers in AD involves analysis of their role in inflammatory signaling pathways. For the purposes of our study, the biomarkers we selected emphasized diagnosis, long-term monitoring of disease progression, prognostic, and pharmacodynamic aspects of AD. Certain biomarkers were grouped in more than one category based on their characteristics.

For diagnosis of AD, serum analysis of IgE can potentially facilitate the classification of patients into intrinsic and extrinsic AD phenotypes which can aid in creating a personalized treatment plan for each patient as the efficacy of many biologics relies on patient phenotype. Measurement of filaggrin gene mutations has the potential to serve as a screening biomarker as these mutations are more frequent with patients that present with early onset AD. Early detection can allow for targeting the disease during earlier stages of pathogenesis. TARC, CTACK, and OX40 have the potential to be monitoring biomarkers as their serum levels correlate with disease severity in patients with AD.

Biomarkers have the potential to limit the variability in the diagnosis and severity assessment of patients with AD in addition to providing insight to treatment response. However, there are limitations to the use of biomarkers in AD. Levels of biomarkers, while elevated in certain patients with AD, are not always elevated in those with the disease. This variability makes the use of certain biomarkers, such as IgE, less applicable for disease monitoring, prognosis, and screening. Additionally, serum levels of biomarkers that are indicative of the pathogenesis of AD can be affected by the presence of other concurrent diseases, such as atopic disorders or other skin diseases, suggesting biomarkers such as TARC and CTACK are not specific for AD. The use of biomarkers could potentially limit the variability in severity assessments of patients with AD, however many studies classify biomarkers as potential measures of severity based on their correlation with clinical severity assessment scores such as EASI and SCORAD, nullifying the precision of biomarkers over clinical assessment for measuring disease severity. Moreover, the overall benefit of measuring serum or tissue levels of biomarkers in patients with AD over clinical examination is limited.

4.16 Conclusion

Atopic dermatitis is a complex inflammatory disease affecting the skin. AD prevalence is growing not only in the US, but also worldwide. AD diagnosis is made based on clinical presentation, but reliance on key biomarkers has the potential to confirm the diagnosis and assess patients' prognosis. However, there are limitations to the development of biomarkers for AD. Individual patient presentation of symptoms may render biomarkers unpredictable for diagnosis as levels of certain biomarkers are not always elevated in patients with AD. In addition, other allergic or inflammatory skin conditions that have effects on biomarker levels could confound use of biomarkers in AD. Currently, there is no specific biomarker proven valuable for AD diagnosis, prognosis, or comorbidity. AD is apparent on the skin and is somewhat readily assessed visually. While there is potential for biomarkers to have a role in AD diagnosis and management, a superiority of their use over clinical assessment has not been established and is a high hurdle to overcome.

References

1. Avena-Woods C. Overview of atopic dermatitis. Am J Manag Care. 2017;23(8 Suppl):S115–S23. [published Online First: 2017/10/06].
2. David Boothe W, Tarbox JA, Tarbox MB. Atopic dermatitis: pathophysiology. In: Springer International Publishing; 2017. pp. 21–37.
3. Čepelak I, Dodig S, Pavić I. Filaggrin and atopic march. Biochem Med. 2019;29(2):214–27. https://doi.org/10.11613/bm.2019.020501.
4. Rebane A, Akdis CA. MicroRNAs: essential players in the regulation of inflammation. J Allergy Clin Immunol. 2013;132(1):15–26. https://doi.org/10.1016/j.jaci.2013.04.011.
5. Deo S, Mistry K, Kakade A, et al. Role played by Th2 type cytokines in IgE mediated allergy and asthma. Lung India. 2010;27:66.
6. Chun PIF, Lehman H. Current and future monoclonal antibodies in the treatment of atopic dermatitis. Clin Rev Allergy Immunol. 2020;59(2):208–19. https://doi.org/10.1007/s12016-020-08802-9.
7. Thijs JL, de Bruin-Weller MS, Hijnen D. Current and future biomarkers in atopic dermatitis. Immunol Allergy Clin North Am. 2017;37(1):51–61. https://doi.org/10.1016/j.iac.2016.08.008 [publishedOnlineFirst:2016/11/26].
8. Thijs J, Van Seggelen W, Bruijnzeel-Koomen C, et al. New developments in biomarkers for atopic dermatitis. J Clin Med. 2015;4(3):479–87. https://doi.org/10.3390/jcm4030479.
9. Furue M, Chiba T, Tsuji G, et al. Atopic dermatitis: immune deviation, barrier dysfunction, IgE autoreactivity and new therapies. Allergol Int. 2017;66(3):398–403. https://doi.org/10.1016/j.alit.2016.12.002.
10. Czarnowicki T, He H, Krueger JG, et al. Atopic dermatitis endotypes and implications for targeted therapeutics. J Allergy Clin Immunol. 2019;143(1):1–11. https://doi.org/10.1016/j.jaci.2018.10.032.
11. Gasser P, Tarchevskaya SS, Guntern P, et al. The mechanistic and functional profile of the therapeutic anti-IgE antibody ligelizumab differs from omalizumab. Nat Commun. 2020;11(1). https://doi.org/10.1038/s41467-019-13815-w.
12. Renert-Yuval Y, Thyssen JP, Bissonnette R, et al. Biomarkers in atopic dermatitis—a review on behalf of the International Eczema Council. J Allergy Clin Immunol. 2021;147(4):1174-90.e1. https://doi.org/10.1016/j.jaci.2021.01.013.
13. Kakinuma T, Nakamura K, Wakugawa M, et al. Thymus and activation-regulated chemokine in atopic dermatitis: serum thymus and activation-regulated chemokine level is closely related with disease activity. J Allergy Clin Immunol. 2001;107(3):535–41. https://doi.org/10.1067/mai.2001.113237.
14. Renert-Yuval Y, Guttman-Yassky E. New treatments for atopic dermatitis targeting beyond IL-4/IL-13 cytokines. Ann Allergy Asthma Immunol. 2020;124(1):28–35. https://doi.org/10.1016/j.anai.2019.10.005.

15. Hong KL, Leung TF, Ma KC, Li AM, Wong Y, Fok TF. Serum levels of cutaneous T-cell attracting chemokine (CTACK) as a laboratory marker of the severity of atopic dermatitis in children. Clin Exp Dermatol. 2004;29(3):293–6. https://doi.org/10.1111/j.1365-2230.2004.01501.
16. Czech W, Krutmann J, Schöpf E, Kapp A. Serum eosinophil cationic protein (ECP) is a sensitive measure for disease activity in atopic dermatitis. Br J Dermatol. 1992;126(4):351–5. https://doi.org2133.1992.tb00677.x.
17. Wu KG, Li TH, Chen CJ, Cheng HI, Wang TY. Correlations of serum Interleukin-16, total IgE, eosinophil cationic protein and total eosinophil counts with disease activity in children with atopic dermatitis. Int J Immunopathol Pharmacol. 2011;24(1):15–23. https://doi.org/10.1177/039463201102400103.
18. Hashimoto S, Nakamura K, Oyama N, et al. Macrophage-derived chemokine (MDC)/CCL22 produced by monocyte derived dendritic cells reflects the disease activity in patients with atopic dermatitis. J Dermatol Sci. 2006;44(2):93–9. https://doi.org/10.1016/j.jdermsci.2006.08.004.
19. Kakinuma T, Saeki H, Tsunemi Y, et al. Increased serum cutaneous T cell-attracting chemokine (CCL27) levels in patients with atopic dermatitis and psoriasis vulgaris. J Allergy Clin Immunol. 2003;111(3):592–7. https://doi.org/10.1067/mai.2003.114.
20. Knol EF, Hijnen D. Atopic dermatitis: a tale of two distinct pathomechanisms that make you itch. Eur J Immunol. 2016;46(11):2512–5. https://doi.org/10.1002/eji.201646708.
21. Liang Y, Chang C, Lu Q. The genetics and epigenetics of atopic dermatitis—filaggrin and other polymorphisms. Clin Rev Allergy Immunol. 2016;51(3):315–28. https://doi.org/10.1007/s12016-015-8508-5.
22. Martin MJ, Estravís M, García-Sánchez A, et al. Genetics and epigenetics of atopic dermatitis: an updated systematic review. Genes. 2020;11(4):442. https://doi.org/10.3390/genes11040442.
23. Ziaali A, Sharifi L, Teimourian S, et al. Clinical features of children with atopic dermatitis according to filaggrin gene variants. Allergol Immunopathol. 2021;49(4):162–6. https://doi.org/10.15586/aei.v49i4.209.
24. Smieszek SP, Welsh S, Xiao C, et al. Correlation of age-of-onset of atopic dermatitis with filaggrin loss-of-function variant status. Sci Rep. 2020;10(1). https://doi.org/10.1038/s41598-020-59627-7.
25. Chiricozzi A, Maurelli M, Peris K, et al. Targeting IL-4 for the treatment of atopic dermatitis. ImmunoTargets Therapy. 2020;9:151–6. https://doi.org/10.2147/itt.s260370.
26. Tenero L, Arturi E, Piazza M, et al. Anti-IL-5 in pediatric allergic diseases. Pediatr Allergy Immunol. 2020;31(S26):14–6. https://doi.org/10.1111/pai.13374.
27. Furue K, Ito T, Tsuji G, et al. The IL -13– OVOL 1– FLG axis in atopic dermatitis. Immunology. 2019;158(4):281–6. https://doi.org/10.1111/imm.13120.
28. Bagnasco D, Ferrando M, Varricchi G, et al. A critical evaluation of anti-IL-13 and anti-IL-4 strategies in severe asthma. Int Arch Allergy Immunol. 2016;170(2):122–31. https://doi.org/10.1159/000447692.
29. Ungar B, Garcet S, Gonzalez J, et al. An integrated model of atopic dermatitis biomarkers highlights the systemic nature of the disease. J Investig Dermatol. 2017;137(3):603–13. https://doi.org/10.1016/j.jid.2016.09.037.
30. Cornelissen C, Marquardt Y, Czaja K, et al. IL-31 regulates differentiation and filaggrin expression in human organotypic skin models. J Allergy Clin Immunol. 2012;129(2):426-33.e8. https://doi.org/10.1016/j.jaci.2011.10.042.
31. Huang E, Ong PY. Severe atopic dermatitis in children. Curr Allergy Asthma Rep. 2018;18(6). https://doi.org/10.1007/s11882-018-0788-4.
32. Tokura Y, Hayano S. Subtypes of atopic dermatitis: from phenotype to endotype. Allergol Int. 2021. https://doi.org/10.1016/j.alit.2021.07.003.
33. Simpson EL, Parnes JR, She D, et al. Tezepelumab, an anti–thymic stromal lymphopoietin monoclonal antibody, in the treatment of moderate to severe atopic dermatitis: a randomized phase 2a clinical trial. J Am Acad Dermatol. 2019;80(4):1013–21. https://doi.org/10.1016/j.jaad.2018.11.059.

34. Kim J, Kim BE, Lee J, et al. Epidermal thymic stromal lymphopoietin predicts the development of atopic dermatitis during infancy. J Allergy Clin Immunol. 2016;137(4):1282-1285.e4. https://doi.org/10.1016/j.jaci.2015.12.1306.
35. Nygaard U, Hvid M, Johansen C, et al. TSLP, IL-31, IL-33 and sST2 are new biomarkers in endophenotypic profiling of adult and childhood atopic dermatitis. J Eur Acad Dermatol Venereol. 2016;30(11):1930–8. https://doi.org/10.1111/jdv.13679.
36. Holm JG, Hurault G, Agner T, et al. Immunoinflammatory biomarkers in serum are associated with disease severity in atopic dermatitis. J Dermatol. 2021;237(4):513–20. https://doi.org/10.1159/000514503.
37. Guttman-Yassky E, Pavel AB, Zhou L, et al. GBR 830, an anti-OX40, improves skin gene signatures and clinical scores in patients with atopic dermatitis. J Allergy Clin Immunol. 2019;144(2):482-93.e7. https://doi.org/10.1016/j.jaci.2018.11.053.
38. Ezzat MH, Sallam MA, Shaheen KY, Abo-El-Haythim RE. Serum OX40 ligand: a potential marker of atopic dermatitis disease severity in children. Egypt J Pediatr Allergy Immunol. 2009;7(1). https://doi.org/10.4314/ejpai.v7i1.
39. Avena-Woods C. Overview of atopic dermatitis. Am J Manag Care. 2017;23(8):S115–23 PMID: 28978208.
40. Hijnen DJ. En route to precision medicine. Br J Dermatol. 2019;180(3):455–6. https://doi.org/10.1111/bjd.17411.
41. Ferreira S, Guttman-Yassky E, Torres T. Selective JAK1 inhibitors for the treatment of atopic dermatitis: focus on upadacitinib and abrocitinib. Am J Clin Dermatol. 2020;21(6):783–98. https://doi.org/10.1007/s40257-020-00548-6.

Chapter 5
Biomarkers in Cutaneous Keratinocyte Carcinomas

Jelena Ostojic and Michael D. Howell

Abstract Approximately 1 in 5 Americans will develop skin cancer in their lifetime. Skin cancer develops when DNA damage triggers mutations in keratinocytes leading to their uncontrolled growth and potential malignant tumor formation. Basal cell carcinoma (BCC) and squamous cell carcinoma (SCC) are the two most common keratinocyte carcinomas and frequently develop in skin areas exposed to harmful ultraviolet radiation (UVR). In addition to UVR, the development of BCC and SCC may be impacted by environmental, behavioral, and genetic risk factors. While the mortality rate for BCC and SCC is lower than melanoma, a significant number of these cancers fall into the aggressive category, capable of invading regional structures, recurring, and metastasizing. These features, combined with the financial burden of skin cancer to both patients and healthcare systems, highlight the importance of skin cancer screening to identify and diagnose those at higher risk of developing skin cancer. One of the challenges in screening for NMSC is the low diagnostic accuracy upon primary examination. Clinically, BCC and SCC are variable and may be difficult to distinguish from benign lesions using visual examination alone; thereby requiring potentially unnecessary biopsies to facilitate the diagnosis. In addition to visual examination, biomarkers may provide a more objective measure to provide clinically relevant information for patients' diagnosis, prognosis, risk/susceptibility assessments, and the response to therapy. This chapter reviews our current understanding of biomarkers that have been identified in BCC and SCC as well as their promise for improving disease diagnosis, pathogenesis, and treatment.

Keywords Biomarkers · Basal cell carcinoma · Non-melanoma skin cancer · Precision medicine · Squamous cell carcinoma

Abbreviations

5-FU 5-Fluorouracil

J. Ostojic · M. D. Howell (✉)
San Diego, CA, USA
e-mail: mhowell@dermtech.com

R. Norman (ed.), *Biomarkers in Dermatology*,
https://doi.org/10.1007/978-3-031-66513-4_5

AK	Actinic keratosis
BCC	Basal cell carcinoma
BD	Bowen's disease
CDC	Center for disease control and prevention
CFB	Complement factor B
CFH	Complement factor H
EB	Epidermolysis bullosa
ERK	Extracellular signal-related kinase
FDA	Food and drug administration
FHL-1	Factor H-like protein-1
HH	Hedgehog
MAC	Membrane attack complex
miRNA	MicroRNAs
NGS	Next generation sequencing
NMSC	Non-melanoma skin cancer
PD	Programmed death
PI3K	Phosphoinositide 3-kinase
PTPRD	Protein tyrosine phosphatase delta (PTPRD)
RISC	RNA-induced silencing complexes
SCC	Squamous cell carcinoma
TADs	Topologically associated domains (TADs)
UVR	Ultraviolet radiation
USPSTF	U.S. preventive services task force

5.1 Context

In the United States, skin cancer is the most common cancer type, with over 5 million cases treated annually and 1 in 5 Americans predicted to develop the disease by the age of 70 [1]. Skin cancer can be classified as melanoma or non-melanoma (NMSC), the latter including basal cell carcinoma (BCC) and cutaneous squamous cell carcinoma (SCC), among others [2]. Melanoma represents 1% of skin cancers, but has historically claimed the majority of skin cancer-related deaths, which has made it the main focus of diagnostic and drug development efforts in the realm of skin malignancies [3, 4]. Compared to melanoma, BCC and SCC have a better outcome, however given their high incidence, a significant number of these cancers fall into the aggressive category, capable of invading regional structures, recurring and metastasizing [5, 6]. Although the overall mortality rate for BCC and SCC is relatively low, morbidity is substantial, including disfigurement, loss of function, chronic pain, adverse psychosocial impact, and high treatment costs [7].

Increasing incidence of skin cancers also represents a heavy financial burden to patients and healthcare systems worldwide [8, 9]. According to the Centers for Disease Control and Prevention (CDC), the costs to treat skin cancer increased 5 times faster than those of other cancers between 2002 and 2011, climbing from 3.6 to upwards of 8 billion dollars; more than 50% of these expenditures are related to BCC and SCC [10, 11]. In addition, these numbers are likely to be underestimates due to common exclusion of non-melanoma skin cancers from national cancer registries [4, 12].

Development of BCC and SCC is impacted by environmental, behavioral, and genetic risk factors, most prominent of which is the environmental exposure to the ultraviolet radiation (UVR) [13–18]. Correlations between chronic UVR exposure and NMSC suggest that changes in sun-related behaviors may be able to prevent a significant portion of cutaneous carcinomas; however, the implementation of preventative measures has been hampered by low public compliance and conflicting evidence on efficacy [19–21]. The U.S. Preventive Services Task Force (USPSTF) cites insufficient evidence to recommend for or against skin cancer screening of the general population [22, 23], while data from countries like Germany and Australia shows that systematic skin cancer screening can be both beneficial and cost-effective [24, 25]. One of the challenges in screening for NMSC is the low diagnostic accuracy upon primary examination. Clinical presentations of NMSC are diverse, and carry considerable phenotypic similarities to benign lesions, resulting in high numbers of unnecessary biopsies [24, 26, 27]. Nonetheless, early diagnosis is key for the successful treatment of skin cancer patients, especially those with aggressive disease. Non-invasive solutions for the evaluation of NMSC lesions have been developed, such as medical imaging or non-invasive tissue collection via adhesive tape stripping. Medical imaging tools used to guide clinical diagnosis and biopsy decisions include dermatoscopy, confocal microscopy, and Raman spectroscopy, among others. Dermatoscopy is used by approximately 81% of US dermatologists when evaluating lesions for melanoma and NMSC [28]. Non-pigmented lesions are generally difficult to diagnose; in fact, the frequencies of correct specific diagnoses of a malignant non-pigmented lesion are 40.2% for unaided expert eye and 51.3% when using dermatoscopy [29]. Confocal microscopy tools show promise in helping with diagnosis and management of skin cancers, however most of these tools require long processing times and specific training in image interpretation, currently limiting their widespread use in clinic [30–32]. Another approach is the collection of stratum corneum via tape stripping [33]. Tape stripping procedure on skin involves applying and then removing adhesive tapes from the lesion of interest. Epidermal cells from the outermost skin layer are removed with the tapes and can be used for the investigation of molecular biomarkers, allowing for both initial assessments and follow-up procedures within the same skin area. Identifying specific molecular biomarkers associated with BCC and SCC, including their aggressive forms, may result in earlier diagnosis and more efficient management of these tumors.

Biomarkers are defined as objective and measurable indicators of normal biological processes, pathogenic processes, responses to an exposure or intervention, including therapeutic interventions [34, 35]. Biomarkers can provide clinically relevant information for patients' diagnosis, prognosis, risk/susceptibility assessments and the response to therapy. Technical advances and cost reductions in the next-generation sequencing (NGS) allow access to unprecedented amounts of information on patients' genomic and molecular profiles, supporting the development of new biomarkers. Indeed, the biomarker-based companion diagnostic market is predicted to have a healthy growth in the foreseeable future, driven by the need to further develop targeted therapies for more patients and fueled by the widespread use of NGS technologies [36, 37]. The impact of these advances is already notable in clinical oncology, with several FDA-approved multi-gene panel tests now available to inform managing decisions for various cancer types, including melanoma [3, 38, 39]. While still in its early phases, the development of molecular biomarkers for BCC and SCC holds promise for improving several aspects of these diseases, from prevention to treatment selection and response.

5.2 Basal Cell Carcinoma (BCC)

BCC is the most common global malignancy; in United States only, its incidence is increasing by 4–8% annually [40]. BCC arises upon malignant transformation of cells in the basal layer of the epidermis and its appendages. While BCCs have low mortality rates, they can cause significant morbidity through local tissue destruction and recurrence [41–43]. Staging, treatment and follow-up decisions for BCCs can be quite complex, depending on patient characteristics, tumor localization, cosmetic outcomes, complications, and comorbidities [44, 45]. Given its high incidence, advances in the management of this ubiquitous cancer have worldwide relevance.

5.2.1 Biomarkers in BCC

5.2.1.1 Prevention and Risk Assessment

UVR

BCC risk is correlated with certain phenotypic, genetic, and environmental factors. Development of BCC is more common in individuals with Fitzpatrick skin types I and II, light eye color, freckles, blonde or red hair, and the inability to tan. Individuals with family history of skin cancer are at a higher risk of developing BCC, as well as those presenting defined genetic disorders, such as basal cell nevus syndrome, xeroderma pigmentosum, and Bazex-Dupré-Christol syndrome [46–48]. Among environmental risk factors, UVR exposure is the most important one. UV photons absorbed by DNA molecules induce the formation of DNA lesions, most common of which are cyclobutane pyrimidine dimers and 6–4 photoproducts [49]. These result in high proportion of C > T and CC > TT substitutions, hallmarks of the UV mutational DNA signature [50]. Certain areas of the DNA double helix are more susceptible to damage, creating the so-called "mutational hotspots"; one such hotspot for UVR-induced damage is commonly found within the P53 gene, a tumor suppressor involved in DNA repair and apoptosis. While P53 is mutated in a number of different tumors, skin cancers display enrichment of UVR-specific mutations in the gene; these appear in more than 60% of BCCs [51–53]. Mutations in P53 are recognized as early events in skin carcinogenesis as they are also frequently found in normal, phenotypically unsuspicious sun-exposed skin [54, 55]. While mutations in P53 are unlikely to predict the evolution of an existing BCC [56], their accumulation in normal skin is indicative of positive clonal selection and an increased risk of skin cancer development [55, 57, 58]. NOTCH signaling is crucial in diverse cellular processes and its dysregulation is linked to malignancy [59]. High frequency of missense and truncating mutations in NOTCH1 (29–50%) and NOTCH2 (26–67%) genes were reported in BCC by two independent exome sequencing studies [52, 53]. NOTCH1 and NOTCH2 are also frequently mutated and linked to positive clonal selection in normal sun-exposed skin, suggesting these to be early events in skin transformation [55, 58]. UVR exposure was also shown to induce significant changes in gene expression, especially for genes involved in cellular stress and inflammation [60]. Genome wide re-arrangements in histone acetylation, changes in DNA methylation or direct mutagenesis of transcriptional factors and regulators can all contribute to UVR-related alterations of the transcriptome [61–63]. Identification of genomic biomarkers of cancer-promoting UV damage, together with phenotypic and environmental data, could be useful to stratify patients who would mostly benefit from routine skin cancer screening and preventative interventions. The ability to non-invasively sample normal skin and detect the underlying genomic changes would greatly enhance the feasibility for this type of screening.

5.2.1.2 Tumor Diagnosis and Profiling

Many histological subtypes of BCC have been described, but the major variants are superficial, nodular, micronodular, infiltrative, and morpheaform. Nodular and superficial are the less aggressive subtypes, however it is not uncommon for tumors to present mixed patterns containing two or more subtypes, usually including at least one with the aggressive attributes [64]. The clinical presentation of basal cell carcinoma is variable and may appear as a flesh-colored dome-shaped papule with visible telangiectasia, a scaly patch with or without central atrophy or even a pigmented lesion with a blue, brown, or black tint. The surface of the lesion is typically rather smooth and shiny, although scar-like plaques, ulcers or yellowish indurated waxy structures may be observed, potentially indicating a more aggressive form of BCC [65]. Clinical presentation of several non-neoplastic skin lesions, including eczema and psoriasis, can be like BCC, potentially delaying medical evaluation and complicating the diagnosis. Conventional biopsy of any suspicious lesion followed by the histopathologic examination is still the gold standard for diagnosing skin cancer, including BCC, leading to a high number of unnecessary invasive interventions [27]. Several studies have evaluated the diagnostic accuracy of biopsies by comparing initial biopsies to excisional specimens of BCC; these studies show that initial biopsies miss features of aggressive cancer subtypes in 11–26% of cases [6, 66, 67]. There is a significant interest in the development of new molecular biomarkers of NMSC, as these have the potential to identify the disease early and greatly reduce the associated morbidity, mortality, and costs.

Hedgehog Pathway

Activation of the Hedgehog (HH) signaling pathway has been shown to play a critical role in the oncogenesis of BCC [68, 69]. In brief, pathway activation is initiated by the cell-surface protein, Smoothened (SMO), which is inhibited by the transmembrane receptor Patched (PTCH1); binding of the HH ligand to PTCH1 prevents the inhibition of SMO, which migrates to the primary cilium and regulates the transcription of GLI transcription factors to activate signaling. Loss-of-function mutations in the PTCH gene or gain-of-function mutations in SMO can lead to constitutive activation of the HH pathway. Germline mutations in the PTCH gene were initially detected in basal cell nevus syndrome patients [70]. Subsequently, approximately 85% of sporadic BCCs were also found to contain mutations in PTCH1 and other genes related to the HH pathway, such as SMO and SUFU [52, 68]. While it seems that the activation of the hedgehog signal transduction pathway may be a necessary event in the development of BCC, mutations of the pathway are frequent in BCCs of different size, histology, or recurrence status [52, 68, 71]. Biomarkers in the HH pathway may help distinguish BCC from benign lesions, but the development of additional markers is needed to account for non-HH drivers or modifiers. Furthermore, given the ambiguity in diagnosing aggressive forms of BCC, identification of genomic biomarkers related to histological subtypes would be highly desirable.

Hippo-YAP Pathway

Yes-associated protein (YAP) is a co-transcriptional activator with a role in regulation of proliferation in normal skin [72]. Upon Hippo signaling activation, YAP is phosphorylated and transported to the cytoplasm where it is bound by 14–3-3σ and can no longer induce the expression of target genes [73]. In primary mouse keratinocytes, YAP activation was shown to accelerate proliferation, suppress differentiation, and inhibit apoptosis [72]. Bonilla et al. carried out a genetic profiling of 293 BCCs and reported recurrent loss-of-function mutations in PTPN14 (23%) and LATS1 (8%) that can promote transcriptional activation of YAP1 [52]. Recurrent mutations were also detected in genes so far unrelated to BCC, such as the serine/threonine protein phosphatase PPP6C, mutated in 15% of the BCCs analyzed [52]. PPP6C promotes phosphorylation-dependent activation of LATS1 and inactivation of YAP [74]. Besides its role in the regulation of the Hippo pathway, PPP6C is also involved in the regulation of the cell cycle, DNA damage repair and cutaneous tumorigenesis [75]. The overall mutational burden of BCC was found to be exceptionally high (65 mutations/Mb) [52], which may complicate the detection of significant mutations in driver genes. Several candidate genes were found to be frequently mutated in BCC, however without reaching statistical significance. These include ARID1A, CASP8, KRAS, NRAS and RAC1, among others [52, 53].

MYCN

MYCN is a member of the MYC family of transcriptional activators, involved in multiple cellular functions such as DNA repair, proliferation, differentiation, and apoptosis [76]. Missense mutations in MYCN have been identified in 30% of BCCs [52], most of these mapping to the MYC box 1 domain, which is involved in the interaction with FBXW7 tumor suppressor [52]. FBXW7 is the substrate-binding component of an ubiquitin ligase complex that promotes proteasome-mediated degradation of N-MYC [77]. Functional studies of the most commonly identified N-MYC substitutions in BCC (T58A, P59L, P60L, and P63L) show that these mutations impair binding to FBXW7, resulting in an increase of N-MYC protein levels [52]. Interestingly, deleterious mutations and loss-of-heterozygosity (LOH) events in the FBXW7 gene occur in 5% and 8% of BCC samples, respectively, indicating that increased N-MYC stability may be advantageous for the development of this carcinoma [52].

TERT Promoter

Telomere repeats cap the ends of chromosomes and are critical to genome integrity; their length is maintained through a tightly regulated process, involving the activity of an essential reverse transcriptase, telomerase [78]. TERT gene encodes the catalytic subunit of telomerase, and its promoter region is considered the most important regulatory element for telomerase expression. Mutations in TERT promoter occur at high frequency in numerous cancers and have been correlated with increased expression, longer telomeres, and poor patient outcomes [79]. TERT promoter mutations are frequent in skin cancers, including BCC, suggesting that the increased expression of telomerase might play an important role in their pathogenesis. Common C > T and CC > TT substitutions reveal the UV signature underlying most of the TERT promoter mutations in cutaneous malignancies [80–82].

DPH3-OXNAD1 Promoter

UV signature mutations in the bidirectional promoter region of DPH3-OXNAD1 were found in 42% of BCCs in one study [83]. Mutations occurred in or adjacent to the ETS/TCF transcription factor binding motif, near the transcription start site. No difference in expression levels of DPH3 or OXNAD1 was reported in the tumors carrying the mutations, so their functional significance still needs to be determined [83].

Kinastin

Kinastin (kinetochore-localized ASTRIN/SPAG5 binding protein (KNSTRN)) encodes a kinetochore-associated protein in the mitotic spindle, crucial for correct chromosomal segregation. Recurrent point mutations in KNSTRN that disrupt chromatid cohesion and promote chromosomal instability have been identified in melanoma, SCC, and more recently BCC [84, 85]. Comparison between 18 advanced (inoperable and > 3 cm in size) and 30 early stage (<2 cm in size) BCCs suggests that KNSTRN mutations may be more common in advanced or aggressive disease, although this remains to be more firmly established by evaluating a larger patient cohort [84].

Non-coding RNAs

MicroRNAs (miRNA) are small non-coding RNAs involved in a variety of biological processes through their roles in the regulation of gene expression [86]. Aberrant activity of miRNAs has been liked to various human diseases, including cancer [87]. Most miRNAs are transcribed into primary miRNAs (pri-miRNAs) and processed into precursor miRNAs (pre-miRNAs) and mature miRNAs by the microprocessor complex [88]. After being incorporated into the RNA-induced silencing complexes (RISC), mature miRNA will interact with their target mRNAs to suppress expression [89]. Compared to healthy controls, BCCs were shown to have altered expression profiles of the microprocessor complex, RISC, and different miRNAs [90–92]. miR-203, proposed to act as a tumor suppressor in BCC, was shown to be downregulated in the tumors following the activation of HH and EGFR/MEK/ERK/c-JUN signaling [93]. A study profiling global miRNA expression in nodular and infiltrative BCCs found 6 miRNAs that showed significantly different expression between the two tumor subtypes [94]. In this cohort, miR-183 was found to have no overlap between nodular and infiltrative tumors, suggesting that distinct miRNA profiles could be one of the variables underlying the differences in the aggressiveness of BCC subtypes [94]. In addition to miRNAs, preliminary studies have shown that other types of regulatory non-coding RNAs, such as circular and long non-coding (LINC) RNAs display different expression patterns in BCCs compared to non-lesional skin [95, 96].

5.2.1.3 Therapy and Follow-Up

BCC treatment should ideally completely remove the tumor to prevent recurrence, correct any loss of function resulting from the tumor, and provide the best cosmetic outcome to the patient. Treatment primarily consists of surgical approaches, although some patients can undergo radiation, topical or systemic therapy. Classification of BCC lesions as low or high-risk shapes the initial treatment decisions, and these are made after consideration of tumor size, location, immune status of the patient, recurrent lesions, and histological analyses [44, 45]. Historically, BCCs were known as having a very low metastatic potential, up to 0.5% [41, 42]. While this is relevant for small tumors, recent data suggests that the risk of metastasis and death can be as high as 6.5% for larger lesions ($\geq$ 2 cm) [97]. The same study found that the head/neck location (OR, 5.3; 95% CI, 1.2–23.2), tumor diameter $\geq$ 4 cm (OR, 11.9; 95% CI, 2.4–59.4), and depth beyond fat (OR, 28.6; 95% CI, 6.7–121) were significant predictors of metastasis and death in large BCCs [97]. In general, smaller lesions (< 2 cm) that are located on the trunk and extremities are considered low risk, whereas large lesions (> 2 cm) are considered high risk. If the lesions are located on the head and neck, the size larger than 1 cm can already indicate a higher risk lesion. Histologic subtypes modulate the risk of recurrence and/or metastasis; nodular and superficial BCCs are considered low risk, whereas aggressive growth patterns of micronodular, infiltrative, or morpheaform subtypes are indicative of high-risk lesions. However, large nodular or superficial lesions can also be difficult to completely clear, which may contribute to the high rate of recurrence; the probability of developing another BCC is 35–75% at 5 years, depending on the number of initial diagnoses [98].

Low-risk superficial BCCs can be treated with topical 5-fluorouracil (5-FU) and Imiquimod 5% creams [99, 100], although there is limited control over complete tumor clearance. Localized adverse reactions are common and may include erythema, pain, edema, crusting, bleeding, and changes in pigmentation. Another treatment option for low-risk BCCs is cryosurgery [101]. It consists of a controlled application of liquid nitrogen to the visible tumor and a small surrounding margin of normal skin. While the procedure is fast, the treated area may be painful and swollen, sometimes leaving hypertrophic scars and permanent pigment alterations. Radiation therapy is used as a primary option or an adjuvant treatment for BCC when surgery is contraindicated [102]. Radiation treatment is a lengthy process and may increase the risk for future skin cancers. Mohs surgery is the gold standard for treating high-risk and recurrent BCCs because of its high cure rate and tissue preservation [65, 103]. Compared to the standard surgical excision, Mohs surgery collects thin tissue layers and evaluates all layer margins, achieving good tumor clearance rates while minimizing the wound size.

Systemic therapy with HH pathway inhibitors (HHI) can be used to treat patients with advanced/recurrent BCC who are not good surgery candidates, or those with metastatic BCC. Currently, two HHIs targeting SMO are approved by the FDA: vismodegib and sonidegib. Objective response rates of 30–45% are usually reported, although a complete response can be achieved in some patients [104, 105]. Considerable toxicity of these agents can lead to treatment discontinuation in up to 55% of patients; the most commonly reported adverse effects included nausea, muscle spasm, alopecia, weight loss, diarrhea, and fatigue [106]. Persistent HHI therapy leads to significant secondary resistance which usually occurs through de novo mutations in SMO, reactivation of the HH pathway through GLI or SUFU, or upregulation of alternative pathways such as PI3K [107–109]. In patients with advanced or metastatic BCC resistant to HHIs, treatment with the antifungal agent itraconazole may be beneficial [110]. In a phase II trial involving 84 patients with advanced BCC, immunotherapy with cemiplimab, a high-affinity human monoclonal antibody directed against programmed death 1 (PD-1) receptor, showed an acceptable toxicity profile and objective responses in 31% of the patients and was recently approved for locally advanced and metastatic BCCs that failed on HHI or for whom an HHI is not an appropriate therapeutic approach [111, 112].

The use of systemic therapies in BCC treatment has been especially important for advanced disease, however it has also raised new questions and challenges to overcome. These include the selection of patients, the effective management of common side effects, timing of treatment discontinuation after apparent complete clinical response to avoid recurrence, and the combined use of systemic therapy after incomplete surgical clearance or radiation treatment of the tumor. It is also still unclear if there is a differential response based on BCC subtype. So far, no clear correlation has been established between the response to systemic therapy and factors such as age, number of sites affected by BCC, or prior treatment with radiation [113]. Clinical decision-making process could be supported by understanding if certain molecular biomarkers, such as mutation profiles or gene expression changes, correlate with therapy response. A diagnostic test indicating the likelihood of response could effectively stratify patients and lower the costs of treatment. Having the ability to non-invasively sample treated lesions and assess genomic changes may allow determining the risk of recurrence and making timely adjustments to treatments, thereby facilitating therapy monitoring and follow-up care.

5.3 Squamous Cell Carcinoma (SCC)

SCC makes up to 20% of all skin cancers, its frequency second only to BCC [114]. Although many SCCs have a favorable outcome when treated with surgery or radiotherapy, these tumors frequently occur on sensitive sites such as face and scalp, carrying significant morbidity. Metastasis occurs in ~5% of cases, accounting for 75% of NMSC and 25% of all skin cancer-related deaths [15, 26]. The past decades have seen a rise in the SCC incidence rates, morbidity and cost, signaling the need for a solid registration system, accurate diagnosing, and effective management [8].

5.3.1 Biomarkers in SCC

5.3.1.1 Prevention and Risk Assessment

UVR

Similarly to BCC, SCC is more common in people with light skin (Fitzpatrick types I and II), poor tanning response, immune suppression and presence of certain genetic pigmentary disorders; however, the leading risk factor is the exposure to UVR and the majority of SCCs have extensive UV signature lesions [115, 116]. Recurrent mutations in P53, FAT1 and genes encoding the NOTCH receptors have been described as early events and likely drivers in the pathogenesis of SCC, although these mutations can exist in phenotypically normal skin decades before the onset of the disease [115–117].

Actinic Keratosis

Excessive UV exposure can trigger the development of actinic keratoses (AKs), precursor lesions of SCC, resulting from the proliferation of atypical epidermal keratinocytes. AKs appear as irregularly shaped and rough papules or patches on sun-damaged skin, and usually follow one of three clinical outcomes: spontaneous regression, persistence, or evolution into SCC [118]. Although most SCCs are found to arise from AK lesions, the likelihood and timing of the transition from AK to SCC is highly variable between individuals, and difficult to reliably predict [118, 119]. AK lesions have been reported to regress in 15–63% of cases, recur 15–53% of cases and progress in 5–20% over the span of several years [118–121]. Due to such broad variability, it is currently recommended to carefully monitor and/or appropriately treat all AKs [122], although this is not always straightforward; management decisions require considerations of available treatments, their cost-effectiveness, and other patient-specific factors. Morphologically, AKs have been classified as grade I, II or III lesions, based on the extent of epidermal involvement with the focal atypia of basal keratinocytes [123]. Traditionally, grade I lesions have been considered 'low grade' with a low probability of progression into SCC. Until recently, the AK grade evolution from 'low' to 'high' was thought necessary for the progression of AK into invasive SCC; however, it has been recently shown that grade I AK (atypical keratinocytes restricted to the basal layer) is commonly associated with invasive SCC and that therefore all types of AK lesions should be regarded as potentially invasive [124, 125]. These findings suggest that early detection and continuous monitoring are important for all lesions, including those with almost invisible clinical presentations in which only local inflammation and altered skin cornification can be appreciated. From a genetic standpoint, AK and SCC exist on a progressive disease spectrum and display similar genetic alterations, making the differentiation between the two conditions challenging. A study comparing normal non–sun-exposed skin, normal sun-exposed skin, AK, and SCC showed progressive abnormal gene expression levels along this spectrum [126]. However, while this study was able to outline an 89-gene classifier sufficient to distinguish between normal and transformed skin, it could not separate AK and SCC, in line with their close genetic relationship [126]. A diverse panel of biomarkers, including mutations, gene expression, and protein accumulation levels may be necessary to clearly mark the separation between AK and SCC and help predict the likelihood of disease progression.

5.3.1.2 Tumor Diagnosis and Profiling

Biopsy and subsequent histological analysis are the commonly used tools in diagnosing SCC, enabling the differentiation between in situ and invasive forms, classification of high- and low-risk lesions and determination of tumor subtypes. SCC in situ is also known as Bowen's disease (BD) and histologically differs from AK in showing full-thickness epidermal dysplasia with hair follicle involvement, complete loss of normal epidermal maturation, and a clear demarcation from adjacent healthy skin [127]. BD is predicted to progress to SCC in 3–5% of cases, however 20% of these cases are eventually reported to be metastatic [128, 129]. Invasive SCCs, in which the malignant keratinocytes invade the underlying dermis at various depths, usually arise from precursor AKs or BDs and several histological subtypes can be distinguished, including common SCC, spindle cell, clear cell, and Bowenoid subtypes [128]. De novo SCCs, which are not derived from a precursor AK or BD lesion, are particularly aggressive forms with high likelihood of metastasis, increased risk of recurrence and overall poor prognosis [130, 131]. As there is no accepted standard system for defining SCC lesions, it remains challenging to accurately estimate risks and predict outcomes for individual patients. Various studies have described protein, gene expression, and mutational patterns in SCC, without reaching a consensus on a biomarker panel that would improve patient management. Development of novel, consistent and reliable biomarker panels for SCC is sorely needed to support diagnostic and prognostic models and aid treatment decisions.

Protein Biomarker Panel for SCC Progression

In the attempt to characterize the progression of SCC, a study by Sun et al. used immunohistochemistry to compare the protein profiles of non-cancerous (normal), pre-cancerous lesions, and SCC samples, by mapping 10 selected proteins in groups of keratins (CK10, CK17), cell–cell adhesion factors (CD44, EZR, membrane E-cadherin, and β-catenin), chaperone proteins (Hsp75 and Hsp90-α), transcription regulator EXOSC10 and mitochondrial redox protein SOD2 [132]. Samples were divided into three groups: 42 normal tissue (non-cancerous regions surrounding the cancer), 34 pre-cancerous lesions (3 Bowen's disease, 24 actinic keratosis, and 7 cutaneous horns), and 51 SCCs. The SCC specimens were further distinguished as well- (18), moderate- (13), and poorly- (20) differentiated subgroups. To a degree, all ten proteins appeared informative in this study cohort. Keratins, cell adhesion proteins and EXOSC10 showed progressive changes in the intensity of immunohistochemical stains between the three test groups, correlating with disease progression, but not SCC differentiation. SOD2 was virtually absent from normal and pre-cancerous tissue but showed a sharp increase in protein levels in SCC (normal vs. SCC, 2–63%, $P < 0.001$; pre-cancerous vs. SCC, 0–63%, $P < 0.001$) and a positive correlation with the tumor differentiation status ($rs = 0.423$, $P < 0.005$). The expression levels of the chaperone proteins Hsp75 and Hsp90-α were correlated with cancer development ($rs = 0.593$, $P < 0.001$, and $rs = 0.660$, $P < 0.001$, respectively) as they both showed increased expression from normal to SCC (7–73%, $P < 0.001$, and 29–100%, $P < 0.001$, respectively) and from pre-cancerous to SCC groups (15–73%, $P < 0.001$, and 65–100%, $P < 0.05$, respectively). Hsp90-α expression was also significantly higher in pre-cancerous than the normal group (29–65%, $P = 0.001$). The strength of Hsp90-α staining in SCC group was associated with differentiation status (rs = 0.389, $P = 0.005$), as the protein expression levels were defined as predominantly (+) or (++) in well and moderately differentiated samples, and mostly (+++) in poorly differentiated SCC samples.

Epidermal Homeostasis

Presence of chronic wounds and disruption of skin homeostasis represent risk factors for the development of aggressive SCC, suggesting that the balance of key players in these processes may contribute to creating a permissive environment crucial for tumor initiation and progression. Epidermolysis bullosa (EB) is a heterogeneous group of inherited skin disorders determined by dysfunction of structural components of the cutaneous basement membrane [133]. Disease is characterized by skin fragility, persistent blistering, and chronic skin trauma. In severe forms of the disease, lesional skin shows defective wound healing, increased bacterial colonization, inflammation with progressive fibrosis and scarring. EB patients are at an increased risk of developing SCC, in particular those suffering from the severe generalized recessive dystrophic EB (RDEB), caused by mutations in the COL7A1 gene that encodes type VII collagen (COL7) [134]. The cumulative risk of developing at least one SCC for patients with RDEB increases with age, being already 67.8% by the age of 35 and attaining 90.1% by the age of 55 [135]. SCCs that develop at sites of chronic wounds and scarring in RDEB have a high propensity of relapse and metastasis, making early detection key for effective treatment decisions [136, 137]. However, early diagnosis of SCC in RDEB patients remains a challenge, especially given the difficulty in histopathologic differentiation of RDEB-SCC from granulation tissue or benign epidermal hyperplasia [137]. Combination of delayed diagnosis and the exceptionally aggressive features of RDEB-SCC contribute to the poor prognosis in these patients; indeed, the USA National EB registry reports the cumulative risk of death from SCC in RDEB patients to be 57.2% by age 35 and 87.3% by age 45 [135]. Structural proteins or enzymes involved in would healing and skin homeostasis, including COL7 and matrix metalloproteinases, have been considered as biomarkers or regulators of SCC carcinogenesis [138, 139]. Patients with dominant EB, that have one normal COL7A1 allele, develop less SCC than RDEB patients, prompting the idea that the increase in the amounts of COL7 may be beneficial in this setting; however, it was also noted that higher-than-physiological levels of COL7 correlated with increased activities of PI3K and MAPK pathways, cell migration and invasion, suggesting caution in the development of such therapeutic interventions [133, 138]. Matrix metalloproteinases (MMPs) are a large family of proteolytic enzymes able to degrade almost all components of the extracellular matrix and basement membranes. Aberrant expression of the MMPs has been described in numerous human diseases, including malignancies of squamous origin [140, 141]. Progressively increasing accumulation of matrix metalloproteinases 7 and 13 (MMP-7, MMP-13) was reported between Bowen disease, non-EB SCCs, and RDEB-SCCs, indicating a possible role for these enzymes in the promotion of cutaneous carcinogenesis and usefulness as markers of SCC progression and aggressiveness [139, 142].

The Complement System

Complement is a part of the innate immune system with roles in the inflammatory response initiation as well as clearing of microbes and apoptotic cells [143]. Complement system consists of three distinct pathways (classical, alternative, and lectin pathways) that converge on the activation of complement C3 resulting in the formation of membrane attack complex (MAC) and lysis of the target cell [143]. The activity of the complement system is in part regulated by cell-bound and soluble inhibitors, which protect cells against complement-mediated lysis. Complement factor H is an important soluble inhibitor of the alternative pathway that exists as two isoforms with similar functions: CFH (150 kDa) and factor H-like protein-1 (FHL-1, 45 kDa) [144]. CFH has been proposed as a biomarker for the progression of SCC following the results of a study that analyzed CFH and FHL-1 expression through qPCR and immunohistochemical stains in SCC, AK, and normal skin [145]. Overexpression of both isoforms in SCC cells relative to normal keratinocytes and increased rates of expression with the progression from AK to invasive SCC was reported in the study [145]. Overexpression of CFH in patients was associated with negative prognosis as it was found to promote proliferation and migration of SCC cells, as well as help their escape from the complement-mediated destruction [145]. Complement factor B (CFB), another important soluble component in the alternative pathway, was also shown to be upregulated by SCC cells in culture and by SCC tumors in vivo [146]. C3 and CFB were found to regulate proliferation and migration of SCC cells and promote growth of SCC xenografts in vivo, suggesting their potential use as disease biomarkers [146]. Increased expression levels of C1r and C1s, components of the classical pathway, were reported in SCC cells in culture and SCC tumor cells in vivo [147]. Conversely, knockdown of C1r and C1s was shown to inhibit activation of the extracellular signal-related kinase (ERK)1/2 and phosphoinositide 3-kinase (PI3K) signaling pathways, promote the apoptosis of SCC cells and suppress vascularization and growth of SCC xenografts in vivo [147], suggesting a role in viability, apoptosis resistance and invasion.

Chromosomal Alterations in SCC

Changes in chromosomal number, insertions, deletions, and translocations are common in many cancers, including SCC, which displays extensive chromosomal istability [148]. LOH studies have shown recurrent regions of loss and gain in SCC, including loss of 3p (65%), 9p (75%), 2q, 8p and gains on 3q, 8q, 9q, and 11q [148].

Substantial chromosomal instability is also seen in AK, with frequent alterations at 3p, 9p, 13q, 17p, and 17q. The extent of chromosomal instability may correlate with the tumor differentiation status, as significantly fewer changes have been identified in well-compared with poorly differentiated SCCs [148]. Tumor suppressor locus CDKN2A on chromosome 9p21 encodes the p16(INK4a) and p14(ARF) genes that function as cell cycle regulatory proteins in the p53 and RB pathways; these are susceptibility genes for a number of cancers, including melanoma and the squamous carcinomas of the head and neck [149]. Chromosomal aberrations and inactivation of the CDKN2A locus by both genetic and epigenetic mechanisms are frequently reported in SCC [116, 148, 150, 151], in line with common LOH events at the 9p region. Within the same region, a frequent microdeletion at 9p23 was reported, found within the gene encoding protein tyrosine phosphatase delta (PTPRD). SCC tumors carrying the PTPRD microdeletion were more likely to be poorly differentiated and associated with a higher metastatic risk [148]. PTPRD may be a candidate tumor suppressor gene in SCC, however given its chromosomal localization, further functional studies are needed to explore this hypothesis.

S100A7

S100A7 (psoriasin) is a calcium-modulated protein, originally identified in psoriatic keratinocytes [152, 153]. Expression of S100A7 is upregulated in many types of squamous cell carcinomas, including lung, oral, bladder, and skin, where it may play a role in carcinogenesis and metastasis [154–156]. Several studies report increased expression levels of S100A7 in highly differentiated SCCs, as well as in precursor lesions, compared to weak or absent expression in less differentiated tumors, suggesting a possible association with the balance of proliferation and differentiation in SCC [154, 156, 157]. Further suggesting the involvement of S100A7 in differentiation is its location within the epidermal differentiation gene cluster on chromosome 1q21; indeed, the upregulation of S100A7 was found to be paralleled by the upregulation of squamous differentiation markers, including keratin-4, keratin-13, TG-1, and involucrin [158, 159].

Histone Methyltransferases

KMT2C and KMT2D encode histone methyltransferases that play a role in the regulation of gene expression through the targeted modification of histone H3. Frequent inactivating mutations in both genes, most displaying a UV signature, were reported in aggressive SCCs and associated with poor prognosis [115, 160]. KMT2C mutations had a significant positive correlation with bone invasion and shorter recurrence-free survival in SCC patients [115]. Tumors harboring KMT2C mutations also had trends toward shorter time to disease recurrence and shorter overall survival in the same study [115]. KMT2D has been reported mutated in other cancers such as cutaneous melanoma (19–29%), esophageal SCC (14–19%), and head and neck SCC (11–16%) [161–163]. Significantly higher rates of mutations in KMT2D were reported for metastatic (62%) relative to non-metastatic cutaneous SCC tumors (31%) [164].

CTCF Insulator Binding Sites

A study by Mueller et al. profiled mutational patterns in 15 SCC metastases and found a pervasive UV signature with uneven distribution of the mutational load in certain regions of the genome, especially insulator elements [165]. Insulators are DNA sequences involved in the regulation of long-range interactions between enhancers and promoters [166], which may affect the expression of multiple genetic loci. The study assessed the main human insulator CTCF and found high prevalence of mutations in its consensus DNA binding motif. CTCF simultaneously binds to multiple consensus-containing DNA sites, thereby approximating distant chromatin regions and forming 3-dimensional DNA loops termed topologically associated domains (TADs) [167]. Changes in CTCF function could alter the transcriptional activity of multiple genes associated within each CTCF-bound TAD loop, which was proposed to play a role in carcinogenesis [168, 169]. CTCF binding motif seems susceptible to UV-induced damage because of its high cytosine and dipyrimidine content; the clustering of UV signature mutations at the CTCF motif was previously described in melanoma and is thought to be due to bound CTCF blocking access of DNA repair enzymes [170, 171]. Interestingly, the study by Mueller et al. found that the mutation density in the CTCF binding motif in metastatic SCC was considerably higher than the one reported in melanoma, and it also exceeded the expected concentration based on the high cytosine and dipyrimidine content [165]. If the identified mutations in consensus motifs disrupt the efficient binding of CTCF in metastatic SCCs, these could potentially result in disruption of the TAD structure and dysregulation of the enclosed genes. Mueller et al. report 422 TADs with mutations in least one relevant CTCF motif, containing a total of 1979 enclosed genes, including 38 oncogenes, 52 tumor suppressor genes, and 11 genes identified as potential tumor drivers [165]. While CTCF mutations were previously shown to be able to significantly change the expression of genes within the affected TADs in melanoma [171], additional functional analyses are needed to determine the potential impact of these mutations in SCC.

5.3.1.3 Therapy and Follow-Up

Based on the initial assessment of the tumor, the primary strategy for SCC treatment is the complete tumor removal with the maximal functional and cosmetic preservation. Accurate histological reports are only one part of the tumor assessment process, and the combination of clinical features and host-specific factors are recognized as important aspects of tumor evaluation and treatment decisions, especially when discriminating between high- and low-risk lesions. The high-risk features of SCCs include tumor size (> 2 cm), tumor depth of invasion (> 2 mm or Clark Level > IV), speed of growth, anatomic location (ear and lip), perineural invasion, and poor differentiation [172, 173]. Lymphovascular invasion (tumor nests around and/or within blood and/or lymphatic vessels) and tumor budding (single tumor cells or small groups of tumor cells ahead of the invasive tumor front) were more recently recognized to be features of adverse outcomes in SCC [174–176].

Conventional surgery with safety margins and MOHS surgery are treatments of choice in patients with primary SCC. MOHS surgery has lower recurrence rates (0–4%) compared to conventional surgery, and it is also indicated in patients with high-risk tumors in order to obtain a complete tumor removal with optimal tissue preservation [177–179]. Non-invasive SCCs are successfully treated with techniques such as curettage, electrodessication, cryosurgery, lasers, and photodynamic therapy (PDT). Also, radiation therapy is a viable alternative treatment for small tumors, or for patients who are not eligible for surgery because of tumor- or patient-related features [180, 181].

Systemic treatments available for SCC patients include targeted therapy to the epidermal growth factor receptor (EGFR), chemotherapy, and anti-PD-1 immunetherapy [182]. EGFR is highly expressed in SCC and two monoclonal antibodies targeting EGFR, cetuximab and panitumumab, were evaluated in clinical trials as first line in patients with advanced or metastatic disease. Objective response rates analyzed in prospective and retrospective studies were reported to be between 28 and 53%, with mostly acceptable safety profiles [183–185]. In a phase II study, an oral anti-EGFR agent, gefitinib, showed overall response rate of 16% and the median progression-free survival of 3.8 months in a cohort of 40 patients with advanced SCC [186]. Chemotherapy agents commonly used for systemic treatment of SCC are cisplatin and 5-fluorouracil (5-FU). Literature review on these agents shows response rates above 50% for platinum monotherapy or in combination with 5-FU [187, 188]; however, only a limited number of studies with small sample size have been conducted to formally evaluate these therapies [189]. Because of the considerable toxicity associated with systemic chemotherapies, their use in advanced SCC is mostly indicated when other therapeutic alternatives are limited or exhausted, and systemic immune therapy is becoming the new standard of care for advanced and metastatic SCC [188, 189].

Generally, SCC has the hallmarks of a tumor that is likely to be responsive to systemic immune therapy: the risk for developing the disease is increased in patients with immunosuppressive conditions and the mutation burden is high, indicating potential expression of tumor neoantigens that attract effector T cells [190–192]. Activated T cells express the PD-1 receptor, and binding of the programmed death (PD)-ligands (PD-L1 or PD-L2) can inhibit T cell proliferation and cytokine production, leading to a reduced immune response to tumors [193]. Expression of PD-L1 has been observed in 35–70% of advanced SCCs and in 58–100% of metastatic SCCs, and could potentially be used as a biomarker in predicting response to immune checkpoint inhibitors [190, 194, 195]. Systemic therapy with cemiplimab is indicated for the treatment of metastatic SCC and for locally advanced SCC not amenable to surgical or radiation treatments [196]. The response rates to cemiplimab for patients with metastatic SCC were 50% in phase I and 47% in phase II trials; similar efficacy was observed in patients with regional metastatic disease and in those with distant metastatic disease [197]. In a recent single-arm phase II trial, 44% of patients with locally advanced SCC showed an objective response to cemiplimab (34 of 78) [198]. Specifically, 13% of patients (10) displayed a complete response and 31% (24) a partial response [198]. For non-responders, further molecular profiling of advanced and metastatic SCCs is needed to identify new biomarkers which would guide therapy selection, facilitate patient monitoring, and accelerate the development of novel targeted therapies.

5.4 Conclusions

Non-melanoma skin cancer is the most commonly diagnosed cancer in the U.S. and represents a substantial public health issue. Advances in sequencing technologies have led to a much deeper understanding of the underlying pathology in NMSC, providing critical information on valuable molecular biomarkers of the disease. Various types of molecular biomarkers, including DNA, RNA, and proteins have been explored in the context of NMSC and some of these have influenced the development or repurposing of targeted therapies, such as the HH inhibitors or the immune checkpoint blockade now used for patients with advanced BCC and SCC. Relevant combinations of new molecular and clinical biomarkers may improve diagnosis and staging of skin tumors, a critical step in structuring the patient management strategy. Environmental exposure to ultraviolet radiation (UVR) is the key etiological factor in the development of skin cancer, however the long lag between the initial skin damage induced by UVR and the onset of skin cancer decreases the perception of UVR danger and hinders preventative efforts. Development of a biomarker panel that accurately reflects UVR damage has been challenging, but also a longstanding goal in the efforts to standardize skin cancer screening. Translation of UVR-related biomarkers into a clinical test providing an objective risk score for the development of skin cancer has the potential to considerably improve skin cancer prevention by efficiently stratifying patients, increasing public compliance with preventative measures and reducing screening costs. Use of non-invasive methods for skin evaluation and sampling will likely play a key role in enabling widespread screening and patient monitoring. Further research into NMSC pathogenesis and the development of novel biomarkers is expected to continue to transform patient care and improve outcomes.

References

1. Rigel DS, Friedman RJ, Kopf AW. Lifetime risk for development of skin cancer in the U.S. population: current estimate is now 1 in 5. J Am Acad Dermatol. 1996;35:1012–13.
2. Types of skin cancer. https://www.aad.org/public/diseases/skin-cancer/types/common.
3. Jørgensen JT. The current landscape of the FDA approved companion diagnostics. Transl Oncol. 2021;14: 101063.
4. Siegel RL, Miller KD, Fuchs HE, Jemal A. Cancer statistics, 2021. CA Cancer J Clin. 2021;71:7–33.
5. Rowe DE, Carroll RJ, Day CL. Prognostic factors for local recurrence, metastasis, and survival rates in squamous cell carcinoma of the skin, ear, and lip. Implications for treatment modality selection. J Am Acad Dermatol. 1992;26:976–90.
6. Kyllo RL, Staser KW, Rosman I, Council ML, Hurst EA. Histopathologic upgrading of nonmelanoma skin cancer at the time of Mohs micrographic surgery: a prospective review. J Am Acad Dermatol. 2019;81:541–7.
7. Burdon-Jones D, Thomas P, Baker R. Quality of life issues in nonmetastatic skin cancer. Br J Dermatol. 2010;162:147–51.
8. Lomas A, Leonardi-Bee J, Bath-Hextall F. A systematic review of worldwide incidence of nonmelanoma skin cancer. Br J Dermatol. 2012;166:1069–80.
9. Smith H, Wernham A, Patel A. When to suspect a non-melanoma skin cancer. BMJ. 2020;368: m692.
10. Ruiz ES, Morgan FC, Zigler CM, Besaw RJ, Schmults CD. Analysis of national skin cancer expenditures in the United States Medicare population, 2013. J Am Acad Dermatol. 2019;80:275–8.
11. Guy GP, Machlin SR, Ekwueme DU, Yabroff KR. Prevalence and costs of skin cancer treatment in the U.S., 2002–2006 and 2007–2011. Am J Prev Med. 2015;48:183–87.
12. Eide MJ, et al. Identification of patients with nonmelanoma skin cancer using health maintenance organization claims data. Am J Epidemiol. 2010;171:123–8.
13. Nikolaou V, Stratigos AJ, Tsao H. Hereditary nonmelanoma skin cancer. Semin Cutan Med Surg. 2012;31:204–10.
14. Welsh MM, et al. Genetic determinants of UV-susceptibility in non-melanoma skin cancer. PLoS ONE. 2011;6:e20019.
15. Leiter U, Eigentler T, Garbe C. Epidemiology of skin cancer. In: Reichrath J, editor. Sunlight, vitamin D and skin cancer. Springer; 2014, pp. 120–40. https://doi.org/10.1007/978-1-4939-0437-2_7.
16. Emri G, et al. Low doses of UVB or UVA induce chromosomal aberrations in cultured human skin cells. J Invest Dermatol. 2000;115:435–40.
17. Xiang F, Lucas R, Hales S, Neale R. Incidence of nonmelanoma skin cancer in relation to ambient UV radiation in white populations, 1978–2012: empirical relationships. JAMA Dermatol. 2014;150:1063–71.
18. Wehner MR, et al. Indoor tanning and non-melanoma skin cancer: systematic review and meta-analysis. BMJ. 2012;345:e5909.
19. Buller DB, et al. Prevalence of sunburn, sun protection, and indoor tanning behaviors among Americans: review from national surveys and case studies of 3 states. J Am Acad Dermatol. 2011;65:S114-123.
20. Centers for Disease Control and Prevention (CDC). Sunburn and sun protective behaviors among adults aged 18–29 years--United States, 2000–2010. MMWR Morb Mortal Wkly Rep. 2012;61:317–22.
21. Trager MH, et al. Advances in prevention and surveillance of cutaneous malignancies. Am J Med. 2020;133:417–23.
22. US Preventive Services Task Force, et al. Screening for skin cancer: US preventive services task force recommendation statement. JAMA 2016;316:429–35.
23. Johansson M, Brodersen J, Gøtzsche PC, Jørgensen KJ. Screening for reducing morbidity and mortality in malignant melanoma. Cochrane Database Syst Rev. 2019;6:CD012352.

24. Breitbart EW, et al. Systematic skin cancer screening in Northern Germany. J Am Acad Dermatol. 2012;66:201–11.
25. Curchin DJ, Harris VR, McCormack CJ, Smith SD. Changing trends in the incidence of invasive melanoma in Victoria, 1985–2015. Med J Aust. 2018;208:265–9.
26. Apalla Z, Nashan D, Weller RB, Castellsagué X. Skin cancer: epidemiology, disease burden, pathophysiology, diagnosis, and therapeutic approaches. Dermatol Ther. 2017;7:5–19.
27. Privalle A, Havighurst T, Kim K, Bennett DD, Xu YG. Number of skin biopsies needed per malignancy: comparing the use of skin biopsies among dermatologists and nondermatologist clinicians. J Am Acad Dermatol. 2020;82:110–6.
28. Murzaku EC, Hayan S, Rao BK. Methods and rates of dermoscopy usage: a cross-sectional survey of US dermatologists stratified by years in practice. J Am Acad Dermatol. 2014;71:393–5.
29. Sinz C, et al. Accuracy of dermatoscopy for the diagnosis of nonpigmented cancers of the skin. J Am Acad Dermatol. 2017;77:1100–9.
30. Que SKT, Grant-Kels JM, Longo C, Pellacani G. Basics of confocal microscopy and the complexity of diagnosing skin tumors: new imaging tools in clinical practice, diagnostic workflows, cost-estimate, and new trends. Dermatol Clin. 2016;34:367–75.
31. Malvehy J, Pellacani G. Dermoscopy, confocal microscopy and other non-invasive tools for the diagnosis of non-melanoma skin cancers and other skin conditions. Acta Derm Venereol. 2017;Suppl 218:22–30.
32. Mu EW, et al. Use of digitally stained multimodal confocal mosaic images to screen for nonmelanoma skin cancer. JAMA Dermatol. 2016;152:1335–41.
33. Olesen CM, et al. Advancement through epidermis using tape stripping technique and Reflectance confocal microscopy. Sci Rep. 2019;9:12217.
34. Research, C. About biomarkers and qualification. FDA 2021.
35. Strimbu K, Tavel JA. What are biomarkers? Curr Opin HIV AIDS. 2010;5:463–6.
36. Companion Diagnostics Market—Global Forecast to 2025 | MarketsandMarkets. https://www.marketsandmarkets.com/Market-Reports/companion-diagnostics-market-155571681.html.
37. MarketsandMarkets. Companion diagnostics market worth $7.3 billion by 2024—exclusive market report by M&M. https://www.prnewswire.com/news-releases/companion-diagnostics-market-worth-7-3-billion-by-2024---exclusive-market-report-by-mm-300918472.html.
38. Colomer R, et al. When should we order a next generation sequencing test in a patient with cancer? EClinicalMedicine. 2020;25.
39. Bernardini R, et al. Personalized medicine: biomarkers and companion diagnostics. Farmeconomia Health Econ Ther Pathw. 2018;19.
40. Lai V, Cranwell W, Sinclair R. Epidemiology of skin cancer in the mature patient. Clin Dermatol. 2018;36:167–76.
41. Ozgediz D, et al. Basal cell carcinoma does metastasize. Dermatol Online J. 2008;14:5.
42. von Domarus H, Stevens PJ. Metastatic basal cell carcinoma. Report of five cases and review of 170 cases in the literature. J Am Acad Dermatol. 1984;10.
43. Kasper M, Jaks V, Hohl D, Toftgård R. Basal cell carcinoma—molecular biology and potential new therapies. J Clin Invest. 2012;122:455–63.
44. Bichakjian CK, et al. Basal cell skin cancer, Version 1.2016, NCCN clinical practice guidelines in oncology. J Natl Compr Cancer Netw JNCCN 2016;14:574–97.
45. Peris K, et al. Diagnosis and treatment of basal cell carcinoma: European consensus-based interdisciplinary guidelines. Eur J Cancer Oxf Engl. 2019;1990(118):10–34.
46. Akbari M, Chen H, Guo G, Legan Z, Ghali G. Basal cell nevus syndrome (Gorlin syndrome): genetic insights, diagnostic challenges, and unmet milestones. Pathophysiol Off J Int Soc Pathophysiol. 2018;25:77–82.
47. DiGiovanna JJ, Kraemer KH. Shining a light on xeroderma pigmentosum. J Invest Dermatol. 2012;132:785–96.
48. AlSabbagh MM, Baqi MA. Bazex-Dupré-Christol syndrome: review of clinical and molecular aspects. Int J Dermatol. 2018;57:1102–6.

49. Sinha RP, Häder D-P. UV-induced DNA damage and repair: a review. Photochem Photobiol Sci. 2002;1:225–36.
50. Brash DE. UV signature mutations. Photochem Photobiol. 2015;91:15–26.
51. Pfeifer GP. Mechanisms of UV-induced mutations and skin cancer. Genome Instab Dis. 2020;1:99–113.
52. Bonilla X, et al. Genomic analysis identifies new drivers and progression pathways in skin basal cell carcinoma. Nat Genet. 2016;48:398–406.
53. Jayaraman SS, Rayhan DJ, Hazany S, Kolodney MS. Mutational landscape of basal cell carcinomas by whole-exome sequencing. J Invest Dermatol. 2014;134:213–20.
54. Jonason AS, et al. Frequent clones of p53-mutated keratinocytes in normal human skin. Proc Natl Acad Sci U S A. 1996;93:14025–9.
55. Martincorena I, et al. High burden and pervasive positive selection of somatic mutations in normal human skin. Science. 2015;348:880–6.
56. Bolshakov S, et al. p53 mutations in human aggressive and nonaggressive basal and squamous cell carcinomas. Clin Cancer Res Off J Am Assoc Cancer Res. 2003;9:228–34.
57. Saini N, et al. UV-exposure, endogenous DNA damage, and DNA replication errors shape the spectra of genome changes in human skin. PLOS Genet. 2021;17:e1009302.
58. Yizhak K, et al. RNA sequence analysis reveals macroscopic somatic clonal expansion across normal tissues. Science 2019;364.
59. Steinbuck MP, Winandy S. A review of notch processing with new insights into ligand-independent notch signaling in T-Cells. Front Immunol. 2018;0.
60. Dawes JM, et al. Genome-wide transcriptional profiling of skin and dorsal root ganglia after ultraviolet-B-induced inflammation. PLoS ONE. 2014;9:e93338.
61. Shen Y, Stanislauskas M, Li G, Zheng D, Liu L. Epigenetic and genetic dissections of UV-induced global gene dysregulation in skin cells through multi-omics analyses. Sci Rep. 2017;7:42646.
62. Sun X, Kim A, Nakatani M, Shen Y, Liu L. Distinctive molecular responses to ultraviolet radiation between keratinocytes and melanocytes. Exp Dermatol. 2016;25:708–13.
63. Holzscheck N, et al. Concomitant DNA methylation and transcriptome signatures define epidermal responses to acute solar UV radiation. Sci Rep. 2020;10:12918.
64. Firnhaber JM. Diagnosis and treatment of basal cell and squamous cell carcinoma. Am Fam Physician. 2012;86:161–8.
65. McDaniel B, Badri T, Steele RB. Basal cell carcinoma. In: StatPearls. StatPearls Publishing; 2021.
66. Wolberink EAW, Pasch MC, Zeiler M, van Erp PEJ, Gerritsen MJP. High discordance between punch biopsy and excision in establishing basal cell carcinoma subtype: analysis of 500 cases. J Eur Acad Dermatol Venereol JEADV 2013;27:985–89.
67. Kamyab-Hesari K, et al. Diagnostic accuracy of punch biopsy in subtyping basal cell carcinoma. J Eur Acad Dermatol Venereol JEADV. 2014;28:250–3.
68. Epstein EH. Basal cell carcinomas: attack of the hedgehog. Nat Rev Cancer. 2008;8:743–54.
69. Tanese K, Emoto K, Kubota N, Fukuma M, Sakamoto M. Immunohistochemical visualization of the signature of activated Hedgehog signaling pathway in cutaneous epithelial tumors. J Dermatol. 2018;45:1181–6.
70. Lam C-W, et al. Novel mutations in the PATCHED gene in basal cell nevus syndrome. Mol Genet Metab. 2002;76:57–61.
71. Reifenberger J, et al. Somatic mutations in the PTCH, SMOH, SUFUH and TP53 genes in sporadic basal cell carcinomas. Br J Dermatol. 2005;152:43–51.
72. Zhang H, Pasolli HA, Fuchs E. Yes-associated protein (YAP) transcriptional coactivator functions in balancing growth and differentiation in skin. Proc Natl Acad Sci U S A. 2011;108:2270–5.
73. Zhao B, et al. Inactivation of YAP oncoprotein by the Hippo pathway is involved in cell contact inhibition and tissue growth control. Genes Dev. 2007;21:2747–61.
74. Sarmasti Emami S, Zhang D, Yang X. Interaction of the Hippo pathway and phosphatases in tumorigenesis. Cancers. 2020;12:E2438.

75. Ohama T. The multiple functions of protein phosphatase 6. Biochim Biophys Acta BBA Mol Cell Res. 2019;1866:74–82.
76. Meyer N, Penn LZ. Reflecting on 25 years with MYC. Nat Rev Cancer. 2008;8:976–90.
77. Welcker M, et al. The Fbw7 tumor suppressor regulates glycogen synthase kinase 3 phosphorylation-dependent c-Myc protein degradation. Proc Natl Acad Sci U S A. 2004;101:9085–90.
78. Wu RA, Upton HE, Vogan JM, Collins K. Telomerase mechanism of Telomere synthesis. Annu Rev Biochem. 2017;86:439–60.
79. Heidenreich B, Kumar R. TERT promoter mutations in telomere biology. Mutat Res. 2017;771:15–31.
80. Pópulo H, et al. TERT promoter mutations in skin cancer: the effects of sun exposure and X-irradiation. J Invest Dermatol. 2014;134:2251–7.
81. Scott GA, Laughlin TS, Rothberg PG. Mutations of the TERT promoter are common in basal cell carcinoma and squamous cell carcinoma. Mod Pathol Off J U S Can Acad Pathol Inc 2014;27:516–23.
82. Griewank KG, et al. TERT promoter mutations are frequent in cutaneous basal cell carcinoma and squamous cell carcinoma. PLoS ONE. 2013;8:e80354.
83. Denisova E, et al. Frequent DPH3 promoter mutations in skin cancers. Oncotarget. 2015;6:35922–30.
84. Jaju PD, et al. Mutations in the Kinetochore gene KNSTRN in basal cell carcinoma. J Invest Dermatol. 2015;135:3197–200.
85. Lee CS, et al. Recurrent point mutations in the kinetochore gene KNSTRN in cutaneous squamous cell carcinoma. Nat Genet. 2014;46:1060–2.
86. Gebert LFR, MacRae IJ. Regulation of microRNA function in animals. Nat Rev Mol Cell Biol. 2019;20:21–37.
87. Paul P, et al. Interplay between miRNAs and human diseases. J Cell Physiol. 2018;233:2007–18.
88. Creugny A, Fender A, Pfeffer S. Regulation of primary microRNA processing. FEBS Lett. 2018;592:1980–96.
89. O'Brien J, Hayder H, Zayed Y, Peng C. Overview of MicroRNA biogenesis, mechanisms of actions, and circulation. Front Endocrinol. 2018;0.
90. Sand M, et al. Expression levels of the microRNA processing enzymes Drosha and dicer in epithelial skin cancer. Cancer Invest. 2010;28:649–53.
91. Sand M, et al. Expression levels of the microRNA maturing microprocessor complex component DGCR8 and the RNA-induced silencing complex (RISC) components argonaute-1, argonaute-2, PACT, TARBP1, and TARBP2 in epithelial skin cancer. Mol Carcinog. 2012;51:916–22.
92. Sand M, et al. Expression of microRNAs in basal cell carcinoma. Br J Dermatol. 2012;167:847–55.
93. Sonkoly E, et al. MicroRNA-203 functions as a tumor suppressor in basal cell carcinoma. Oncogenesis. 2012;1:e3.
94. Heffelfinger C, et al. Correlation of global MicroRNA expression with basal cell carcinoma subtype. G3 Bethesda Md 2012;2:279–86.
95. Sand M, et al. Long-noncoding RNAs in basal cell carcinoma. Tumour Biol J Int Soc Oncodevelopmental Biol Med 2016;37:10595–608.
96. Sand M, et al. Circular RNA expression in basal cell carcinoma. Epigenomics. 2016;8:619–32.
97. Morgan FC, et al. Factors predictive of recurrence, metastasis, and death from primary basal cell carcinoma 2 cm or larger in diameter. J Am Acad Dermatol. 2020;83:832–8.
98. Wehner MR, et al. Timing of subsequent new tumors in patients who present with basal cell carcinoma or cutaneous squamous cell carcinoma. JAMA Dermatol. 2015;151:382–8.
99. Kamath P, Darwin E, Arora H, Nouri K. A review on imiquimod therapy and discussion on optimal management of basal cell carcinomas. Clin Drug Investig. 2018;38:883–99.
100. Naik MP, Mehta A, Abrol S, Kumar S, Gupta VS. Topical 5% 5-fluorouracil in the treatment of multifocal basal cell carcinoma of the face: a novel chemotherapeutic approach. Orbit Amst Neth. 2016;35:352–4.

101. Buckley D, Marczuk C, Kennedy T. Cryosurgery for basal cell carcinoma treated in primary care. Ir J Med Sci. 2020;189:1183–7.
102. Cheraghi N, Cognetta A, Goldberg D. Radiation therapy in dermatology: non-melanoma skin cancer. J Drugs Dermatol JDD. 2017;16:464–9.
103. Drucker AM, et al. Treatments of primary basal cell carcinoma of the skin: a systematic review and network meta-analysis. Ann Intern Med. 2018;169:456–66.
104. Sekulic A, et al. Efficacy and safety of vismodegib in advanced basal-cell carcinoma. N Engl J Med. 2012;366:2171–9.
105. Migden MR, et al. Treatment with two different doses of sonidegib in patients with locally advanced or metastatic basal cell carcinoma (BOLT): a multicentre, randomised, double-blind phase 2 trial. Lancet Oncol. 2015;16:716–28.
106. Basset-Séguin N, et al. Vismodegib in patients with advanced basal cell carcinoma: primary analysis of STEVIE, an international, open-label trial. Eur J Cancer Oxf Engl. 2017;1990(86):334–48.
107. Pricl S, et al. Smoothened (SMO) receptor mutations dictate resistance to vismodegib in basal cell carcinoma. Mol Oncol. 2015;9:389–97.
108. Sharpe HJ, et al. Genomic analysis of smoothened inhibitor resistance in basal cell carcinoma. Cancer Cell. 2015;27:327–41.
109. Basset-Seguin N, Sharpe HJ, de Sauvage FJ. Efficacy of Hedgehog pathway inhibitors in basal cell carcinoma. Mol Cancer Ther. 2015;14:633–41.
110. Sohn GK, et al. Topical itraconazole for the treatment of basal cell carcinoma in patients with basal cell nevus syndrome or high-frequency basal cell carcinomas: a phase 2, open-label, placebo-controlled Trial. JAMA Dermatol. 2019;155:1078–80.
111. Stratigos AJ, et al. Cemiplimab in locally advanced basal cell carcinoma after hedgehog inhibitor therapy: an open-label, multi-centre, single-arm, phase 2 trial. Lancet Oncol. 2021;22:848–57.
112. Romero D. Cemiplimab is a new option in BCC. Nat Rev Clin Oncol. 2021;18:400–400.
113. Chang ALS, et al. Expanded access study of patients with advanced basal cell carcinoma treated with the Hedgehog pathway inhibitor, vismodegib. J Am Acad Dermatol. 2014;70:60–9.
114. Voiculescu V, et al. From normal skin to squamous cell carcinoma: a quest for novel biomarkers. Dis Markers. 2016;2016:4517492.
115. Pickering CR, et al. Mutational landscape of aggressive cutaneous squamous cell carcinoma. Clin Cancer Res Off J Am Assoc Cancer Res. 2014;20;6582–92.
116. Inman GJ, et al. The genomic landscape of cutaneous SCC reveals drivers and a novel azathioprine associated mutational signature. Nat Commun. 2018;9:3667.
117. South AP, et al. NOTCH1 mutations occur early during cutaneous squamous cell carcinogenesis. J Invest Dermatol. 2014;134:2630–8.
118. Criscione VD, et al. Actinic keratoses: natural history and risk of malignant transformation in the veterans affairs topical tretinoin chemoprevention trial. Cancer. 2009;115:2523–30.
119. Werner RN, et al. The natural history of actinic keratosis: a systematic review. Br J Dermatol. 2013;169:502–18.
120. Siegel JA, Korgavkar K, Weinstock MA. Current perspective on actinic keratosis: a review. Br J Dermatol. 2017;177:350–8.
121. Casari A, Chester J, Pellacani G. Actinic keratosis and non-invasive diagnostic techniques: an update. Biomedicines. 2018;6:E8.
122. Werner RN, et al. Evidence- and consensus-based (S3) guidelines for the treatment of actinic keratosis—international league of dermatological societies in cooperation with the European dermatology forum—short version. J Eur Acad Dermatol Venereol JEADV. 2015;29:2069–79.
123. Zalaudek I, et al. Morphologic grading and treatment of facial actinic keratosis. Clin Dermatol. 2014;32:80–7.
124. Fernández-Figueras MT, et al. Actinic keratosis with atypical basal cells (AK I) is the most common lesion associated with invasive squamous cell carcinoma of the skin. J Eur Acad Dermatol Venereol JEADV. 2015;29:991–7.

125. Schmitz L, et al. Cutaneous squamous cell carcinomas are associated with basal proliferating actinic keratoses. Br J Dermatol. 2019;180:916–21.
126. Padilla RS, Sebastian S, Jiang Z, Nindl I, Larson R. Gene expression patterns of normal human skin, actinic keratosis, and squamous cell carcinoma: a spectrum of disease progression. Arch Dermatol. 2010;146:288–93.
127. Majores M, Bierhoff E. Actinic keratosis, Bowen's disease, keratoacanthoma and squamous cell carcinoma of the skin. Pathol. 2015;36:16–29.
128. Yanofsky VR, Mercer SE, Phelps RG. Histopathological variants of cutaneous squamous cell carcinoma: a review. J Skin Cancer. 2011;2011:210813.
129. Cox NH, Eedy DJ, Morton CA. Guidelines for management of Bowen's disease: 2006 update. Br J Dermatol. 2007;156:11–21.
130. Sabin SR, Goldstein G, Rosenthal HG, Haynes KK. Aggressive squamous cell carcinoma originating as a Marjolin's ulcer. Dermatol Surg Off Publ Am Soc Dermatol Surg Al 2004;30, 229–30.
131. Cassarino DS, Derienzo DP, Barr RJ. Cutaneous squamous cell carcinoma: a comprehensive clinicopathologic classification–part two. J Cutan Pathol. 2006;33:261–79.
132. Sun Y, et al. A panel of biomarkers for skin squamous cell carcinoma: various functional entities and differential responses to resveratrol. Int J Clin Exp Pathol. 2019;12:1363–77.
133. Fine J-D, et al. Inherited epidermolysis bullosa: updated recommendations on diagnosis and classification. J Am Acad Dermatol. 2014;70:1103–26.
134. Has C, Nyström A, Saeidian AH, Bruckner-Tuderman L, Uitto J. Epidermolysis bullosa: molecular pathology of connective tissue components in the cutaneous basement membrane zone. Matrix Biol J Int Soc Matrix Biol 2018;71–72:313–29.
135. Fine J-D, Johnson LB, Weiner M, Li K-P, Suchindran C. Epidermolysis bullosa and the risk of life-threatening cancers: the National EB Registry experience, 1986–2006. J Am Acad Dermatol. 2009;60:203–11.
136. Montaudié H, Chiaverini C, Sbidian E, Charlesworth A, Lacour J-P. Inherited epidermolysis bullosa and squamous cell carcinoma: a systematic review of 117 cases. Orphanet J Rare Dis. 2016;11:117.
137. Mellerio JE, et al. Management of cutaneous squamous cell carcinoma in patients with epidermolysis bullosa: best clinical practice guidelines. Br J Dermatol. 2016;174:56–67.
138. Pourreyron C, et al. High levels of type VII collagen expression in recessive dystrophic epidermolysis bullosa cutaneous squamous cell carcinoma keratinocytes increases PI3K and MAPK signalling, cell migration and invasion. Br J Dermatol. 2014;170:1256–65.
139. Kivisaari AK, et al. Matrix metalloproteinase-7 activates heparin-binding epidermal growth factor-like growth factor in cutaneous squamous cell carcinoma. Br J Dermatol. 2010;163:726–35.
140. Cabral-Pacheco GA, et al. The roles of matrix metalloproteinases and their inhibitors in human diseases. Int J Mol Sci. 2020;21:9739.
141. Yuan S, et al. Elevated matrix metalloproteinase 7 expression promotes the proliferation, motility and metastasis of tongue squamous cell carcinoma. BMC Cancer. 2020;20:33.
142. Kivisaari AK, et al. Transformation-specific matrix metalloproteinases (MMP)-7 and MMP-13 are expressed by tumour cells in epidermolysis bullosa-associated squamous cell carcinomas. Br J Dermatol. 2008;158:778–85.
143. Ricklin D, Hajishengallis G, Yang K, Lambris JD. Complement: a key system for immune surveillance and homeostasis. Nat Immunol. 2010;11:785–97.
144. Zipfel PF, Skerka C. FHL-1/reconectin: a human complement and immune regulator with cell-adhesive function. Immunol Today. 1999;20:135–40.
145. Riihilä PM, et al. Complement factor H: a biomarker for progression of cutaneous squamous cell carcinoma. J Invest Dermatol. 2014;134:498–506.
146. Riihilä P, et al. Complement component C3 and complement factor B promote growth of cutaneous squamous cell carcinoma. Am J Pathol. 2017;187:1186–97.
147. Riihilä P, et al. Tumour-cell-derived complement components C1r and C1s promote growth of cutaneous squamous cell carcinoma. Br J Dermatol. 2020;182:658–70.

148. Purdie KJ, et al. Single nucleotide polymorphism array analysis defines a specific genetic fingerprint for well-differentiated cutaneous SCCs. J Invest Dermatol. 2009;129:1562–8.
149. Chan SH, Chiang J, Ngeow J. CDKN2A germline alterations and the relevance of genotype-phenotype associations in cancer predisposition. Hered Cancer Clin Pract. 2021;19:21.
150. Kubo Y, Urano Y, Matsumoto K, Ahsan K, Arase S. Mutations of the INK4a locus in squamous cell carcinomas of human skin. Biochem Biophys Res Commun. 1997;232:38–41.
151. Brown VL, et al. P16INK4a and p14ARF tumor suppressor genes are commonly inactivated in cutaneous squamous cell carcinoma. J Invest Dermatol. 2004;122:1284–92.
152. Madsen P, et al. Molecular cloning, occurrence, and expression of a novel partially secreted protein 'psoriasin' that is highly up-regulated in psoriatic skin. J Invest Dermatol. 1991;97:701–12.
153. Kulski JK, Lim CP, Dunn DS, Bellgard M. Genomic and phylogenetic analysis of the S100A7 (Psoriasin) gene duplications within the region of the S100 gene cluster on human chromosome 1q21. J Mol Evol. 2003;56:397–406.
154. Ostergaard M, et al. Proteome profiling of bladder squamous cell carcinomas: identification of markers that define their degree of differentiation. Cancer Res. 1997;57:4111–7.
155. Tripathi SC, et al. Nuclear S100A7 is associated with poor prognosis in head and neck cancer. PLoS ONE. 2010;5:e11939.
156. Kesting MR, et al. Psoriasin (S100A7) up-regulation in oral squamous cell carcinoma and its relation to clinicopathologic features. Oral Oncol. 2009;45:731–6.
157. Alowami S, Qing G, Emberley E, Snell L, Watson PH. Psoriasin (S100A7) expression is altered during skin tumorigenesis. BMC Dermatol. 2003;3:1.
158. Martinsson H, Yhr M, Enerbäck C. Expression patterns of S100A7 (psoriasin) and S100A9 (calgranulin-B) in keratinocyte differentiation. Exp Dermatol. 2005;14:161–8.
159. Qi Z, et al. The characteristics and function of S100A7 induction in squamous cell carcinoma: heterogeneity, promotion of cell proliferation and suppression of differentiation. PLoS ONE. 2015;10:e0128887.
160. Shen Y, Ha W, Zeng W, Queen D, Liu L. Exome sequencing identifies novel mutation signatures of UV radiation and trichostatin A in primary human keratinocytes. Sci Rep. 2020;10:4943.
161. Hodis E, et al. A landscape of driver mutations in melanoma. Cell. 2012;150:251–63.
162. Gao Y-B, et al. Genetic landscape of esophageal squamous cell carcinoma. Nat Genet. 2014;46:1097–102.
163. Chung CH, et al. Genomic alterations in head and neck squamous cell carcinoma determined by cancer gene-targeted sequencing. Ann Oncol Off J Eur Soc Med Oncol. 2015;26:1216–23.
164. Yilmaz AS, et al. Differential mutation frequencies in metastatic cutaneous squamous cell carcinomas versus primary tumors. Cancer. 2017;123:1184–93.
165. Mueller SA, et al. Mutational patterns in metastatic cutaneous squamous cell carcinoma. J Invest Dermatol. 2019;139:1449-1458.e1.
166. Melnikova LS, Georgiev PG, Golovnin AK. The functions and mechanisms of action of insulators in the genomes of higher eukaryotes. Acta Naturae. 2020;12:15–33.
167. Braccioli L, de Wit E. CTCF: a Swiss-army knife for genome organization and transcription regulation. Essays Biochem. 2019;63:157–65.
168. Kemp CJ, et al. CTCF haploinsufficiency destabilizes DNA methylation and predisposes to cancer. Cell Rep. 2014;7:1020–9.
169. Hnisz D, et al. Activation of proto-oncogenes by disruption of chromosome neighborhoods. Science. 2016;351:1454–8.
170. Sabarinathan R, Mularoni L, Deu-Pons J, Gonzalez-Perez A, López-Bigas N. Nucleotide excision repair is impaired by binding of transcription factors to DNA. Nature. 2016;532:264–7.
171. Poulos RC, et al. Functional mutations form at CTCF-Cohesin binding sites in melanoma due to uneven nucleotide excision repair across the motif. Cell Rep. 2016;17:2865–72.
172. Jambusaria-Pahlajani A, et al. Evaluation of AJCC tumor staging for cutaneous squamous cell carcinoma and a proposed alternative tumor staging system. JAMA Dermatol. 2013;149:402–10.

173. Jennings L, Schmults CD. Management of high-risk cutaneous squamous cell carcinoma. J Clin Aesthetic Dermatol. 2010;3:39–48.
174. Krediet JT, et al. Prognostic value of the area and density of lymphatic vessels in cutaneous squamous cell carcinoma. J Dtsch Dermatol Ges J Ger Soc Dermatol JDDG 2016;14:1114–21.
175. Fujimoto M, et al. Tumor budding is an objective high-risk factor associated with metastasis and poor clinical prognosis in cutaneous squamous cell carcinoma sized <4 cm. Am J Surg Pathol. 2019;43:975–83.
176. Karayannopoulou G, Euvrard S, Kanitakis J. Tumour budding correlates with aggressiveness of cutaneous squamous-cell carcinoma. Anticancer Res. 2016;36:4781–5.
177. Chren M-M, et al. Tumor recurrence 5 years after treatment of cutaneous basal cell carcinoma and squamous cell carcinoma. J Invest Dermatol. 2013;133:1188–96.
178. Brantsch KD, et al. Analysis of risk factors determining prognosis of cutaneous squamous-cell carcinoma: a prospective study. Lancet Oncol. 2008;9:713–20.
179. Marrazzo G, Zitelli JA, Brodland D. Clinical outcomes in high-risk squamous cell carcinoma patients treated with Mohs micrographic surgery alone. J Am Acad Dermatol. 2019;80:633–8.
180. Porceddu SV. Prognostic factors and the role of adjuvant radiation therapy in non-melanoma skin cancer of the head and neck. Am Soc Clin Oncol Educ Book Am Soc Clin Oncol Annu Meet 2015;e513–18. https://doi.org/10.14694/EdBook_AM.2015.35.e513.
181. Stratigos AJ, et al. European interdisciplinary guideline on invasive squamous cell carcinoma of the skin: part 2. Treatment. Eur J Cancer Oxf Engl. 2020;1990(128):83–102.
182. Ribero S, Stucci LS, Daniels GA, Borradori L. Drug therapy of advanced cutaneous squamous cell carcinoma: is there any evidence? Curr Opin Oncol. 2017;29:129–35.
183. Maubec E, et al. Phase II study of cetuximab as first-line single-drug therapy in patients with unresectable squamous cell carcinoma of the skin. J Clin Oncol Off J Am Soc Clin Oncol. 2011;29:3419–26.
184. Foote MC, et al. Phase II study of single-agent panitumumab in patients with incurable cutaneous squamous cell carcinoma. Ann Oncol Off J Eur Soc Med Oncol. 2014;25:2047–52.
185. Montaudié H, et al. Cetuximab is efficient and safe in patients with advanced cutaneous squamous cell carcinoma: a retrospective, multicentre study. Oncotarget. 2020;11:378–85.
186. William WN, et al. Gefitinib for patients with incurable cutaneous squamous cell carcinoma: a single-arm phase II clinical trial. J Am Acad Dermatol. 2017;77:1110-1113.e2.
187. Behshad R, Garcia-Zuazaga J, Bordeaux JS. Systemic treatment of locally advanced nonmetastatic cutaneous squamous cell carcinoma: a review of the literature. Br J Dermatol. 2011;165:1169–77.
188. Gellrich FF, et al. Medical treatment of advanced cutaneous squamous-cell carcinoma. J Eur Acad Dermatol Venereol JEADV. 2019;33(Suppl 8):38–43.
189. Claveau J, et al. Multidisciplinary management of locally advanced and metastatic cutaneous squamous cell carcinoma. Curr Oncol. 2020;27:e399–407.
190. Patel R, Chang ALS. Immune checkpoint inhibitors for treating advanced cutaneous squamous cell carcinoma. Am J Clin Dermatol. 2019;20:477–82.
191. Rizvi NA, et al. Cancer immunology. Mutational landscape determines sensitivity to PD-1 blockade in non-small cell lung cancer. Science 2015;348:124–28.
192. Le DT, et al. Mismatch repair deficiency predicts response of solid tumors to PD-1 blockade. Science. 2017;357:409–13.
193. García-Pedrero JM, et al. Tumor programmed cell death ligand 1 expression correlates with nodal metastasis in patients with cutaneous squamous cell carcinoma of the head and neck. J Am Acad Dermatol. 2017;77:527–33.
194. Amoils M, et al. PD-L1 expression and tumor-infiltrating lymphocytes in high-risk and metastatic cutaneous squamous cell carcinoma. Otolaryngol Head Neck Surg Off J Am Acad Otolaryngol Head Neck Surg. 2018;160:93–99.
195. Slater NA, Googe PB. PD-L1 expression in cutaneous squamous cell carcinoma correlates with risk of metastasis. J Cutan Pathol. 2016;43:663–70.
196. Lee A, Duggan S, Deeks ED. Correction to: cemiplimab: a review in advanced cutaneous squamous cell carcinoma. Drugs. 2020;80:939.

197. Migden MR, et al. PD-1 blockade with cemiplimab in advanced cutaneous squamous-cell carcinoma. N Engl J Med. 2018;379:341–51.
198. Migden MR, et al. Cemiplimab in locally advanced cutaneous squamous cell carcinoma: results from an open-label, phase 2, single-arm trial. Lancet Oncol. 2020;21:294–305.

Chapter 6
Skin Biomarkers of Neurodegenerative Diseases

Lauren Reilly, Connor Bargar, Dominic Bunn, and Shu G. Chen

Abstract Neurodegenerative diseases encompass several neurological disorders such as prion diseases, synucleinopathies, tauopathies, Huntington's disease, amyotrophic lateral sclerosis, and frontotemporal dementia. Currently, definitive diagnosis of neurodegenerative diseases often requires postmortem detection of their characteristic misfolded protein aggregates in the central nervous system (CNS). Therefore, a pressing need exists to identify biomarkers of protein misfolding early using specimens outside the CNS. Human skin is the body's largest organ with extensive nerve innervation, allowing for easy punch biopsies to be collected premortem. Over the last few decades, extensive research has been done to search for skin biomarkers of misfolded protein aggregates for neurodegenerative diseases. Methodological developments to detect misfolded protein aggregates in the skin include conventional immunoassays and novel proteopathic seed amplification assays. Although still in its early stages, the diagnostic potential of skin biomarker assays has been demonstrated in a multitude of recent studies. The identification of biomarkers within easily accessible peripheral tissues, like the skin, would greatly improve the process of diagnosing these diseases, monitoring disease progression, and assessing the efficacy of clinical trials of potential therapeutic options. The following is an overview of the research in the ongoing investigation of skin biomarkers as viable indicators of neurodegenerative diseases.

Keywords Biomarker · Neurodegenerative disease · Immunohistochemistry · Real-time quaking-induced conversion · Protein misfolding cyclic amplification · Prion disease · Huntington's disease · Tauopathies · Skin · Synucleinopathies · Amyotrophic lateral sclerosis · Frontotemporal dementia

L. Reilly · C. Bargar · D. Bunn · S. G. Chen (✉)
Department of Pathology, Case Western Reserve University School of Medicine, 2103 Cornell Road, Cleveland, OH 44106-7288, USA
e-mail: shuchen@uab.edu

S. G. Chen
Department of Pathology, University of Alabama at Birmingham, 1720 Second Avenue South, Birmingham, AL 35294-2182, USA

R. Norman (ed.), *Biomarkers in Dermatology*,
https://doi.org/10.1007/978-3-031-66513-4_6

6.1 Introduction

The term neurodegenerative disease describes a wide array of disorders in which the deterioration of neurons and glial cells in the central nervous system (CNS) leads to cognitive and motor impairments. A major hallmark of these diseases is the accumulation of misfolded protein aggregates in the brain. Currently, the definitive diagnosis of neurodegenerative diseases often requires the detection of misfolded protein aggregates in postmortem CNS samples obtained through autopsies. Interestingly, these protein aggregates have also been found in the cerebrospinal fluid (CSF), a brain-derived fluid accessible through lumbar puncture of living patients, thus they could serve as a CSF biomarker of neurodegenerative diseases. Although CSF presents as a viable biomarker reservoir, the invasive nature of the lumbar puncture done to collect the CSF requires specialized clinical settings. Moreover, lumbar puncture is not a feasible procedure for all patients due to the contraindications and complications in certain conditions. Finally, CSF collection may not be fully justified for early diagnosis during routine outpatient visits. Therefore, identification of a biomarker in more easily accessible peripheral tissues, like the skin, would significantly enhance the clinical practice of diagnosing neurodegenerative diseases.

The human skin is the largest organ of the body, covering the entire surface with extensive nerve innervations, allowing for skin punch biopsies to be easily taken from living patients. Newly emerged evidence has suggested that protein misfolding readily occurs in the skin and may be an early event during the pathogenesis of CNS neurodegeneration. Several experimental techniques have been used to distinguish skin samples of patients with the diseases from those of healthy individuals, including positive immunoreactivity through immunohistochemical (IHC) staining and amplified detection of protein aggregates through proteopathic seed amplification assays such as Real-Time Quaking-Induced Conversion (RT-QuIC). The results of these analyses have provided promising evidence for the merit of skin biomarkers of misfolded proteins as indicators of neurodegenerative diseases, which can eventually be used to help in the diagnosis of diseases, monitoring of their progression, and assessment of clinical trials or therapeutic options for patients affected by these devastating brain disorders.

6.2 An Overview of Protein Biomarkers for Neurodegenerative Diseases

Despite the broad range of neurodegenerative diseases, each having its unique and specific pathogenic mechanisms, these diseases are closely related through the misfolding of proteins that share similar biochemical properties. Therefore, the biomarkers for common neurodegenerative disorders can be categorized based on the types of protein inclusions and symptoms seen in each disorder. The following forms of neurodegenerative diseases will be covered in this review: prion diseases, synucleinopathies, tauopathies, Huntington's Disease (HD), Amyotrophic Lateral Sclerosis (ALS), and Frontotemporal Dementia (FTD).

Pathological prions, the normal isoform of which is cellular prion protein (PrP^C), are composed of the misfolded scrapie isoform as the protease-resistant prion protein (PrP^{Sc}) and can cause a variety of transmissible neurodegenerative diseases called transmissible spongiform encephalopathies (TSEs) [1]. TSEs that occur in animals include scrapie in sheep and goats, chronic wasting disease in cervids, and bovine spongiform encephalopathy (BSE), also known as mad cow disease in cattle [2, 3]. The most common human form of TSEs is sporadic Creutzfeldt–Jakob disease (sCJD), a disorder that is thought to be caused by the spontaneous misfolding of PrP^C. A genetic version of CJD, familial CJD, also exists and is transmitted through inheritance [4]. Iatrogenic CJD is yet another form that is transmitted via injection of contaminated biologicals or transfer of infected nervous tissue through surgery [4]. Research has shown that a new variant form of CJD (vCJD) can be transmitted through contaminated blood and through the consumption of meat from cattle with BSE [5, 6]. In prion disease, the presence of PrP^{Sc} induces misfolding of PrP^C to cause the formation of more PrP^{Sc} into insoluble protein aggregates, which leads to neuronal dysfunction, cell death, and astrogliosis [7]. The resulting brain lesions, which often have a sponge-like appearance caused by vacuolation called spongiform degeneration, are accompanied by rapid and progressive dementia, hallucinations, and systemic motor complications.

Synucleinopathies are a category of neurodegenerative diseases defined by the abnormal accumulation of the protein α-synuclein (α-syn) primarily in neurons. Accumulation of α-syn is caused by either an inherited mutation of its corresponding gene, *SNCA*, or environmental and other risk factors causing the aggregation of α-syn in affected cells [8]. In some of these diseases, α-syn can aggregate and assemble into amyloid-like fibrils, which form inclusions called Lewy bodies within the neurons [9]. These α-syn aggregates are cytotoxic, disrupting cellular homeostasis and causing neuron injury and cell death in the brain [10]. Common symptoms of synucleinopathies are motor dysfunction in the form of parkinsonism and impaired cognition. There are three synucleinopathies which include Parkinson's disease (PD), dementia with Lewy bodies (DLB), and multiple system atrophy (MSA). All three diseases present with overlapping symptoms and pathology of abnormal α-syn accumulation, but PD is the most common and, therefore, is the most extensively researched.

In tauopathies, the protein tau is misfolded and hyperphosphorylated (p-tau), causing it to aggregate into insoluble inclusions within the neurons, usually in a form called neurofibrillary tangles (NFTs) [11]. Tau is a protein involved in the stabilization and assembly of microtubules within the axons of neurons. The microtubule dysregulation and presence of the cytotoxic NFTs result in loss of axonal integrity and neurotransmission, leading to neuron death. The most common tauopathy is Alzheimer's disease (AD) with pathological hallmarks including intracellular NFT inclusions and extracellular inclusions called amyloid plaques, made of the amyloid-β (Aβ) peptide formed from abnormal cleavage of the amyloid precursor protein [12]. The amyloid plaques contribute to astrogliosis and cytokine release resulting in neuroinflammation. Together, NFTs and amyloid plaques are associated with neuronal injury and cell death resulting in dementia and psychological issues. However, how these two types of protein aggregates interact is still under debate. Other tauopathies may present similar symptoms to AD but differ in severity and other features. Another tauopathy is the behavioral variant frontotemporal dementia, otherwise known as Pick's disease [13]. Pick's disease is defined by the presence of specialized tau-positive inclusions within the neurons called Pick bodies, which differ from the NFTs in AD since they only consist of the three-repeat isoforms of tau, unlike NFTs, which contain a mixture of both three- and four-repeat tau isoforms [13–15]. The tau inclusions in Pick's disease, like in AD, are linked to neurodegeneration leading to dementia and distinctive behavioral changes. Two other tauopathies are corticobasal degeneration (CBD) and progressive supranuclear palsy (PSP), but the inclusions found in these two disorders are made of four-repeat tau isoforms [14, 15].

Huntington's disease (HD) is an inherited autosomal dominant neurodegenerative disorder caused by a genetic mutation where there is an expansion of the repeated CAG sequence found within the *HTT* gene on chromosome 4 [16]. The encoded protein huntingtin (Htt) is thought to play a role in neurodevelopment [17]. The expanded polyglutamine tract from the mutation causes Htt to misfold into insoluble, cytotoxic aggregates within the neurons, causing a disruption of neuron processes and synaptic transmission [17]. The loss of neuronal function causes the recognizable HD symptoms, the most notable of which are involuntary movements known as chorea, incoordination, behavioral issues, and cognitive decline [18].

Amyotrophic lateral sclerosis (ALS) is a neurodegenerative disease in which motor neurons deteriorate, resulting in movement issues, variable cognitive decline, and eventual muscle atrophy and weakness [19]. Several autosomal dominant inherited mutations have been linked to familial ALS, the most notable of which are mutations in the *TARDBP, FUS*, and *C9orf72* genes, all of which result in the misfolding of their respective proteins, causing the formation of inclusions within the neurons [19, 20]. However, approximately 90% of ALS cases are sporadic, where the disease spontaneously manifests with unknown etiology [19]. The *TARDP* gene encodes for the transactive response DNA-binding protein 43 (TDP-43), and the *FUS* gene encodes for the fusion in sarcoma (FUS) protein, both of which act as regulators of gene expression and RNA splicing [19]. TDP-43 protein aggregates have been found in both sporadic and familial ALS within inclusions in neurons and glial cells [21]. The FUS protein has also been shown to aggregate in a similar manner to TDP-43 [19]. The C9orf72 gene encodes for the protein C9orf72 involved in the RNA processing and metabolism pathways, both of which can be negatively impacted by the mutations of the C9orf72 gene known to promote TDP-43 inclusion formation [20]. The formation of these protein aggregations within the cytoplasm of motor neurons causes loss of neuronal function and eventual cell death. Frontotemporal dementia (FTD) is also associated with ALS since neurons within the frontal and temporal lobes can be infiltrated and affected by the TDP-43 protein inclusions, which also can be induced by the presence of the *C9orf72* gene mutations as in ALS [20, 22]. Individuals with FTD present with cognitive decline, psychiatric disorders, and behavioral changes.

The misfolded protein aggregates in the CNS described above can, in theory, serve as biomarkers that are distinctive for each disease, but in practice, these aggregates are largely inaccessible to laboratory assessments for research and diagnostic purposes. It is thus unfortunate that currently, a definitive diagnosis of neurodegenerative diseases is often made postmortem when samples of the CNS can be taken, which is not feasible to identify individuals with the ongoing diseases. CSF samples from living individuals have been discovered to contain the misfolded proteins as a surrogate marker of brain cell injury or death associated with neurodegenerative diseases, but the disadvantages of the CSF collection process via the invasive lumbar puncture are a deterrent [23–25]. Recently, exciting new research has led to the examination of neurodegenerative biomarkers within the peripheral tissues such as the skin. The skin is the largest organ of the body, with vast surface access, extensive nerve innervation, and fast healing and regeneration, thus enabling sample collection at multiple times and in multiple locations without long-lasting risks.

In contrast to CSF, skin sample collection through punch biopsy is much less invasive, more receptive, more compatible with the complications associated with neurodegenerative diseases, and much more amenable to collection at regular clinics. Studies of skin biomarkers have shown early promises of detecting the peripheral presence of the misfolded protein aggregates in the skin. These skin biomarkers could be the first step in establishing a viable peripheral method for the diagnosis of neurodegenerative diseases, which could impact every aspect of neurodegenerative disease research.

6.3 Detection of Misfolded Proteins Through Immunological Methods

6.3.1 Prion Diseases

The diagnosis of prion diseases, such as CJD, begins with the initial clinical examination of the cardinal neurological symptoms, which is then confirmed through immunohistochemical (IHC) staining and Western blotting of the postmortem CNS tissue in which the presence of PrP^{Sc}, and its protease-resistant products resulting from its presence, are found [26]. IHC staining and Western blotting of skin samples have been attempted in order to detect the presence of PrP^{Sc} and its protease-resistant byproducts.

Initial IHC staining of skin samples was done in studies on animal prion diseases such as BSE and scrapie. First, IHC staining of the skin samples of cattle revealed normal PrP^{C} in basal keratinocytes (KCs) and sebaceous glands [27, 28]. Then, hamsters infected with experimental prions and sheep infected with natural scrapie showed the presence of PrP^{Sc} in the nerve fibers of sebaceous glands [29]. PrP^{Sc} was also detected in the skin, from the stratum basale to stratum granulosum and surrounding the nerve fibers of the epidermis and along the basal side of the epithelium of the sweat glands in sheep naturally infected with scrapie [30].

The presence of PrP^{C} and PrP^{Sc} in the skin of animals suggests the possibility of using IHC staining for the detection of PrP^{C} and PrP^{Sc} in the epidermis of human subjects with sCJD as well. Indeed, detection of PrP^{C} through IHC staining has proven to be successful in several studies of the skin from autopsy and biopsy samples of those with sCJD. PrP^{C} was ultimately found within KCs and infiltrating mononuclear cells within the epidermis, within hair follicles, and in the basement membrane of several cutaneous structures such as the dermal papilla, eccrine glands, sebaceous glands, arrector pili muscles, and peripheral dermal nerves [31–33]. However, despite the fact that PrP^{C} can be readily detected in the human epidermis with IHC staining, indicating locations where PrP^{Sc} could possibly congregate, no evidence of consistent detection of PrP^{Sc} has been observed in skin samples through IHC staining within both sCJD and vCJD patients [34]. Instead, Western blotting has provided more promising evidence of PrP^{Sc} detection within the skin.

In animal studies, Western blot analysis of skin PrP^{Sc} has notably been determined to be positive at ~20 kDa in the skin of hamster models in the late preclinical stages of scrapie, along with evidence of PrP^{Sc} in naturally infected sheep [29]. The discovered protein bands increased in intensity as the disease progressed, thus showing that PrP^{Sc} is detectable in skin tissues and is dependent on the stages of the disease. Human studies have also shown promise of PrP^{Sc} detection through Western blotting when PrP^{Sc} in the postmortem skin sample from an individual with vCJD was detected following enrichment of the protein sample with sodium phosphotungstate precipitation [6]. Further research into skin PrP^{Sc} detection through Western blotting in human cases includes an alternative approach, found to have worked in studies on scrapie-infected sheep, where the samples were treated with proteinase K (PK) [34]. Due to the PK-resistant nature of PrP^{Sc}, this method would result in the specific detection of PrP^{Sc} on the Western blots. This method was not entirely successful as skin biopsies from many areas of the body, including the torso, forearm, apex of the head, ear, and leg, taken from individuals with sCJD and vCJD, were found to have a majority of negative signals for PrP^{Sc}. Only one sample of each form of the disease showed weakly positive signals. Another approach, where the samples were treated with both PK and peptide N-glycosidase F to increase the sensitivity of the sample to the anti-C antibody being used, showed one case of sCJD and one case of vCJD having slightly stronger positive signals [34].

Western blotting is clearly more effective than IHC staining in detecting skin PrP^{Sc} in human prion diseases as it has yielded some results, unlike the latter. However, Western blotting detection of the PrP^{Sc} in the skin of sCJD patients remains challenging. The fact that PrP^{Sc} can be detected in some CJD samples, however, does suggest that skin is a promising peripheral tissue for prion diseases, but Western blotting alone is not the best procedure, likely due to a lack of sufficient antibody sensitivity.

6.3.2 Synucleinopathies

The distinctive accumulation of α-syn aggregates within the brain is a hallmark of synucleinopathies. IHC staining and immunofluorescence, which are efficient in localizing α-syn aggregates as the phosphorylated form (p-α-syn) at the serine 129 site of α-syn in brain samples, have been used to reveal these aggregates as biomarkers in the skin. Initial IHC staining and immunofluorescence of autopsied skin samples from individuals with the synucleinopathies PD and DLB have shown variable success and sometimes inconsistent results, with a sensitivity range of 10–93% for PD and a sensitivity of 40% for DLB [35–37]. Notably, another study found zero sensitivity in autopsied skin samples for p-α-syn accumulation in either PD or DLB [38], while a different study also reported no detection in the skin samples of MSA [35].

IHC staining of skin punch biopsy samples from living individuals with synucleinopathies has confirmed the trend of positive results and findings of p-α-syn within the cutaneous structures. For example, p-α-syn has been discovered to accumulate in over 58% of the skin samples taken from living patients with PD [39]. Skin samples from living individuals with MSA show some positive results for α-syn accumulation as well [37, 40]. Intriguingly, IHC staining has also shown positive results for p-α-syn in skin samples from living patients with idiopathic rapid eye movement sleep behavior disorder (iRBD), who are vulnerable to develop synucleinopathies some years later [41]. A large majority of individuals with iRBD show positive IHC staining and immunofluorescence for p-α-syn, which implies that p-α-syn could potentially be discovered in skin tissues before the symptoms of synucleinopathies begin in iRBD patients and could provide an explanation for why some iRBD patients develop synucleinopathies [37, 41].

From these results, it would seem that IHC staining is a potential method for the detection of p-α-syn in the postmortem and antemortem skin of patients with synucleinopathies. The presence of α-syn aggregation in the skin indicates that the cutaneous nerves are being infiltrated. The aggregates can result in morphological and functional changes of the cutaneous autonomic nervous system, which could be yet another measurable skin biomarker in addition to the IHC staining.

IHC staining and immunofluorescence of cutaneous nerves have shown morphological changes. Some of these changes include reduced intraepidermal and pilomotor nerve fiber densities in individuals with PD, a decrease in somatic as well as autonomic skin innervations in individuals with Lewy body-based disorders, and the presence of α-syn in intraepidermal nerve fibers and autonomic nerves throughout the dermis [42–45]. Accumulations of α-syn have consistently been found in the cutaneous nerve fibers positive for tyrosine hydroxylase, which is typically used as a biomarker for dopaminergic neuronal loss in PD, implying there is some relationship between the neuronal biomarker in the CNS and its function in the peripheral tissues [45]. Skin fiber neuropathy, denervation, and dysfunctional postganglionic sympathetic adrenergic/cholinergic and parasympathetic functions such as cutaneous vasomotor control, thermoregulation, and sweating have also been found in individuals with synucleinopathies [42, 43, 46]. The presence of p-α-syn in the cutaneous nerve fibers of the epidermis, and its effects on the functionality of the cutaneous nerve fibers, indicates that examination of skin biopsies could be a viable biomarker detection method for synucleinopathies, most interestingly in the most commonly studied synucleinopathy of PD. Overall, IHC staining and immunofluorescence have detected the presence of p-α-syn accumulations in the skin autonomic nerve fibers in patients living with different synucleinopathies: PD, DLB, and MSA [40, 45, 47, 48].

6.3.3 Tauopathies

Tauopathies are diverse but are known to have the common biomarker of p-tau aggregates, usually in the form of NFTs in the brain. Other biomarkers specific to the type of tauopathy can also distinguish the diseases, such as the Aβ aggregation presentation as amyloid plaques in AD brains. Identification of these known biomarkers in the peripheral system through IHC staining of the skin samples has proven to be productive in finding the misfolded protein accumulations in tauopathies.

In Rodriguez-Leyva et al. [49], IHC staining and immunofluorescence of skin punch biopsies of living AD patients showed higher levels of p-tau, which was confirmed through Western blotting. The Western blotting also showed that p-tau found in the skin has a similar molecular weight to the p-tau found in other known locations of AD pathology, suggesting that the biomarker to p-tau in the skin could be the equivalent to p-tau in neurons. Other studies have also discovered the presence of p-tau protein deposits in the skin fibroblasts and epithelial cells of living individuals with AD, PSP, and CBD through the use of IHC and Western blotting [50–52]. More immunostaining of the skin, especially from individuals with AD, has been explored in both premortem and postmortem tissue samples to find other protein biomarkers of tauopathies.

Through the use of immunocytochemical methods, Aβ protein deposits have been found in the skin harvested during the autopsy of subjects with sporadic and familial AD [53]. Similar findings have been found through immunocytochemical methods in the skin and skin fibroblasts from living AD individuals, where increased Aβ protein deposits have even been identified in the skin cells of presymptomatic subjects [54–57]. Akerman et al. [58] specifically found, along with the presence of $A\beta_{40}$ and $A\beta_{42}$, that the epidermis contained $A\beta_{34}$, an intermediate of the $A\beta_{40}$ and $A\beta_{42}$ degradation pathway, implying that the Aβ deposits seen in the skin via immunocytochemistry are similar to the pathogenic deposits normally seen in the AD brains.

6.3.4 *Huntington's Disease*

The current search for peripheral biomarkers in HD by IHC staining and immunofluorescence focuses primarily on identifying mutated huntingtin (mtHtt) within the skin. Cytotoxicity resulting from mtHtt accumulation causes the degradation of the nerves seen in HD. Through Western blotting, immunofluorescence, and confocal laser scanning microscopy, De Rooij et al. [59] found that normal Htt is present in the cytoplasm and the nucleus, with the exclusion of the nucleoli, in human skin fibroblasts indicating the expression of the protein within the peripheral skin cells. In a study on the skin of the R6/2 mouse model of HD, IHC staining, immunofluorescence, and Western blotting detected aggregation of mtND2, which is the model equivalent of mtHtt in the mice, within the skin, providing evidence for the capability of mtHtt to accumulate in peripheral tissues [60]. Upregulation of Htt and the increased presence of mtHtt aggregates have been found in the skin fibroblasts from living HD patients [61]. From these results, it is clear that the mtHtt aggregates are present in the skin of individuals with HD and may potentially serve as a biomarker for the disease.

6.3.5 *Amyotrophic Lateral Sclerosis and Frontotemporal Dementia*

FUS and TDP-43 are proteins that accumulate in the cytoplasm of motor neurons during sporadic ALS and FTD. Analysis of several skin biopsies with IHC staining and immunofluorescence microscopy has shown some distinguishable differences between skin samples of ALS and FTD patients and those of healthy controls. IHC studies have found that there is strong FUS expression in the epidermis of sporadic ALS patients, which increases as the disease progresses [62]. TDP-43 has also been found to be elevated in the skin of ALS individuals through IHC staining and immunofluorescence of skin biopsies [63, 64]. Ren et al. [65] attempted to discern how phosphorylated TDP-43 deposits in the nerve fibers of the skin affect neuropathy in eighteen ALS and eighteen control skin biopsies. Those with ALS show a higher degree of small-fiber neuropathy and a lower degree of sweat gland nerve fiber density when compared to the healthy controls. Within a few of these same ALS patients, phosphorylated TDP-43 was found to have accumulated in the skin tissue. This could indicate that TDP-43 accumulation can potentially correlate to the dysfunctional nerve innervation of the skin in ALS, making the accumulation of TDP-43 a potential peripheral biomarker for ALS.

Additional studies have found that immunoreactive TDP-43 positive cells are present in skin biopsies of ALS patients, and these appeared to increase as the disease progressed [66]. This could be due to an increase in the synthesis of or a decrease in the degradation of TDP-43. Wang et al. [63] determined that there was elevated immunoreactive TDP-43 in the epidermis of skin samples in familial ALS patients with the A315T mutation. Since TDP-43 is normally present in the nuclei of cells of healthy individuals and in the cytoplasm of those with ALS or FTD as inclusions, fibroblasts and keratinocytes from sporadic and familial ALS individuals were used to generate tissue-engineered skin samples to see where TDP-43 would be within the cells [67]. It was found through immunofluorescence that there are TDP-43 aggregates in the cytoplasm of both sporadic and familial ALS engineered tissue models. To confirm these findings, IHC was performed on skin biopsies from sporadic ALS patients. TDP-43 inclusions were found in the cytoplasm of the skin fibroblasts confirming that the cytoplasmic TDP-43 seen in the neurons of sporadic and familial ALS individuals can also occur in the peripheral tissues. Other studies have confirmed that accumulations of pathological TDP-43 can occur in the epidermis and within the cutaneous autonomic nerves of sporadic ALS patients, potentially providing an easily accessible, peripheral biomarker for ALS [65, 66, 68, 69].

6.4 Detection of Protein Aggregates Through Proteopathic Seed Amplification Assays

While IHC staining immunofluorescence have proven to be effective in identifying skin biomarkers for neurodegenerative diseases, it has several limitations, as reviewed by Matos et al. [70]. First, handling and fixation of the specimen needs to be done with significant care to avoid losing antigenicity. Second, the selection of the antibody detection systems can be difficult and expensive, which makes it difficult to produce large quantities of IHC specimens for viewing. Lastly, specimens can present with variations in antibody sensitivity and specificity. Due to these disadvantages, a novel approach has been developed in the form of proteopathic seed amplification assays.

Proteopathic seed amplification assays take advantage of the prion-like, self-templating nature of the protein aggregates found in neurodegenerative diseases. In these assays, a specimen is incubated with the soluble protein monomers in conditions meant to induce the generation of aggregates [71, 72]. If the specimen contains a proteopathic seed capable of causing the aggregations of the soluble monomers, the monomers will assemble into oligomers and fibrils. The presence of these fibrils, when generated within a certain reaction time frame, can reveal if the tested sample is positive for the proteopathic seeds that would cause the aggregation, thus indicating the disease status of the test sample. This amplification of protein aggregation can be very efficient as positive detection can be achieved with very few seed particles present in the tested sample [71].

The two main forms of the proteopathic seed amplification assay are the protein misfolding cyclic amplification (PMCA) and Real-Time Quaking-Induced Conversion (RT-QuIC) assays [71, 72]. The PMCA was first developed to amplify the misfolded PrP^{Sc} in prion diseases [71]. In the original PMCA assay, a prion sample with PrP^{Sc} was incubated and polymerized with PrP^{C} in a noninfected brain homogenate. Through sonication, the aggregates formed would be broken down to promote further aggregation. Western blotting would then be conducted along with a PK treatment to identify the newly amplified, misfolded PrP^{Sc}. The more recently developed RT-QuIC assay uses a similar procedure to PMCA, except the breakdown of the protein aggregates during RT-QuIC is done through automated shaking instead of sonication and with the addition of the fluorescent dye thioflavin T, which increases in fluorescence signal as the aggregation progresses, allowing observation of the aggregation process for real-time monitoring [72]. The automation and real-time monitoring makes it possible to run the RT-QuIC assay on multiple samples simultaneously through the multi-well plates used today (Fig. 6.1). Both of these assays are highly sensitive and amplify the minute amounts of aggregating seeds within a sample in order to produce large quantities of newly generated aggregates and fibrils of the misfolded proteins to enable robust detection.

6.4.1 Prion Diseases

Serial protein misfolding cyclic amplification (sPMCA) is a form of PMCA that amplifies the targeted misfolded protein through a series of seeded polymerizations [73]. The use of sPMCA, followed by subsequent Western blotting, has been used for PrP^{Sc} detection in the skin. PrP^{Sc} is present both before clinical symptoms and at the start of brain spongiosis in the skin of scrapie-infected hamsters and transgenic mice infected with sCJD [74]. The sPMCA technique has shown more promising results than Western blotting alone, and other studies have already started using this technique to research prion disease treatment methods in transgenic mice [73]. More impressively, RT-QuIC has shown a distinct advantage in the monitoring of the presence of PrP^{Sc} in skin samples due to its automated fluorescence-based detection.

RT-QuIC has mainly been used to diagnose CJD through CSF and CNS tissue samples but has shown evidence of prion biomarkers in the skin as well [75]. Using RT-QuIC, Orrú et al. [34] examined biopsied skin samples from living sCJD and vCJD patients and found PrP^{Sc} positive results. Each patient with either form of the disease had at least one skin sample show positivity for PrP^{Sc}, with skin samples from the area around the ear most notably having a 94% positive result while the non-CJD controls showed no signals.

PrP^{Sc} detection in sCJD skin samples through RT-QuIC has continued to be explored both in humans and transgenic mice, along with further research on scrapie prions in hamsters, using samples taken postmortem and from live animals, and a majority of the samples show positive results for PrP^{Sc} while maintaining negative results for the control groups [33, 74, 76, 77]. Interestingly, in transgenic mice studies, RT-QuIC has proven to detect PrP^{Sc} in the skin before clinical symptoms are present, indicating the possible use of RT-QuIC as an early diagnostic technique [74]. Studies focused on skin samples from living human subjects with sCJD have shown a high sensitivity and specificity of prion detection by RT-QuIC, ranging from 89 to 100% sensitivity and 100% specificity, and in some cases, the skin showed even higher sensitivity than the comparable CSF samples taken from the same individuals [33,

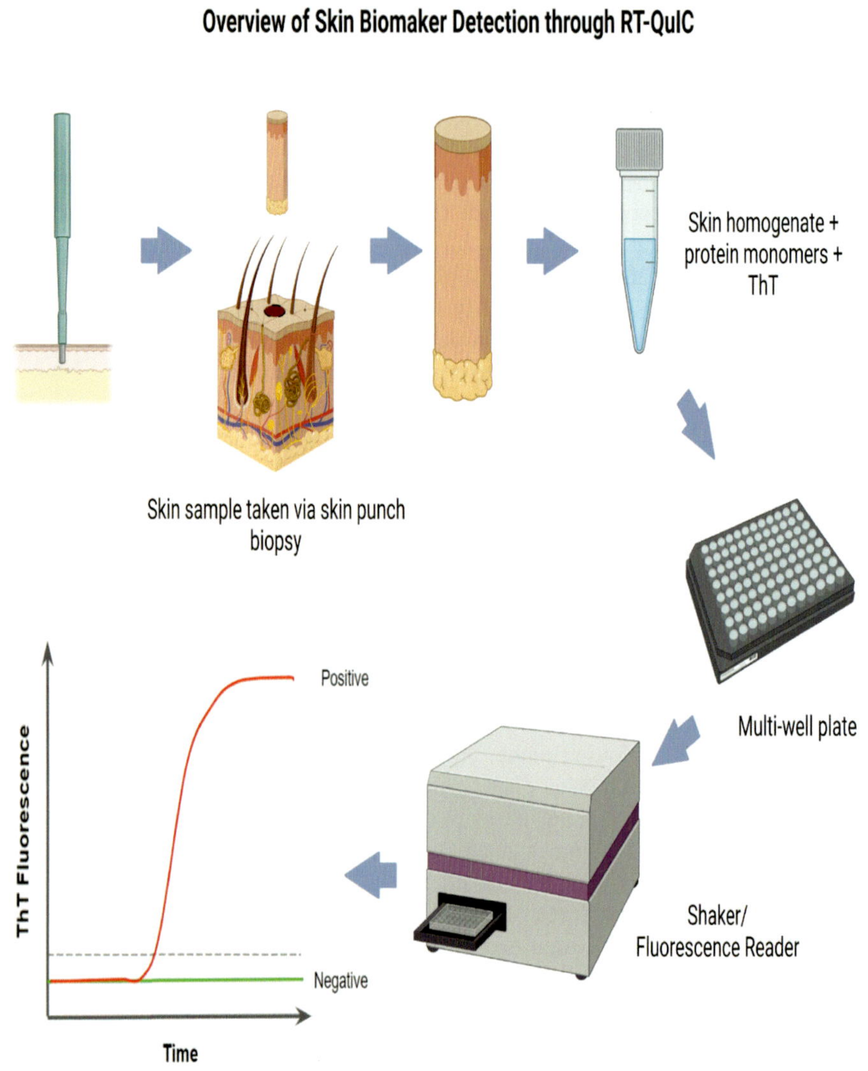

Fig. 6.1 Schematic diagram of skin biomarker detection through RT-QuIC assay. Skin samples can be obtained by punch biopsy. Skin homogenate is prepared to mix with recombinant protein monomers and ThT. The resulting mixture is dispensed into reaction wells of a 96-well plate. The plate is then incubated while shaking in an automated plate reader. ThT fluorescence is monitored in real time, shown for one positive and one negative reactions, respectively. *Graph created with BioRender.com*

76, 77]. Given the current research, it appears that RT-QuIC is the most consistent and accurate method to detect the PrP^{Sc} biomarker in the skin of individuals with prion diseases.

6.4.2 *Synucleinopathies*

RT-QuIC seeding assays have been shown to detect α-syn aggregates in multiple synucleinopathies with a reported average sensitivity of 85% to 97% and specificity of 80% to 100% in CSF samples [78–80]. Manne et al. [81] found there was a 96% sensitivity and specificity to identify PD individuals through the α-syn RT-QuIC assay run on scalp skin samples from autopsied individuals with PD. Further studies have successfully identified the presence of α-syn aggregates in autopsied skin tissues and have shown a sensitivity range of 88.9–100% for DLB, 88.9–100% for PD, and 67% for MSA, as well as a specificity range of 96.3–98% [82, 83]. It has been hypothesized that the sensitivity for MSA is lower since it is associated with a different conformational strain of α-syn, which could also explain why MSA may present negative results for p-α-syn IHC staining in the cutaneous nerves as reported in one study [84]. Wang et al. [82] also ran PMCA on the autopsy abdominal skin samples from PD cadavers and found a sensitivity of 82% and specificity of 96%.

Recent studies have also shown that RT-QuIC can accurately identify the presence of α-syn aggregates in the skin punch biopsies taken from living patients with synucleinopathies as well, showing promise for this technique as a diagnostic tool [82, 83, 85]. Donadio et al. [85] conducted an RT-QuIC assay on skin samples from thirty-eight patients living with probable PD, DLB, or MSA. The results demonstrated that RT-QuIC analysis done on skin biopsy samples had an average 86% sensitivity and 80% specificity for identifying synucleinopathies, which was greater than the paired CSF RT-QuIC assay sensitivity of 78% from the same patients. Results from other RT-QuIC studies done on living subjects showed similarly high sensitivity and specificity results, reporting a range of 76.9–95% sensitivity and 97.5–100% specificity of PD, as well as one study reporting an 89.3% sensitivity and 97.5% specificity for DLB [82, 83]. It is of note that Wang et al. [82] also conducted a PMCA assay on the cervical and leg skin biopsy tissue of patients living with PD and reported an 80% sensitivity and 90% specificity.

In both postmortem and antemortem skin samples, proteopathic seed amplification assays have shown a high sensitivity and specificity for identifying synucleinopathies. Therefore, RT-QuIC of skin samples appears to be the most promising method in the peripheral identification of synucleinopathies.

6.4.3 Tauopathies

RT-QuIC seeding studies for tauopathies for the detection of tau accumulations in the skin have yet to be conducted. Currently, all completed analyses for the detection of tau aggregates have been performed on brain and CSF samples [15, 75, 86–88]. Salvadores et al. [86] performed a PMCA assay dedicated to the detection of Aβ aggregation in the CSF of living AD patients. Through the amplification of the misfolded protein, an overall sensitivity of 90% and specificity of 92% were discovered. In Kraus et al. [15], RT-QuIC assay seeded with human AD brain homogenates showed high sensitivity and specificity for both the three and four repeated tau isoforms seen in NFTs. On average, the sensitivity and specificity for the detection of tau and Aβ aggregation in AD and Pick's disease CSF samples have been high [75, 87, 88].

Due to the shared properties of the skin and the CNS biomarkers in tauopathies, such as the phosphorylated tau, and the positive findings seen in studies on CSF, RT-QuIC assays may in future be used for the diagnosis of tauopathies through peripheral skin samples, but additional research still needs to be done.

6.4.4 Huntington's Disease

At the time of this publication, there are no published studies on the use of either proteopathic seed amplification assays in the analysis of brain, CSF, or skin of HD patients. However, due to the abundant success PMCA and RT-QuIC assays have in the detection of misfolded protein aggregates, theoretically, a seeding activity could be done with the intent of detecting the misfolded mtHtt protein. If positive results are shown in the analysis of the CNS tissue, then CSF and skin testing will soon follow.

6.4.5 Amyotrophic Lateral Sclerosis and Frontotemporal Dementia

Limited research has been done on RT-QuIC analysis of ALS or FTD. Scialò et al. [89] focuses on the detection of TDP-43 aggregates in the CSF of thirty-six FTD or ALS patients. The result of the assay showed a high sensitivity of 94% and a specificity of 85%, indicating the method could contribute to the diagnosis of ALS or FTD. The utilization of RT-QuIC to detect TDP-43 aggregates in the peripheral tissues like the skin is still awaiting further research.

6.4.6 Biomarkers in Blood and Other Peripheral Tissues

Skin is arguably the most desirable peripheral tissue for sample collection, serving as a sample pool for misfolded protein biomarkers, which can be used in diagnostic processes and advancements of neurodegenerative disease research. However, other peripheral specimens have started to be examined for biomarkers of neurodegeneration. Most notably, blood, olfactory mucosa, and several other peripheral tissues have become strong interests of study.

6.4.7 Blood

Blood has been shown to contain biomarkers for all the previously listed neurodegenerative diseases, with special attention to prion disease, synucleinopathies, and tauopathies. In plasma, the normal PrP^{C} isoform can be detected, which led researchers to question if the PrP^{C} plasma levels would be altered in patients with sCJD, vCJD, and iatrogenic CJD [90]. The plasma PrP^{C} levels have shown through immunoassays to decrease in vCJD and increase in sCJD and iatrogenic CJD, the reasoning for why this occurs still needs to be explored [90, 91]. Bougard et al. [92] found that in a blinded PMCA assay, small amounts of PrP^{Sc} could be identified in plasma samples taken from 256 vCJD patients with a reported 100% sensitivity and specificity. Concha-Marambio et al. [93] recently conducted another PMCA assay using vCJD primate model blood samples, and the results suggest that PMCA could be used to identify the PrP^{Sc} in the blood. Both of these studies provide strong evidence to suggest that blood could potentially be used in proteopathic amplification seed assays to detect prions in humans.

Erythrocytes are a physiological source of α-syn in the blood; approximately 99% of all α-syn in the blood is found in red blood cells (RBCs) [94]. This makes blood, specifically RBCs, of interest as a potential biomarker for the state of α-syn during synucleinopathies. Through immunoassay, Foulds et al. [95] found that there is an overall increase in the amount of p-α-syn in the plasma of individuals living with PD, along with a steady increase in total-α-syn as the disease progresses, which could be used to potentially monitor the progression of PD in individuals. Furthermore, amounts of insoluble α-syn oligomers are reportedly higher in enzyme-linked immunosorbent assays performed on RBCs of PD and MSA patients, with a sensitivity of 79.0% and specificity of 64.7%, suggesting that α-syn aggregation may be detected in the blood [96].

The blood of individuals with tauopathies has shown increased neurofilament light chain protein (NfL) levels, which is released when there is neuronal and axonal injury, therefore making it a possible biomarker of neurodegeneration [97]. An elevation in plasma NfL reportedly occurs in AD, PSP, and Pick's disease [98–101]. Elevated levels of p-tau have also been reported to occur in the plasma of humans with AD, as it was reported in the Palmqvist et al. [102] study where 1402 individual plasma samples, 121 of which came from participants with AD, were observed through immunoassays. Additionally, fluctuations of the $A\beta_{42}$ to $A\beta_{40}$ ratio in the blood is a debated biomarker that requires further study as there is continued debate on whether there is a significant difference in the plasma of patients with tauopathies [103–105].

The blood and blood vessels have also been shown to contain potential HD, ALS, and FTD biomarkers. Blood vessels harvested from HD cadavers have been found to contain mtHtt through IHC staining [106]. The plasma of patients living with HD has also shown an increase in NfL indicative of the neuronal damage occurring during HD [107, 108]. NfL levels in the blood are also elevated in blood samples from individuals living with FTD or ALS [109, 110]. More research should be done on the potential of blood biomarkers in HD, ALS, and FTD.

6.4.8 Other Peripheral Tissues

Olfactory mucosa (OM) is another peripheral tissue of interest for use as a peripheral biomarker for neurodegenerative diseases, as it is easily obtainable through scrapings of the inner nasal mucosa. This tissue has been utilized mainly in the study of prion diseases, synucleinopathies, and tauopathies in living patients. Zanusso et al. [111] discovered the consistent presence of PrP^{Sc} in the nasal septum and olfactory mucosa through IHC staining of samples taken during the autopsy of nine individuals with sCJD. Subsequent studies used RT-QuIC assays to determine that olfactory mucosa, taken through nasal brushings of living sCJD patients, contained high amounts of PrP^{Sc}, which was used in the identification of the patients with sCJD with a sensitivity range of 90–97% and a specificity of 100% [112, 113]. The OM has also been shown to have accumulations of α-syn in synucleinopathies, which has been demonstrated mainly through the use of the RT-QuIC assays. RT-QuIC assays of the OM taken from patients living with either MSA, PD, or DLB have shown the detection of α-syn aggregates [114, 115]. These studies suggest that the RT-QuIC assay of OM samples can discriminate between diseased and healthy subjects, with one study finding a sensitivity of 81.4% and specificity of 92.1% for DLB patients [115]. IHC staining and other immunoassays of OM samples from living individuals with tauopathies displayed increased Aβ levels indicating biomarkers of the tauopathy AD may also be discovered in this peripheral tissue [116, 117]. The submandibular gland (SMG) is an additional peripheral tissue that can be biopsied in living individuals, and research suggests it contains the misfolded protein biomarkers of synucleinopathies. IHC staining of SMG biopsies, taken from patients with either PD or DLB, have shown positive results for p-α-syn [38, 118]. Recently, RT-QuIC assays results have suggested α-syn aggregates can be found in the SMG of autopsied individuals with PD [119, 120]. In Manne et al. [120], RT-QuIC assay results presented the ability to distinguish the SMG samples of patients with either PD or DLB and from healthy individuals with a reported 100% sensitivity and a 94% specificity. Moreover, deposition of p-α-syn has been detected in the gastrointestinal tract by IHC staining including the sigmoid colon (SC) [121, 122], which is also a clinically accessible site for biopsy. Bargar et al. [119] recently reported RT-QuIC detection of α-syn aggregates in the SC, as well as the SMG and skin from autopsied cases of PD, but not from the control cases. The quantitative analyses of α-syn aggregates in paired PD autopsy tissues of the SC, SMG, and skin revealed significant α-syn seeding activity in all of these peripheral tissues, at a level much less than that in the brain but still can be readily detected by the ultrasensitive RT-QuIC assay [123]. Overall, these studies provide early support for the proposition that the skin and other peripheral tissues may be used as biopsy sites for the detection of abnormal protein aggregation in certain neurodegenerative diseases.

6.5 Conclusions

The search for peripheral biomarkers for neurodegenerative diseases is an ongoing process that has yielded promising results in both immunological and proteopathic seed amplification assays. The neurodegenerative diseases reviewed here each have distinctive, characteristic protein aggregates found in the CNS and CSF, and these protein aggregates may also be found in the skin, thus serving as valuable peripheral biomarkers.

Skin biomarkers of prion diseases present as PrP^{Sc} accumulations within the cutaneous tissues. IHC and Western blot analyses of skin samples from all forms of CJD and animal prion disease have shown to be insufficient in detecting PrP^{Sc}. RT-QuIC analysis of these samples, however, has proven to successfully detect PrP^{Sc} aggregates in skin samples with high sensitivity and specificity, indicating its potential as a future diagnostic method. In synucleinopathies, IHC staining and immunofluorescence of skin samples from patients have revealed the presence of p-α-syn in dermal nerves. RT-QuIC of skin samples of synucleinopathies has demonstrated high specificity and sensitivity, thus likely serving as an accurate peripheral diagnostic method for synucleinopathies. In tauopathies, p-tau deposits have been found in the skin through IHC, immunofluorescence, and Western blotting of biopsy and autopsy skin samples. RT-QuIC has shown promise for CSF analysis in tauopathies, which hopefully will lead to its use in skin analysis as well. Through immunofluorescence and Western blotting, mtHtt has successfully been found in the cytoplasm and nucleus of skin fibroblasts and as aggregates in the skin of HD patients. Although research on the use of proteopathic seed assays in HD is in its early stages, based on the method's success in other diseases like synucleinopathies and prion disease, there is hope that it can be retrofitted to measure mtHtt in potentially the CSF and skin of individuals afflicted with HD. IHC staining and immunofluorescence have revealed the presence of FUS and TDP-43 cytoplasmic accumulations in the antemortem and postmortem skin of individuals with ALS and FTD. As it is with tauopathies and HD, RT-QuIC analysis of ALS and FTD skin samples still needs to be explored further before any conclusions can be made on its effectiveness as a peripheral biomarker determinant. However, the positive results seen in the CSF samples support a positive outlook for the novel technique. A representation of these results and a comparative analysis of brain and CSF biomarkers can be seen in Table 6.1.

In summary, the discovery of peripheral biomarkers is the key to resolve the diagnostic limitations in neurodegenerative diseases. Skin is the largest, most easily accessible, and most resilient source of peripheral biomarkers, making it a perfect specimen reservoir for the difficult to diagnose neurodegenerative disorders. The investigation of the skin biomarkers of neurodegenerative diseases has shown great promise and, in some cases, can most likely be used as a valuable tool to aid the diagnosis and research for treatment options in the coming years.

Table 6.1 Summary of neurodegenerative disease detection in different tissues

	Brain		CSF		Skin		Other Tissues	
	Immuno-logical	RT-QuIC/ PMCA	Immuno-logical	RT-QuIC/ PMCA	Immuno-logical	RT-QuIC/ PMCA	Immunological	RT-QuIC/ PMCA
Prion diseases								
sCJD	+	+	+	+	+	+	+ (blood, OM)	+ (OM)
vCJD	+	+	+	+	+	+	+ (blood	+ (blood)
Synucleinopathies								
PD	+	+	+	+	+	+	+ (blood, SMG)	+ (OM, SMG)
DLB	+	+	+	+	+	+	+ (SMG)	+ (OM, SMG)
MSA	+	+	+	+	+	+	+ (blood)	+ (OM)
Tauopathies								
AD	+	+	+	+	+	NA	+ (blood, OM)	NA
Pick's disease	+	+	+	+	+	NA	+ (blood)	NA
PSP	+	+	+	+	+	NA	+ (blood)	NA
CBD	+	+	+	+	+	NA	+ (blood)	NA
HD	+	NA	+	NA	+	NA	+ (blood)	NA
ALS	+	NA	+	+	+	NA	+ (blood)	NA
FTD	+	NA	+	+	+	NA	+ (blood)	NA

References are cited in parentheses for the detection of biomarkers in the brain [15, 33, 34, 74–79, 84, 87–89, 123–146], CSF [75, 76, 78–80, 83–89, 147–171], skin [6, 15, 31–89] and other tissues [90–122]. +, indicates there has been detection of biomarkers in the tissue. NA indicates that to our knowledge no studies on the detection of biomarkers have been published at the time of this publication. Immunological methods used include immunohistochemistry, immunocytochemistry, Western blotting, and enzyme-linked immunosorbent assays

References

1. Collinge J. Molecular neurology of prion disease. J Neurol Neurosurg Psychiatry. 2005;76(7):906–19. https://doi.org/10.1136/jnnp.2004.048660.
2. Jeffrey M, González L. Pathology and pathogenesis of bovine spongiform encephalopathy and scrapie. Curr Top Microbiol Immunol. 2004;284:65–97. https://doi.org/10.1007/978-3-662-08441-0_3.
3. Williams ES. Chronic wasting disease. Vet Pathol. 2005;42(5):530–49. https://doi.org/10.1354/vp.42-5-530.
4. Bishop MT, Will RG, Manson JC. Defining sporadic Creutzfeldt-Jakob disease strains and their transmission properties. Proc Natl Acad Sci U S A. 2010;107(26):12005–10. https://doi.org/10.1073/pnas.1004688107.
5. Andréoletti O, Litaise C, Simmons H, Corbière F, Lugan S, Costes P, et al. Highly efficient prion transmission by blood transfusion. PLoS Pathog. 2012;8(6):e1002782. https://doi.org/10.1371/journal.ppat.1002782.
6. Notari S, Moleres FJ, Hunter SB, Belay ED, Schonberger LB, Cali I, et al. Multiorgan detection and characterization of protease-resistant prion protein in a case of variant CJD examined in the United States. PLoS ONE. 2010;5(1):e8765. https://doi.org/10.1371/journal.pone.0008765.
7. Soto C, Satani N. The intricate mechanisms of neurodegeneration in prion diseases. Trends Mol Med. 2011;17(1):14–24. https://doi.org/10.1016/j.molmed.2010.09.001.
8. Goedert M, Jakes R, Spillantini MG. The synucleinopathies: twenty years on. J Parkinsons Dis. 2017;7(s1):S51–69. https://doi.org/10.3233/jpd-179005.
9. Mahul-Mellier A-L, Burtscher J, Maharjan N, Weerens L, Croisier M, Kuttler F, et al. The process of Lewy body formation, rather than simply α-synuclein fibrillization, is one of the major drivers of neurodegeneration. Proc Natl Acad Sci U S A. 2020;117(9):4971–82. https://doi.org/10.1073/pnas.1913904117.
10. Stefanis L. A-synuclein in Parkinson's disease. Cold Spring Harb Perspect Med. 2012;2(2): a009399. https://doi.org/10.1101/cshperspect.a009399.
11. Hernández F, Avila J. Tauopathies. Cell Mol Life Sci. 2007;64(17):2219–33. https://doi.org/10.1007/s00018-007-7220-x.
12. Selkoe DJ. Alzheimer's disease results from the cerebral accumulation and cytotoxicity of amyloid ß-protein. J Alzheimers Dis. 2001;3(1):75–80. https://doi.org/10.3233/jad-2001-3111.
13. Pressman PS, Miller BL. Diagnosis and management of behavioral variant frontotemporal dementia. Biol Psychiatry. 2014;75(7):574–81. https://doi.org/10.1016/j.biopsych.2013.11.006.
14. Buée Scherrer V, Hof PR, Buée L, Leveugle B, Vermersch P, Perl DP, et al. Hyperphosphorylated tau proteins differentiate corticobasal degeneration and Pick's disease. Acta Neuropathol. 1996;91(4):351–9. https://doi.org/10.1007/s004010050436.
15. Kraus A, Saijo E, Metrick MA 2nd, Newell K, Sigurdson CJ, Zanusso G, et al. Seeding selectivity and ultrasensitive detection of tau aggregate conformers of Alzheimer disease. Acta Neuropathol. 2019;137(4):585–98. https://doi.org/10.1007/s00401-018-1947-3.
16. Papoutsi M, Labuschagne I, Tabrizi SJ, Stout JC. The cognitive burden in Huntington's disease: pathology, phenotype, and mechanisms of compensation: the cognitive burden in Hd. Mov Disord. 2014;29(5):673–83. https://doi.org/10.1002/mds.25864.
17. Hatters DM. Protein misfolding inside cells: the case of huntingtin and Huntington's disease. IUBMB Life. 2008;60(11):724–8. https://doi.org/10.1002/iub.111.
18. Walker FO. Huntington's disease. Lancet. 2007;369(9557):218–28. https://doi.org/10.1016/s0140-6736(07)60111-1.
19. Kiernan MC, Vucic S, Cheah BC, Turner MR, Eisen A, Hardiman O, et al. Amyotrophic lateral sclerosis. Lancet. 2011;377(9769):942–55. https://doi.org/10.1016/s0140-6736(10)61156-7.
20. Balendra R, Isaacs AM. C9orf72-mediated ALS and FTD: multiple pathways to disease. Nat Rev Neurol. 2018;14(9):544–58. https://doi.org/10.1038/s41582-018-0047-2.

21. Miki Y, Mori F, Seino Y, Tanji K, Yoshizawa T, Kijima H, et al. Colocalization of Bunina bodies and TDP-43 inclusions in a case of sporadic amyotrophic lateral sclerosis with Lewy body-like hyaline inclusions: possible origin of Bunina bodies. Neuropathology. 2018;38(5):521–8. https://doi.org/10.1111/neup.12484.
22. Weishaupt JH, Hyman T, Dikic I. Common molecular pathways in amyotrophic lateral sclerosis and frontotemporal dementia. Trends Mol Med. 2016;22(9):769–83. https://doi.org/10.1016/j.molmed.2016.07.005.
23. Gaetani L, Paolini Paoletti F, Bellomo G, Mancini A, Simoni S, Di Filippo M, et al. CSF and blood biomarkers in neuroinflammatory and neurodegenerative diseases: implications for treatment. Trends Pharmacol Sci. 2020;41(12):1023–37. https://doi.org/10.1016/j.tips.2020.09.011.
24. Milà-Alomà M, Suárez-Calvet M, Molinuevo JL. Latest advances in cerebrospinal fluid and blood biomarkers of Alzheimer's disease. Ther Adv Neurol Disord. 2019;12. https://doi.org/10.1177/1756286419888819.
25. Parnetti L, Gaetani L, Eusebi P, Paciotti S, Hansson O, El-Agnaf O, et al. CSF and blood biomarkers for Parkinson's disease. Lancet Neurol. 2019;18(6):573–86. https://doi.org/10.1016/s1474-4422(19)30024-9.
26. Connor A, Wang H, Appleby BS, Rhoads DD. Clinical laboratory tests used to aid in diagnosis of human prion disease. J Clin Microbiol. 2019;57(10). https://doi.org/10.1128/JCM.00769-19.
27. Pammer J, Suchy A, Rendl M, Tschachler E. Cellular prion protein expressed by bovine squamous epithelia of skin and upper gastrointestinal tract. Lancet. 1999;354(9191):1702–3. https://doi.org/10.1016/s0140-6736(99)02800-7.
28. Peralta OA, Eyestone WH. Quantitative and qualitative analysis of cellular prion protein (PrPC) expression in bovine somatic tissues. Prion. 2009;3(3):161–70. https://doi.org/10.4161/pri.3.3.9772.
29. Thomzig A, Schulz-Schaeffer W, Wrede A, Wemheuer W, Brenig B, Kratzel C, et al. Accumulation of pathological prion protein PrPSc in the skin of animals with experimental and natural scrapie. PLoS Pathog. 2007;3(5):e66. https://doi.org/10.1371/journal.ppat.0030066.
30. Garza MC, Monzón M, Marín B, Badiola JJ, Monleón E. Distribution of peripheral PrPSc in sheep with naturally acquired scrapie. PLoS ONE. 2014;9(5): e97768. https://doi.org/10.1371/journal.pone.0097768.
31. Pammer J, Weninger W, Tschachler E. Human keratinocytes express cellular prion-related protein in vitro and during inflammatory skin diseases. Am J Pathol. 1998;153(5):1353–8. https://doi.org/10.1016/s0002-9440(10)65720-3.
32. Honda H, Matsuzono K, Satoh K, Fujisawa M, Suzuki SO, Furuyama C, et al. Detection of cutaneous prion protein deposits could help diagnose GPI-anchorless prion disease with neuropathy. Eur J Neurol. 2021;28(6):2133–7. https://doi.org/10.1111/ene.14720.
33. Honda H, Mori S, Watanabe A, Sasagasako N, Sadashima S, Đồng T, et al. Abnormal prion protein deposits with high seeding activities in the skeletal muscle, femoral nerve, and scalp of an autopsied case of sporadic Creutzfeldt-Jakob disease. Neuropathology. 2021;41(2):152–8. https://doi.org/10.1111/neup.12717.
34. Orrú CD, Yuan J, Appleby BS, Li B, Li Y, Winner D, et al. Prion seeding activity and infectivity in skin samples from patients with sporadic Creutzfeldt-Jakob disease. Sci Transl Med. 2017;9(417):eaam7785. https://doi.org/10.1126/scitranslmed.aam7785.
35. Ikemura M, Saito Y, Sengoku R, Sakiyama Y, Hatsuta H, Kanemaru K, et al. Lewy body pathology involves cutaneous nerves. J Neuropathol Exp Neurol. 2008;67(10):945–53. https://doi.org/10.1097/nen.0b013e318186de48.
36. Miki Y, Tomiyama M, Ueno T, Haga R, Nishijima H, Suzuki C, et al. Clinical availability of skin biopsy in the diagnosis of Parkinson's disease. Neurosci Lett. 2010;469(3):357–9. https://doi.org/10.1016/j.neulet.2009.12.027.
37. Al-Qassabi A, Tsao T-S, Racolta A, Kremer T, Cañamero M, Belousov A, et al. Immunohistochemical detection of synuclein pathology in skin in idiopathic rapid eye movement sleep behavior disorder and parkinsonism. Mov Disord. 2020;36(4):895–904. https://doi.org/10.1002/mds.28399.

38. Beach TG, Adler CH, Sue LI, Vedders L, Lue L, White CL Iii, et al. Multi-organ distribution of phosphorylated alpha-synuclein histopathology in subjects with Lewy body disorders. Acta Neuropathol. 2010;119(6):689–702. https://doi.org/10.1007/s00401-010-0664-3.
39. Rodríguez-Leyva I, Calderón-Garcidueñas AL, Jiménez-Capdeville ME, Rentería-Palomo AA, Hernandez-Rodriguez HG, Valdés-Rodríguez R, et al. α-Synuclein inclusions in the skin of Parkinson's disease and parkinsonism. Ann Clin Transl Neurol. 2014;1(7):471–8. https://doi.org/10.1002/acn3.78.
40. Brumberg J, Kuzkina A, Lapa C, Mammadova S, Buck A, Volkmann J, et al. Dermal and cardiac autonomic fiber involvement in Parkinson's disease and multiple system atrophy. Neurobiol Dis. 2021;153:105332. https://doi.org/10.1016/j.nbd.2021.105332.
41. Antelmi E, Donadio V, Incensi A, Plazzi G, Liguori R. Skin nerve phosphorylated α-synuclein deposits in idiopathic REM sleep behavior disorder. Neurology. 2017;88(22):2128–31. https://doi.org/10.1212/wnl.0000000000003989.
42. Wang N, Gibbons CH, Lafo J, Freeman R. α-Synuclein in cutaneous autonomic nerves. Neurology. 2013;81(18):1604–10. https://doi.org/10.1212/wnl.0b013e3182a9f449.
43. Donadio V, Incensi A, Cortelli P, Giannoccaro MP, Jaber MA, Baruzzi A, et al. Skin sympathetic fiber α-synuclein deposits: a potential biomarker for pure autonomic failure. Neurology. 2013;80(8):725–32. https://doi.org/10.1212/wnl.0b013e3182825127.
44. Doppler K, Ebert S, Uçeyler N, Trenkwalder C, Ebentheuer J, Volkmann J, et al. Cutaneous neuropathy in Parkinson's disease: a window into brain pathology. Acta Neuropathol. 2014;128(1):99–109. https://doi.org/10.1007/s00401-014-1284-0.
45. Donadio V, Incensi A, Rizzo G, Capellari S, Pantieri R, Stanzani Maserati M, et al. A new potential biomarker for dementia with Lewy bodies: skin nerve α-synuclein deposits. Neurology. 2017;89(4):318–26. https://doi.org/10.1212/wnl.0000000000004146.
46. Donadio V, Incensi A, Leta V, Giannoccaro MP, Scaglione C, Martinelli P, et al. Skin nerve α-synuclein deposits: a biomarker for idiopathic Parkinson disease. Neurology. 2014;82(15):1362–9. https://doi.org/10.1212/wnl.0000000000000316.
47. Zange L, Noack C, Hahn K, Stenzel W, Lipp A. Phosphorylated α-synuclein in skin nerve fibres differentiates Parkinson's disease from multiple system atrophy. Brain. 2015;138(8):2310–21. https://doi.org/10.1093/brain/awv138.
48. Donadio V, Incensi A, El-Agnaf O, Rizzo G, Vaikath N, Del Sorbo F, et al. Skin α-synuclein deposits differ in clinical variants of synucleinopathy: an in vivo study. Sci Rep. 2018;8(1):14246. https://doi.org/10.1038/s41598-018-32588-8.
49. Rodriguez-Leyva I, Santoyo M, Chii E, Medina-Mier V, Torres B, Casteanedo J, Jimenez-Capdeville M. Presence of phosphorylated tau protein in the skin of Alzheimer's disease patients. J Mol Biomark Diagn. 2015;s6:005. https://doi.org/10.4172/2155-9929.s6-005.
50. Jong Y-JI, Ford SR, Seehra K, Malave VB, Baenziger NL. Alzheimer's disease skin fibroblasts selectively express a bradykinin signaling pathway mediating tau protein Ser phosphorylation. FASEB J. 2003;17(15):2319–21. https://doi.org/10.1096/fj.02-1147fje.
51. Ibáñez-Salazar A, Bañuelos-Hernández B, Rodríguez-Leyva I, Chi-Ahumada E, Monreal-Escalante E, Jiménez-Capdeville ME, et al. Oxidative stress modifies the levels and phosphorylation state of tau protein in human fibroblasts. Front Neurosci. 2017;11:495. https://doi.org/10.3389/fnins.2017.00495.
52. Dugger BN, Hoffman BR, Scroggins A, Serrano GE, Adler CH, Shill HA, et al. Tau immunoreactivity in peripheral tissues of human aging and select tauopathies. Neurosci Lett. 2019;696:132–9. https://doi.org/10.1016/j.neulet.2018.12.031.
53. Joachim CL, Mori H, Selkoe DJ. Amyloid beta-protein deposition in tissues other than brain in Alzheimer's disease. Nature. 1989;341(6239):226–30. https://doi.org/10.1038/341226a0.
54. Citron M, Vigo-Pelfrey C, Teplow DB, Miller C, Schenk D, Johnston J, et al. Excessive production of amyloid beta-protein by peripheral cells of symptomatic and presymptomatic patients carrying the Swedish familial Alzheimer disease mutation. Proc Natl Acad Sci U S A. 1994;91(25):11993–7. https://doi.org/10.1073/pnas.91.25.11993.
55. Johnston JA, Cowburn RF, Norgren S, Wiehager B, Venizelos N, Winblad B, et al. Increased β-amyloid release and levels of amyloid precursor protein (APP) in fibroblast cell lines from

family members with the Swedish Alzheimer's disease APP670/671 mutation. FEBS Lett. 1994;354(3):274–8. https://doi.org/10.1016/0014-5793(94)01137-0.
56. Scheuner D, Eckman C, Jensen M, Song X, Citron M, Suzuki N, et al. Secreted amyloid β–protein similar to that in the senile plaques of Alzheimer's disease is increased in vivo by the presenilin 1 and 2 and APP mutations linked to familial Alzheimer's disease. Nat Med. 1996;2(8):864–70. https://doi.org/10.1038/nm0896-864.
57. Bhattacharya A, Izzo A, Mollo N, Napolitano F, Limone A, Margheri F, et al. Inhibition of 37/67kDa laminin-1 receptor restores APP maturation and reduces amyloid-β in human skin fibroblasts from familial Alzheimer's disease. J Pers Med. 2020;10(4):232. https://doi.org/10.3390/jpm10040232.
58. Akerman SC, Hossain S, Shobo A, Zhong Y, Jourdain R, Hancock MA, et al. Neurodegenerative disease-related proteins within the epidermal layer of the human skin. J Alzheimers Dis. 2019;69(2):463–78. https://doi.org/10.3233/jad-181191.
59. De Rooij KE, Dorsman JC, Smoor MA, Den Dunnen JT, Van Ommen GJ. Subcellular localization of the Huntington's disease gene product in cell lines by immunofluorescence and biochemical subcellular fractionation. Hum Mol Genet. 1996;5(8):1093–9. https://doi.org/10.1093/hmg/5.8.1093.
60. Disatnik M-H, Joshi AU, Saw NL, Shamloo M, Leavitt BR, Qi X, et al. Potential biomarkers to follow the progression and treatment response of Huntington's disease. J Exp Med. 2016;213(12):2655–69. https://doi.org/10.1084/jem.20160776.
61. Pierzynowska K, Gaffke L, Cyske Z, Węgrzyn G. Genistein induces degradation of mutant huntingtin in fibroblasts from Huntington's disease patients. Metab Brain Dis. 2019;34(3):715–20. https://doi.org/10.1007/s11011-019-00405-4.
62. Oketa Y, Higashida K, Fukasawa H, Tsukie T, Ono S. Abundant FUS-immunoreactive pathology in the skin of sporadic amyotrophic lateral sclerosis. Acta Neurol Scand. 2013;128(4):257–64. https://doi.org/10.1111/ane.12114.
63. Wang X, Zhou S, Ding X, Ma M, Zhang J, Zhou Y, et al. Activation of ER stress and autophagy induced by TDP-43 A315T as pathogenic mechanism and the corresponding histological changes in skin as potential biomarker for ALS with the mutation. Int J Biol Sci. 2015;11(10):1140–9. https://doi.org/10.7150/ijbs.12657.
64. Yang S, Zhang KY, Kariawasam R, Bax M, Fifita JA, Ooi L, et al. Evaluation of skin fibroblasts from amyotrophic lateral sclerosis patients for the rapid study of pathological features. Neurotox Res. 2015;28(2):138–46. https://doi.org/10.1007/s12640-015-9532-1.
65. Ren Y, Liu W, Li Y, Sun B, Li Y, Yang F, et al. Cutaneous somatic and autonomic nerve TDP-43 deposition in amyotrophic lateral sclerosis. J Neurol. 2018;265(8):1753–63. https://doi.org/10.1007/s00415-018-8897-5.
66. Suzuki M, Mikami H, Watanabe T, Yamano T, Yamazaki T, Nomura M, et al. Increased expression of TDP-43 in the skin of amyotrophic lateral sclerosis. Acta Neurol Scand. 2010;122(5):367–72. https://doi.org/10.1111/j.1600-0404.2010.01321.x.
67. Paré B, Touzel-Deschênes L, Lamontagne R, Lamarre M-S, Scott F-D, Khuong HT, et al. Early detection of structural abnormalities and cytoplasmic accumulation of TDP-43 in tissue-engineered skins derived from ALS patients. Acta Neuropathol Commun. 2015;3(1):5. https://doi.org/10.1186/s40478-014-0181-z.
68. Abe K, Ohkubo T, Yokota T. TDP-43 in the skin of amyotrophic lateral sclerosis patients. J Med Dent Sci. 2017;64(1):9–17. https://doi.org/10.11480/jmds.640102.
69. Romano N, Catalani A, Lattante S, Belardo A, Proietti S, Bertini L, et al. ALS skin fibroblasts reveal oxidative stress and ERK1/2-mediated cytoplasmic localization of TDP-43. Cell Signal. 2020;70:109591. https://doi.org/10.1016/j.cellsig.2020.109591.
70. de Matos LL, Trufelli DC, de Matos MGL, da Silva Pinhal MA. Immunohistochemistry as an important tool in biomarkers detection and clinical practice. Biomark Insights. 2010;5:9–20. https://doi.org/10.4137/bmi.s2185.
71. Ferreira N do C, Caughey B. Proteopathic seed amplification assays for neurodegenerative disorders. Clin Lab Med. 2020;40(3):257–70. https://doi.org/10.1016/j.cll.2020.04.002.

72. Candelise N, Baiardi S, Franceschini A, Rossi M, Parchi P. Towards an improved early diagnosis of neurodegenerative diseases: the emerging role of in vitro conversion assays for protein amyloids. Acta Neuropathol Commun. 2020;8(1):117. https://doi.org/10.1186/s40478-020-00990-x.
73. Ding M, Teruya K, Zhang W, Lee HW, Yuan J, Oguma A, et al. Decrease in skin prion-seeding activity of prion-infected mice treated with a compound against human and animal prions: a first possible biomarker for prion therapeutics. Mol Neurobiol. 2021. https://doi.org/10.1007/s12035-021-02418-6.
74. Wang Z, Manca M, Foutz A, Camacho MV, Raymond GJ, Race B, et al. Early preclinical detection of prions in the skin of prion-infected animals. Nat Commun. 2019;10(1):247. https://doi.org/10.1038/s41467-018-08130-9.
75. Manca M, Kraus A. Defining the protein seeds of neurodegeneration using real-time quaking-induced conversion assays. Biomolecules. 2020;10(9):1233. https://doi.org/10.3390/biom10091233.
76. Xiao K, Yang X-H, Zhou W, Chen C, Appleby BS, Zou W-Q, et al. Skin RT-QuIC assays are more sensitive than CSF RT-QuIC in prion detection for Chinese probable sporadic Creutzfeldt-Jakob disease. Res Square. 2020. https://doi.org/10.21203/rs.3.rs-92251/v1.
77. Mammana A, Baiardi S, Rossi M, Franceschini A, Donadio V, Capellari S, et al. Detection of prions in skin punch biopsies of Creutzfeldt-Jakob disease patients. Ann Clin Transl Neurol. 2020;7(4):559–64. https://doi.org/10.1002/acn3.51000.
78. Groveman BR, Orrù CD, Hughson AG, Raymond LD, Zanusso G, Ghetti B, et al. Rapid and ultra-sensitive quantitation of disease-associated α-synuclein seeds in brain and cerebrospinal fluid by αSyn RT-QuIC. Acta Neuropathol Commun. 2018;6:7. https://doi.org/10.1186/s40478-018-0508-2.
79. Rossi M, Candelise N, Baiardi S, Capellari S, Giannini G, Orrù CD, et al. Ultrasensitive RT-QuIC assay with high sensitivity and specificity for Lewy body-associated synucleinopathies. Acta Neuropathol. 2020;140(1):49–62. https://doi.org/10.1007/s00401-020-02160-8.
80. Orrù CD, Ma TC, Hughson AG, Groveman BR, Srivastava A, Galasko D, et al. A rapid α-synuclein seed assay of Parkinson's disease CSF panel shows high diagnostic accuracy. Ann Clin Transl Neurol. 2021;8(2):374–84. https://doi.org/10.1002/acn3.51280.
81. Manne S, Kondru N, Jin H, Serrano GE, Anantharam V, Kanthasamy A, et al. Blinded RT-QuIC analysis of α-synuclein biomarker in skin tissue from Parkinson's disease patients. Mov Disord. 2020;35(12):2230–9. https://doi.org/10.1002/mds.28242.
82. Wang Z, Becker K, Donadio V, Siedlak S, Yuan J, Rezaee M, et al. Skin α-synuclein aggregation seeding activity as a novel biomarker for Parkinson disease. JAMA Neurol. 2021;78(1):30–40. https://doi.org/10.1001/jamaneurol.2020.3311.
83. Mammana A, Baiardi S, Quadalti C, Rossi M, Donadio V, Capellari S, et al. RT-QuIC detection of pathological α-synuclein in skin punches of patients with Lewy body disease. Mov Disord. 2021. https://doi.org/10.1002/mds.28651.
84. Shahnawaz M, Mukherjee A, Pritzkow S, Mendez N, Rabadia P, Liu X, et al. Discriminating α-synuclein strains in Parkinson's disease and multiple system atrophy. Nature. 2020;578(7794):273–7. https://doi.org/10.1038/s41586-020-1984-7.
85. Donadio V, Wang Z, Incensi A, Rizzo G, Fileccia E, Vacchiano V, et al. In vivo diagnosis of synucleinopathies: a comparative study of skin biopsy and RT-QuIC: a comparative study of skin biopsy and RT-QuIC. Neurology. 2021;96(20):e2513–24. https://doi.org/10.1212/wnl.0000000000011935.
86. Salvadores N, Shahnawaz M, Scarpini E, Tagliavini F, Soto C. Detection of misfolded Aβ oligomers for sensitive biochemical diagnosis of Alzheimer's disease. Cell Rep. 2014;7(1):261–8. https://doi.org/10.1016/j.celrep.2014.02.031.
87. Saijo E, Groveman BR, Kraus A, Metrick M, Orrù CD, Hughson AG, et al. Ultrasensitive RT-QuIC seed amplification assays for disease-associated tau, α-synuclein, and prion aggregates. Methods Mol Biol. 2019;1873:19–37. https://doi.org/10.1007/978-1-4939-8820-4_2.
88. Metrick MA 2nd, Ferreira N do C, Saijo E, Kraus A, Newell K, Zanusso G, et al. A single ultrasensitive assay for detection and discrimination of tau aggregates of Alzheimer and

Pick diseases. Acta Neuropathol Commun. 2020;8(1):22. https://doi.org/10.1186/s40478-020-0887-z.

89. Scialò C, Tran TH, Salzano G, Novi G, Caponnetto C, Chiò A, et al. TDP-43 real-time quaking induced conversion reaction optimization and detection of seeding activity in CSF of amyotrophic lateral sclerosis and frontotemporal dementia patients. Brain Commun. 2020;2(2):fcaa142. https://doi.org/10.1093/braincomms/fcaa142.
90. Llorens F, Villar-Piqué A, Schmitz M, Diaz-Lucena D, Wohlhage M, Hermann P, et al. Plasma total prion protein as a potential biomarker for neurodegenerative dementia: diagnostic accuracy in the spectrum of prion diseases. Neuropathol Appl Neurobiol. 2020;46(3):240–54. https://doi.org/10.1111/nan.12573.
91. Fagge T, Barclay GR, Macgregor I, Head M, Ironside J, Turner M. Variation in concentration of prion protein in the peripheral blood of patients with variant and sporadic Creutzfeldt-Jakob disease detected by dissociation enhanced lanthanide fluoroimmunoassay and flow cytometry. Transfusion. 2005;45(4):504–13. https://doi.org/10.1111/j.0041-1132.2005.04342.x.
92. Bougard D, Brandel J-P, Belondrade M, Beringue V, Segarra C, Fleury H, et al. Detection of prions in the plasma of presymptomatic and symptomatic patients with variant Creutzfeldt-Jakob disease. Sci Transl Med. 2016;8(370):370ra182–370ra182. https://doi.org/10.1126/scitranslmed.aag1257.
93. Concha-Marambio L, Chacon MA, Soto C. Preclinical detection of prions in blood of nonhuman primates infected with variant Creutzfeldt-Jakob disease. Emerg Infect Dis. 2020;26(1):34–43. https://doi.org/10.3201/eid2601.181423.
94. Barbour R, Kling K, Anderson JP, Banducci K, Cole T, Diep L, et al. Red blood cells are the major source of alpha-synuclein in blood. Neurodegener Dis. 2008;5(2):55–9. https://doi.org/10.1159/000112832.
95. Foulds PG, Diggle P, Mitchell JD, Parker A, Hasegawa M, Masuda-Suzukake M, et al. A longitudinal study on α-synuclein in blood plasma as a biomarker for Parkinson's disease. Sci Rep. 2013;3(1):2540. https://doi.org/10.1038/srep02540.
96. Wang X, Yu S, Li F, Feng T. Detection of α-synuclein oligomers in red blood cells as a potential biomarker of Parkinson's disease. Neurosci Lett. 2015;599:115–9. https://doi.org/10.1016/j.neulet.2015.05.030.
97. Zetterberg H. Neurofilament light: a dynamic cross-disease fluid biomarker for neurodegeneration. Neuron. 2016;91(1):1–3. https://doi.org/10.1016/j.neuron.2016.06.030.
98. Mattsson N, Andreasson U, Zetterberg H, Blennow K, Alzheimer's Disease Neuroimaging Initiative. Association of plasma neurofilament light with neurodegeneration in patients with Alzheimer disease. JAMA Neurol. 2017;74(5):557–66. https://doi.org/10.1001/jamaneurol.2016.6117.
99. Rojas JC, Karydas A, Bang J, Tsai RM, Blennow K, Liman V, et al. Plasma neurofilament light chain predicts progression in progressive supranuclear palsy. Ann Clin Transl Neurol. 2016;3(3):216–25. https://doi.org/10.1002/acn3.290.
100. Steinacker P, Anderl-Straub S, Diehl-Schmid J, Semler E, Uttner I, von Arnim CAF, et al. Serum neurofilament light chain in behavioral variant frontotemporal dementia. Neurology. 2018;91(15):e1390–401. https://doi.org/10.1212/wnl.0000000000006318.
101. Ashton NJ, Leuzy A, Lim YM, Troakes C, Hortobágyi T, Höglund K, et al. Increased plasma neurofilament light chain concentration correlates with severity of post-mortem neurofibrillary tangle pathology and neurodegeneration. Acta Neuropathol Commun. 2019;7(1):5. https://doi.org/10.1186/s40478-018-0649-3.
102. Palmqvist S, Janelidze S, Quiroz YT, Zetterberg H, Lopera F, Stomrud E, et al. Discriminative accuracy of plasma phospho-tau217 for Alzheimer disease vs other neurodegenerative disorders. JAMA. 2020;324(8):772–81. https://doi.org/10.1001/jama.2020.12134.
103. Xiang Y, Bu X-L, Liu Y-H, Zhu C, Shen L-L, Jiao S-S, et al. Physiological amyloid-beta clearance in the periphery and its therapeutic potential for Alzheimer's disease. Acta Neuropathol. 2015;130(4):487–99. https://doi.org/10.1007/s00401-015-1477-1.
104. Janelidze S, Stomrud E, Palmqvist S, Zetterberg H, van Westen D, Jeromin A, et al. Plasma β-amyloid in Alzheimer's disease and vascular disease. Sci Rep. 2016;6:26801. https://doi.org/10.1038/srep26801.

105. Lin C-H, Yang S-Y, Horng H-E, Yang C-C, Chieh J-J, Chen H-H, et al. Plasma biomarkers differentiate Parkinson's disease from atypical parkinsonism syndromes. Front Aging Neurosci. 2018;10:123. https://doi.org/10.3389/fnagi.2018.00123.
106. Sciacca G, Cicchetti F. Mutant huntingtin protein expression and blood-spinal cord barrier dysfunction in huntington disease. Ann Neurol. 2017;82(6):981–94. https://doi.org/10.1002/ana.25107.
107. Byrne LM, Rodrigues FB, Johnson EB, Wijeratne PA, De Vita E, Alexander DC, et al. Evaluation of mutant huntingtin and neurofilament proteins as potential markers in Huntington's disease. Sci Transl Med. 2018;10(458):eaat7108. https://doi.org/10.1126/scitranslmed.aat7108.
108. Johnson EB, Byrne LM, Gregory S, Rodrigues FB, Blennow K, Durr A, et al. Neurofilament light protein in blood predicts regional atrophy in Huntington disease. Neurology. 2018;90(8):e717–23. https://doi.org/10.1212/wnl.0000000000005005.
109. Meeter LH, Kaat LD, Rohrer JD, van Swieten JC. Imaging and fluid biomarkers in frontotemporal dementia. Nat Rev Neurol. 2017;13(7):406–19. https://doi.org/10.1038/nrneurol.2017.75.
110. Poesen K, De Schaepdryver M, Stubendorff B, Gille B, Muckova P, Wendler S, et al. Neurofilament markers for ALS correlate with extent of upper and lower motor neuron disease. Neurology. 2017;88(24):2302–9. https://doi.org/10.1212/wnl.0000000000004029.
111. Zanusso G, Ferrari S, Cardone F, Zampieri P, Gelati M, Fiorini M, et al. Detection of pathologic prion protein in the olfactory epithelium in sporadic Creutzfeldt-Jakob disease. N Engl J Med. 2003;348(8):711–9. https://doi.org/10.1056/nejmoa022043.
112. Orrú CD, Bongianni M, Tonoli G, Ferrari S, Hughson AG, Groveman BR, et al. A test for Creutzfeldt-Jakob disease using nasal brushings. N Engl J Med. 2014;371(6):519–29. https://doi.org/10.1056/nejmoa1315200.
113. Bongianni M, Orrù C, Groveman BR, Sacchetto L, Fiorini M, Tonoli G, et al. Diagnosis of human prion disease using real-time quaking-induced conversion testing of olfactory mucosa and cerebrospinal fluid samples. JAMA Neurol. 2017;74(2):155–62. https://doi.org/10.1001/jamaneurol.2016.4614.
114. De Luca CMG, Elia AE, Portaleone SM, Cazzaniga FA, Rossi M, Bistaffa E, et al. Efficient RT-QuIC seeding activity for α-synuclein in olfactory mucosa samples of patients with Parkinson's disease and multiple system atrophy. Transl Neurodegener. 2019;8(1):24. https://doi.org/10.1186/s40035-019-0164-x.
115. Perra D, Bongianni M, Novi G, Janes F, Bessi V, Capaldi S, et al. Alpha-synuclein seeds in olfactory mucosa and cerebrospinal fluid of patients with dementia with Lewy bodies. Brain Commun. 2021;3(2):fcab045. https://doi.org/10.1093/braincomms/fcab045.
116. Ayala-Grosso CA, Pieruzzini R, Diaz-Solano D, Wittig O, Abrante L, Vargas L, et al. Amyloid-aβ peptide in olfactory mucosa and mesenchymal stromal cells of mild cognitive impairment and Alzheimer's disease patients: amyloid in olfactory mucosa of Alzheimer disease. Brain Pathol. 2015;25(2):136–45. https://doi.org/10.1111/bpa.12169.
117. Lampinen R, Fazaludeen MF, Avesani S, Örd T, Penttilä E, Lehtola J-M, et al. Disease specific alterations in the olfactory mucosa of patients with Alzheimer's disease. bioRxiv. 2020. https://doi.org/10.1101/2020.11.24.395947.
118. Adler CH, Dugger BN, Hinni ML, Lott DG, Driver-Dunckley E, Hidalgo J, et al. Submandibular gland needle biopsy for the diagnosis of Parkinson disease. Neurology. 2014;82(10):858–64. https://doi.org/10.1212/wnl.0000000000000204.
119. Bargar C, Wang W, Gunzler SA, LeFevre A, Wang Z, Lerner A, et al. Streamlined alpha-synuclein RT-QuIC assay for various biospecimens in Parkinson's disease and dementia with Lewy bodies. Acta Neuropathol Commun. 2021;9:62. https://doi.org/10.1186/s40478-021-01175-w.
120. Manne S, Kondru N, Jin H, Anantharam V, Huang X, Kanthasamy A, et al. α-Synuclein real-time quaking-induced conversion in the submandibular glands of Parkinson's disease patients. Mov Disord. 2020;35(2):268–78. https://doi.org/10.1002/mds.27907.

121. Corbillé AG, Letournel F, Kordower JH, Lee J, Shanes E, Neunlist M, et al. Evaluation of alpha-synuclein immunohistochemical methods for the detection of Lewy-type synucleinopathy in gastrointestinal biopsies. Acta Neuropathol Commun. 2016;4:35. https://doi.org/10.1186/s40478-016-0305-8.
122. Beach TG, Corbillé AG, Letournel F, Kordower JH, Kremer T, Munoz DG, et al. Multicenter assessment of immunohistochemical methods for pathological alpha-synuclein in sigmoid colon of autopsied Parkinson's Disease and control subjects. J Parkinsons Dis. 2016;6(4):761–70. https://doi.org/10.3233/JPD-160888.
123. Safar JG, Geschwind MD, Deering C, Didorenko S, Sattavat M, Sanchez H, et al. Diagnosis of human prion disease. Proc Natl Acad Sci U S A. 2005;102(9):3501–6. https://doi.org/10.1073/pnas.0409651102.
124. Williams L, Brown P, Ironside J, Gibson S, Will R, Ritchie D, et al. Clinical, neuropathological and immunohistochemical features of sporadic and variant forms of Creutzfeldt-Jakob disease in the squirrel monkey (Saimiri sciureus). J Gen Virol. 2007;88(Pt 2):688–95. https://doi.org/10.1099/vir.0.81957-0.
125. Liberski PP, Streichenberger N, Giraud P, Soutrenon M, Meyronnet D, Sikorska B, et al. Ultrastructural pathology of prion diseases revisited: brain biopsy studies. Neuropathol Appl Neurobiol. 2005;31(1):88–96. https://doi.org/10.1111/j.1365-2990.2004.00595.x.
126. Roberts RF, Wade-Martins R, Alegre-Abarrategui J. Direct visualization of alpha-synuclein oligomers reveals previously undetected pathology in Parkinson's disease brain. Brain. 2015;138(Pt 6):1642–57. https://doi.org/10.1093/brain/awv040.
127. Nishimura M, Tomimoto H, Suenaga T, Nakamura S, Namba Y, Ikeda K, et al. Synaptophysin and chromogranin A immunoreactivities of Lewy bodies in Parkinson's disease brains. Brain Res. 1994;634(2):339–44. https://doi.org/10.1016/0006-8993(94)91940-2.
128. Mochizuki A, Komatsuzaki Y, Shoji S. Association of Lewy bodies and glial cytoplasmic inclusions in the brain of Parkinson's disease. Acta Neuropathol. 2002;104(5):534–7. https://doi.org/10.1007/s00401-002-0582-0.
129. Iseki E, Marui W, Akiyama H, Uéda K, Kosaka K. Degeneration process of Lewy bodies in the brains of patients with dementia with Lewy bodies using α-synuclein-immunohistochemistry. Neurosci Lett. 2000;286(1):69–73. https://doi.org/10.1016/S0304-3940(00)01090-9.
130. Marui W, Iseki E, Nakai T, Miura S, Kato M, Uéda K, et al. Progression and staging of Lewy pathology in brains from patients with dementia with Lewy bodies. J Neurol Sci. 2002;195(2):153–9. https://doi.org/10.1016/S0022-510X(02)00006-0.
131. Yamamoto R, Iseki E, Murayama N, Minegishi M, Marui W, Togo T, et al. Correlation in Lewy pathology between the claustrum and visual areas in brains of dementia with Lewy bodies. Neurosci Lett. 2007;415(3):219–24. https://doi.org/10.1016/j.neulet.2007.01.029.
132. Tu PH, Galvin JE, Baba M, Giasson B, Tomita T, Leight S, et al. Glial cytoplasmic inclusions in white matter oligodendrocytes of multiple system atrophy brains contain insoluble alpha-synuclein. Ann Neurol. 1998;44(3):415–22. https://doi.org/10.1002/ana.410440324.
133. Nishie M, Mori F, Fujiwara H, Hasegawa M, Yoshimoto M, Iwatsubo T, et al. Accumulation of phosphorylated alpha-synuclein in the brain and peripheral ganglia of patients with multiple system atrophy. Acta Neuropathol. 2004;107(4):292–8. https://doi.org/10.1007/s00401-003-0811-1.
134. Duda JE, Giasson BI, Gur TL, Montine TJ, Robertson D, Biaggioni I, et al. Immunohistochemical and biochemical studies demonstrate a distinct profile of α-synuclein permutations in multiple system atrophy. J Neuropathol Exp Neurol. 2000;59(9):830–41. https://doi.org/10.1093/jnen/59.9.830.
135. Snowden J, Neary D, Mann D. Frontotemporal lobar degeneration: clinical and pathological relationships. Acta Neuropathol. 2007;114(1):31–8. https://doi.org/10.1007/s00401-007-0236-3.
136. van Eersel J, Bi M, Ke YD, Hodges JR, Xuereb JH, Gregory GC, et al. Phosphorylation of soluble tau differs in Pick's disease and Alzheimer's disease brains. J Neural Transm (Vienna). 2009;116(10):1243–51. https://doi.org/10.1007/s00702-009-0293-y.

137. Yasuhara O, Matsuo A, Tooyama I, Kimura H, McGeer EG, McGeer PL. Pick's disease immunohistochemistry: new alterations and Alzheimer's disease comparisons. Acta Neuropathol. 1995;89(4):322–30. https://doi.org/10.1007/BF00309625.
138. Nishimura T, Ikeda K, Akiyama H, Kondo H, Kato M, Li F, et al. Immunohistochemical investigation of tau-positive structures in the cerebral cortex of patients with progressive supranuclear palsy. Neurosci Lett. 1995;201(2):123–6. https://doi.org/10.1016/0304-3940(95)12151-X.
139. Piras A, Collin L, Grüninger F, Graff C, Rönnbäck A. Autophagic and lysosomal defects in human tauopathies: analysis of post-mortem brain from patients with familial Alzheimer disease, corticobasal degeneration and progressive supranuclear palsy. Acta Neuropathol Commun. 2016;4(1):22. https://doi.org/10.1186/s40478-016-0292-9.
140. Sapp E, Schwarz C, Chase K, Bhide PG, Young AB, Penney J, et al. Huntingtin localization in brains of normal and Huntington's disease patients. Ann Neurol. 1997;42(4):604–12. https://doi.org/10.1002/ana.410420411.
141. DiFiglia M, Sapp E, Chase KO, Davies SW, Bates GP, Vonsattel JP, et al. Aggregation of huntingtin in neuronal intranuclear inclusions and dystrophic neurites in brain. Science. 1997;277(5334):1990–3. https://doi.org/10.1126/science.277.5334.1990.
142. Hasegawa M, Arai T, Nonaka T, Kametani F, Yoshida M, Hashizume Y, et al. Phosphorylated TDP-43 in frontotemporal lobar degeneration and amyotrophic lateral sclerosis. Ann Neurol. 2008;64(1):60–70. https://doi.org/10.1002/ana.21425.
143. Arai T, Hasegawa M, Akiyama H, Ikeda K, Nonaka T, Mori H, et al. TDP-43 is a component of ubiquitin-positive tau-negative inclusions in frontotemporal lobar degeneration and amyotrophic lateral sclerosis. Biochem Biophys Res Commun. 2006;351(3):602–11. https://doi.org/10.1016/j.bbrc.2006.10.093.
144. Green AJE. RT-QuIC: a new test for sporadic CJD. Pract Neurol. 2019;19(1):49–55. https://doi.org/10.1136/practneurol-2018-001935.
145. Peden AH, McGuire LI, Appleford NEJ, Mallinson G, Wilham JM, Orrú CD, et al. Sensitive and specific detection of sporadic Creutzfeldt-Jakob disease brain prion protein using real-time quaking-induced conversion. J Gen Virol. 2012;93(Pt 2):438–49. https://doi.org/10.1099/vir.0.033365-0.
146. De Luca CMG, Elia AE, Portaleone SM, et al. Efficient RT-QuIC seeding activity for α-synuclein in olfactory mucosa samples of patients with Parkinson's disease and multiple system atrophy. Transl Neurodegener. 2019;8:24. https://doi.org/10.1186/s40035-019-0164-x.
147. Schmitz M, Lüllmann K, Zafar S, Ebert E, Wohlhage M, Oikonomou P, et al. Association of prion protein genotype and scrapie prion protein type with cellular prion protein charge isoform profiles in cerebrospinal fluid of humans with sporadic or familial prion diseases. Neurobiol Aging. 2014;35(5):1177–88. https://doi.org/10.1016/j.neurobiolaging.2013.11.010.
148. Wong BS, Green AJ, Li R, Xie Z, Pan T, Liu T, et al. Absence of protease-resistant prion protein in the cerebrospinal fluid of Creutzfeldt-Jakob disease. J Pathol. 2001;194(1):9–14. https://doi.org/10.1002/path.872.
149. Torres M, Cartier L, Matamala JM, Hernández N, Woehlbier U, Hetz C. Altered prion protein expression pattern in CSF as a biomarker for Creutzfeldt-Jakob disease. PLoS ONE. 2012;7(4): e36159. https://doi.org/10.1371/journal.pone.0036159.
150. Parnetti L, Chiasserini D, Persichetti E, Eusebi P, Varghese S, Qureshi MM, et al. Cerebrospinal fluid lysosomal enzymes and alpha-synuclein in Parkinson's disease: CSF lysosomal enzymes in Parkinson's disease. Mov Disord. 2014;29(8):1019–27. https://doi.org/10.1002/mds.25772.
151. Majbour NK, Vaikath NN, van Dijk KD, Ardah MT, Varghese S, Vesterager LB, et al. Oligomeric and phosphorylated alpha-synuclein as potential CSF biomarkers for Parkinson's disease. Mol Neurodegener. 2016;11(1):7. https://doi.org/10.1186/s13024-016-0072-9.
152. Tokuda T, Qureshi MM, Ardah MT, Varghese S, Shehab SAS, Kasai T, et al. Detection of elevated levels of α-synuclein oligomers in CSF from patients with Parkinson disease. Neurology. 2010;75(20):1766–72. https://doi.org/10.1212/WNL.0b013e3181fd613b.

153. Lim X, Yeo JM, Green A, Pal S. The diagnostic utility of cerebrospinal fluid alpha-synuclein analysis in dementia with Lewy bodies—a systematic review and meta-analysis. Parkinsonism Relat Disord. 2013;19(10):851–8. https://doi.org/10.1016/j.parkreldis.2013.06.008.
154. van Steenoven I, Majbour NK, Vaikath NN, Berendse HW, van der Flier WM, van de Berg WDJ, et al. α-Synuclein species as potential cerebrospinal fluid biomarkers for dementia with lewy bodies: CSF α-Synuclein species as biomarkers for DLB. Mov Disord. 2018;33(11):1724–33. https://doi.org/10.1002/mds.111.
155. Mondello S, Constantinescu R, Zetterberg H, Andreasson U, Holmberg B, Jeromin A. CSF α-synuclein and UCH-L1 levels in Parkinson's disease and atypical parkinsonian disorders. Parkinsonism Relat Disord. 2014;20(4):382–7. https://doi.org/10.1016/j.parkreldis.2014.01.011.
156. Foulds PG, Yokota O, Thurston A, Davidson Y, Ahmed Z, Holton J, et al. Post mortem cerebrospinal fluid α-synuclein levels are raised in multiple system atrophy and distinguish this from the other α-synucleinopathies, Parkinson's disease and Dementia with Lewy bodies. Neurobiol Dis. 2012;45(1):188–95. https://doi.org/10.1016/j.nbd.2011.08.003.
157. Meredith JE Jr, Sankaranarayanan S, Guss V, Lanzetti AJ, Berisha F, Neely RJ, et al. Characterization of novel CSF Tau and ptau biomarkers for Alzheimer's disease. PLoS ONE. 2013;8(10):e76523. https://doi.org/10.1371/journal.pone.0076523.
158. Welge V, Fiege O, Lewczuk P, Mollenhauer B, Esselmann H, Klafki H-W, et al. Combined CSF tau, p-tau181 and amyloid-beta 38/40/42 for diagnosing Alzheimer's disease. J Neural Transm (Vienna). 2009;116(2):203–12. https://doi.org/10.1007/s00702-008-0177-6.
159. Wallin AK, Blennow K, Andreasen N, Minthon L. CSF biomarkers for Alzheimer's Disease: levels of beta-amyloid, tau, phosphorylated tau relate to clinical symptoms and survival. Dement Geriatr Cogn Disord. 2006;21(3):131–8. https://doi.org/10.1159/000090631.
160. Wagshal D, Sankaranarayanan S, Guss V, Hall T, Berisha F, Lobach I, et al. Divergent CSF τ alterations in two common tauopathies: Alzheimer's disease and progressive supranuclear palsy. J Neurol Neurosurg Psychiatry. 2015;86(3):244–50. https://doi.org/10.1136/jnnp-2014-308004.
161. Borroni B, Gardoni F, Parnetti L, Magno L, Malinverno M, Saggese E, et al. Pattern of Tau forms in CSF is altered in progressive supranuclear palsy. Neurobiol Aging. 2009;30(1):34–40. https://doi.org/10.1016/j.neurobiolaging.2007.05.009.
162. Arai H, Morikawa Y, Higuchi M, Matsui T, Clark CM, Miura M, et al. Cerebrospinal fluid tau levels in neurodegenerative diseases with distinct tau-related pathology. Biochem Biophys Res Commun. 1997;236(2):262–4. https://doi.org/10.1006/bbrc.1997.6908.
163. Green AJ, Harvey RJ, Thompson EJ, Rossor MN. Increased tau in the cerebrospinal fluid of patients with frontotemporal dementia and Alzheimer's disease. Neurosci Lett. 1999;259(2):133–5. https://doi.org/10.1016/S0304-3940(98)00904-5.
164. Urakami K, Wada K, Arai H, Sasaki H, Kanai M, Shoji M, et al. Diagnostic significance of tau protein in cerebrospinal fluid from patients with corticobasal degeneration or progressive supranuclear palsy. J Neurol Sci. 2001;183(1):95–8. https://doi.org/10.1016/S0022-510X(00)00480-9.
165. Mitani K, Furiya Y, Uchihara T, Ishii K, Yamanouchi H, Mizusawa H, et al. Increased CSF tau protein in corticobasal degeneration. J Neurol. 1998;245(1):44–6. https://doi.org/10.1007/s004150050173.
166. Wild EJ, Boggio R, Langbehn D, Robertson N, Haider S, Miller JRC, et al. Quantification of mutant huntingtin protein in cerebrospinal fluid from Huntington's disease patients. J Clin Invest. 2015;125(5):1979–86. https://doi.org/10.1172/JCI80743.
167. Kasai T, Tokuda T, Ishigami N, Sasayama H, Foulds P, Mitchell DJ, et al. Increased TDP-43 protein in cerebrospinal fluid of patients with amyotrophic lateral sclerosis. Acta Neuropathol. 2009;117(1):55–62. https://doi.org/10.1007/s00401-008-0456-1.
168. Majumder V, Gregory JM, Barria MA, Green A, Pal S. TDP-43 as a potential biomarker for amyotrophic lateral sclerosis: a systematic review and meta-analysis. BMC Neurol. 2018;18(1). https://doi.org/10.1186/s12883-018-1091-7.

169. Steinacker P, Hendrich C, Sperfeld AD, Jesse S, von Arnim CAF, Lehnert S, et al. TDP-43 in cerebrospinal fluid of patients with frontotemporal lobar degeneration and amyotrophic lateral sclerosis. Arch Neurol. 2008;65(11):1481–7. https://doi.org/10.1001/archneur.65.11.1481.
170. Bougard D, Bélondrade M, Mayran C, Bruyère-Ostells L, Lehmann S, Fournier-Wirth C, et al. Diagnosis of methionine/valine variant Creutzfeldt-Jakob disease by protein misfolding cyclic amplification. Emerg Infect Dis. 2018;24(7):1364–6. https://doi.org/10.3201/eid2407.172105.
171. Barria MA, Lee A, Green AJ, Knight R, Head MW. Rapid amplification of prions from variant Creutzfeldt-Jakob disease cerebrospinal fluid. J Pathol Clin Res. 2018;4(2):86–92. https://doi.org/10.1002/cjp2.90.

Chapter 7
Defining Diagnosis in Neurodegeneration Through the Search of Biomarkers in Skin

Ildefonso Rodríguez-Leyva, Sandra A. Niño, and María E. Jiménez-Capdeville

Abstract Birth control, population aging, and medicine have made life expectancy longer. However, this has facilitated an increase in the presence of neurodegenerative diseases, which are proteinopathies that cause a functional deterioration of those who suffer them, mainly affecting cognition and motor skills, manifesting as dementia, parkinsonian syndromes, motor neuron disease, behavioral and movement disorders. The in-life diagnosis of these processes remains a real challenge, so the search for biomarkers that allow us to approach the risk of suffering from these processes becomes mandatory. The skin, having a neuroectodermal origin, must share a protein synthesis program like that of nervous tissue, so it could be an ideal site to find the characteristic alterations of synucleinopathies (Parkinson's disease) and tauopathies (Alzheimer's disease), the two epidemiologically most important proteinopathies by incidence and prevalence in the world. Modification of proteins that were functionally and structurally useful to cells will eventually lead to the formation of aggregates that in neurons are recognized as the main characteristic for these pathologies: Lewy bodies (with α-synuclein for Parkinson's disease) and neurofibrillary tangles (with Tau for Alzheimer's disease). We have demonstrated different patterns of distribution of these proteins in the skin of affected subjects, and in this chapter, we tell the story that summarizes ten years of teamwork to achieve a goal, to demonstrate that the skin can be a site of neurodegeneration labeling.

Keywords Neurodegeneration · Parkinson's disease · Alpha-synuclein · Alzheimer's disease · Tau protein

---

I. Rodríguez-Leyva
Department of Neurology, Hospital "Ignacio Morones Prieto", San Luis Potosí, México

S. A. Niño · M. E. Jiménez-Capdeville (✉)
Department of Biochemistry, Facultad de Medicina, Universidad Autónoma de San Luis Potosí. Av. V. Carranza 2405 Col. Los Filtros, 78210 San Luis Potosí, México
e-mail: mejimenez@uaslp.mx

R. Norman (ed.), *Biomarkers in Dermatology*,
https://doi.org/10.1007/978-3-031-66513-4_7

7.1 Introduction

The incidence and prevalence of neurodegenerative diseases have considerably escalated in the world, as the mean age of the living population increases due to better health conditions. Neurodegeneration can be defined as a progressive process associated to the accumulation of proteins that are no longer functional because they are abnormally shaped. Their misfolding and aggregation to form polymers impairs most cellular functions, including energy production and spending. Gradually, dysfunction precipitates the death of the affected neurons and glial cells. The main clinical manifestations are the presence of dementia, parkinsonism, and other movement disorders (chorea), behavioral disturbances and disease of the upper motor neuron [1].

The importance of neurodegenerative diseases has grown as life expectancy increases. Alzheimer's disease is the most common cause of dementia, and it is considered that 60–80% of all cases are due to this neurodegenerative process that possibly started up to 20 years before the disease manifests itself and the diagnosis is made. Dementia or significant cognitive impairment is characterized by deficits of several cognitive areas: memory, judgment, orientation, attention. Although some of those alterations can be associated to normal aging, they become part of a dementia process when they surpass certain defined limits [2]. It is estimated that between 15 and 20% of subjects over the age of 65 have already minimal cognitive impairment (MCI) and that in the following five years, a third of them will develop Alzheimer's disease [3]. Parkinson's disease is, on the other hand, the second-most prevalent neurodegenerative disease, and its main characteristics are recognized with the initials TRAP (tremor, rigidity, akinesia, and postural instability). It is preceded by a constellation of non-motor symptoms that can last for more than a decade before the disease is identified [4].

The impact of early pathology falls on structures that will explain the main manifestations associated with the affected systems. For example, in Alzheimer's disease, the hippocampus and cortex present accumulations of misfolded proteins, which are related to the usual amnesia that the patients report as early symptom. By contrast, the alteration of the dopaminergic nigrostriatal pathway, characterized by protein accumulations called Lewy bodies explain the motor manifestations of the Parkinson's disease patient. However, these diseases may have common characteristics rather than just differences. They are the first and second neurodegenerative diseases in the world, both have age as the most critical risk factor, DNA damage and mitochondrial dysfunction that favors oxidative damage is related to both diseases [5].

Currently, the definitive diagnosis of neurodegenerative diseases is made until the pathologists have the postmortem brains in their hands. Several years ago, we began the search for a biomarker that would be accessible, inexpensive, and that allowed us to address the etiology of the problem with greater precision and specificity. In this chapter, we summon up our findings on the traces of neurodegenerative diseases in the skin.

7.2 Biomarkers of Neurodegeneration

A biomarker is the objectively measurable and evaluable characteristic of a normal biological process, pathological or pharmacological response to a therapeutic intervention. The biomarkers for the central nervous system (CNS) can be clinical, imaging, biochemical, genetic, proteomic, or pathological. They serve to confirm the diagnosis, make epidemiological projections, predictive tests, monitor disease progression after diagnosis, develop medications, measure response to treatment, and for the study of brain–behavior relationships [6].

Since it is recognized that neurodegenerative diseases such as Alzheimer's and Parkinson's disease begin possibly years before they manifest clinically, it is required a pre-symptomatic diagnosis, which could give diagnostic certainty, due to considerable variability in symptoms, signs and cyclical episodes that can characterize each of these conditions. Diagnosis is crucial to establish and follow current therapeutic strategies, to ameliorate specific manifestations of each situation, to improve the quality of life, to recognize neuroprotective measures and truly modifying therapies for the disease.

Some patients have a neurodegenerative problem associated with a vascular one, and it is also possible that a patient with Alzheimer's disease has manifestations of Parkinson's disease and has several proteinopathies concomitantly. Furthermore, it could help to recognize the heterogeneity of presentation in the population according to their genetics, race, origin, and risk factors to which they have been exposed [7, 8].

The fundamental characteristics of neurodegenerative diseases are the neuropathology and the pathophysiological mechanisms of their presentation. Features as neuronal, glial, and synaptic loss as well as each proteinopathy that characterizes it. A biomarker should correlate its expression with the progression of the disease and with the clinical scales that measure its clinical manifestations. It should not only allow monitoring the current state of the disease, but also serve as preclinical validation especially for subjects exposed to risk factors or with genetic load. Ideally, the biomarker should be inexpensive, non-invasive, easy to use, technically validated [9, 10].

Clos and collaborators proposed that neurodegenerative diseases could be studied in the skin, given their close relationship of origin, physiological and pathological activity, what they called "brain-skin connection,". They insist on how amyloidosis in other organs may be related to the presence of protein aggregates in the skin and may even mark the possibility that α-synuclein is transmitted from neuron to neuron in nervous tissue and that amyloidosis of nervous tissue in Alzheimer's disease may manifest in the skin. In fact, some therapies for Parkinson's disease (rotigotine) and Alzheimer's disease (rivastigmine) are applied to the skin to perform its pharmacological action in the brain [11]. This valuable work motivated and inspired our search of skin biomarkers for neurodegenerative diseases.

7.3 Proteinopathy of Parkinson's Disease

Initially, we looked for the presence of α-synuclein in the skin of patients with Parkinson's disease, knowing that the characteristic marker of this disease is the presence of Lewy bodies, which are unusual deposits formed by aggregates of the alpha-synuclein protein, together with other proteins such as ubiquitin [12].

Synuclein is expressed in three forms: α, β, and γ. α and β synuclein are found in synaptic vesicles of nerve endings in the CNS. Synuclein ϒ is found in the nerve endings of the peripheral nervous system. [13]. α-Synuclein is found in the extracellular space and not only at the nuclear and cytoplasmic level, while in Parkinson's disease, it has also been demonstrated at the mitochondria, where it modifies functionality and composition [14]. Its presence in CSF decreases in patients with synucleinopathies (Parkinson's disease, Lewy body dementia) as compared to controls or patients with AD, so it has been proposed as a candidate biomarker for these pathologies, although the results remain controversial [15] α-Synuclein has several isoforms; the healthy functional protein usually has 140 amino acids. At the same time, the ones composed of 112 and 126, which result from the deletion of exons 3 and 5 respectively, are associated with LBD, besides a fourth 98 amino acid isoform associated with a predominantly frontal LBD. α-Synuclein is encoded in the synuclein gene (SNCA) located on chromosome 4q21. Its conformation is characterized by six repeated sequences that make up five amphipathic helices in the middle of the N-terminal, which is very similar to apolipoproteins [16]. The central domain is highly amyloidogenic, especially the fragment corresponding to amino acids 61–95, which seems to be the critical area for the initiation of fibrillation of this protein with the conformation of beta sheets that will be the characteristic of neurodegeneration [17]. Although the function of α-Synuclein is unknown with certainty, it is associated with stabilization and trafficking in the synaptic membrane and is a critical modulator in the functioning of dopaminergic synaptic vesicles. Among the multiple functions in which has been found to participate, it has an important role in synaptic vesicle recycling, neurotransmitter synthesis and release, and synaptic plasticity. Therefore, many of these functions are altered in synucleinopathies [18].

The alteration of the α-synuclein conformation to form beta sheets, the fibrillary aggregation, leads to the conformation of the inclusion conglomerates called Lewy bodies. cytoplasmic alpha-synuclein aggregation may decrease the amount of protein available for any nuclear or cytoplasmic role it may play, contributing to a loss-of-function, namely changes in the release of synaptic vesicles, mitochondrial dysfunction, pore formation, production of reactive oxygen species, with neuronal dysfunction and apoptosis [19–21].

The biomarkers proposed to detect the presence of a synucleinopathy are multiple, many are performed only in specialized centers, but many do not help the clinician to differentiate PD from parkinsonism. These techniques track dopaminergic activity in imaging studies such as PET or SPECT through markers of dopaminergic neurons such as VMAT2, 123I-FP-CIT, DAT, 11C-PK11195 [22].

The Magnetic Resonance Image is highly suggestive for differentiating some parkinsonism such as the PSP with the images of "morning glory," the one hummingbird and the sign of "Mickey Mouse" and for the multiple systems atrophy (MSA) that of "Hot Cross Bun" and the "putaminal ring" [23].

7.4 Proteinopathy in Alzheimer's Disease

Surely multiple factors intervene to favor the presence of the disease. Of course, the individual's genetics, as well as childhood aggressions and adversities (from prenatal exposure to hormones, birth weight, head circumference, height), educational level, individual intelligence, brain and body growth, and multiple environmental exposures (such as trauma, schooling, viral infections, socio-economic and cultural level) [24].

It was calculated in 2016 that there was a prevalence of 47 million subjects with dementia worldwide. By 2050, it is expected to be 130 million with Alzheimer's disease. This pathology is considered the cause of dementia in 76% of cases, followed by vascular, Parkinson–Dementia complex, dementia with Lewy bodies, frontotemporal dementia that average 5% of dementia etiologies. The prevalence of dementia in more than 60 years is calculated between 5 and 8% of the population (depending on the geographic area referred to). The cumulative incidence of dementia in subjects over 60 years of age is estimated to be 52.8 per 1000 population, with variability between 11.5 for Nigeria and 97.8 for the United States of America. Knowing what the real modifiable risk factors are and having biomarkers to help us detect them early to provide better management may soon make a difference in future [25].

Alzheimer's disease causes the most common dementia in the world. The characteristic proteinopathies of this pathology are the Tau (expressed in the neurofibrillary tangles (NFT) at the intraneuronal level), and the beta-amyloid protein (expressed extracellularly in the so-called senile plaques). NFTs formed by helical protein filaments (PHF) in the cytoplasm of neurons affect the microtubular system of the neuronal cytoskeleton. The central involvement occurs at the hippocampal and tonsillar level, in addition to the frontal, temporal, and parietal association cortices [26, 27].

The microtubule-associated protein (Tau) belongs to a family of factors that polymerize tubulin dimers and stabilize microtubules, expressing themselves in neurons and having an essential role in their plasticity. It is also present in neuronal nuclei, where it plays an essential role in regulation of gene expression. It is made up of 441 amino acids encoded in chromosome 17q21 and has six main isoforms, depending on the presence of 3 or 4 repeats (3R or 4R). It has 85 possible phosphorylation sites, which are targets of up to 20 protein kinases. Hyperphosphorylation leads to aggregation, and according to the isoforms that become aggregated, four groups of neurodegenerations have been identified. (a) Class 1. All the isoforms are aggregated. This accumulation has six isoforms. This profile is characteristic of Alzheimer's disease. (b) Class II. Tau isoforms that encode aggregates containing exon 10, corresponding to basal cortical degeneration, progressive supranuclear paralysis (PSP), and manifestations without a neurodegenerative disorder characterized by cognitive and extrapyramidal disorders (dementia with argyrophilic grains) with behavioral changes (personality) that may be grouped within frontotemporal dementias. (c) Class III: corresponding to the loss of coding of the sequence of aggregates of exon 10, characteristic of frontotemporal dementia, previously known as Pick's disease, (d) Class IV: Tau isoform that lacks exons 2, 3 and 10 and related to myotonic dystrophy (MD) type I of onset in adulthood, cognitive, cardiac, intestinal, endocrine disorders. MD is an autosomal dominant disorder, often also associated with the characteristics of frontotemporal dementia. The presence of the Tau protein could be detected in the CSF, and its study could determine the differentiation with other forms of dementia such as Creutzfeldt Jacob's disease (CJD) and other forms of dementia such as LBD and frontotemporal dementia [28].

The aggregation of helical filaments that accumulate in the hippocampus gives the primary manifestation of Alzheimer's dementia, which is amnesia. This progressive process has been divided into stages by Braak and collaborators. Initially, it mainly affects the entorhinal cortex (stage I), the CA1 region of the hippocampus (stage II), later the limbic structures, such as the subiculum and the hippocampal region (stage III). The amygdala, the thalamus, and the claustrum (stage IV), to finally spread throughout the neocortex, first the sensory areas, then the motor areas and finally the associative ones (stage V) [29, 30].

Our question and reason for the study was whether we could compare brain pathology with what happens in cutaneous expression that would help us better serve patients with neurodegenerative diseases, and if there would be a way to stratify the expression in a similar way as it happens in the brain.

7.5 Skin Immunohistochemistry

With the conviction that Parkinson's disease synucleinopathy is a systemic manifestation, we sought its presence on the skin of patients with Parkinson's disease and control subjects comparable in demographic characteristics. Initially, we took a biopsy of the dorsal region at the lumbar level and in the retro-auricular region.

We register our research at the NIH (code NCT01380899). After multiple tests of failure and error, we were finally able to visualize the presence of α-synuclein in the skin of the affected subjects with a clear difference from the controls by means of immunohistochemistry. Previously, Miki and collaborators had reported the presence of α-synuclein in autopsied chest skin of 2 out of 20 subjects with PD, obtained by a 6 mm punch and not in the skin of the foot, where they also looked for it [31].

Prior authorization from the institutional Research and Ethics Committee and signature of the informed consent by the tutor or the research subject, 4 mm skin biopsies were taken at the retro atrial level 3 cm behind the insertion of the auricle, to patients and control subjects. The tissue was fixed in paraffin and subjected to immunohistochemistry and immunofluorescence techniques. Antibodies directed to different epitopes of the Tau and α-synuclein proteins were used and analyzed by light and confocal microscopy. In some subjects, the contralateral biopsies were homogenized to identify the presence of proteins of interest employing Western blotting. Through the digital analysis of microphotographs of the immune stains, the percentage of the positive area was obtained for each immunostaining.

In 2011, we made our first presentation at an international dermatology congress [32]. At the Annual Congress of the American Academy of Neurology, we presented our initial results on the platform; we had the idea that the skin could be an ideal site for early Parkinson's disease detection [33]. Also, in the same year before our first publication, Donadio and collaborators reported the presence of α-synuclein in the nerve endings (thin fibers) of the skin of the cervical region and the foot, in subjects with IPD (idiopathic Parkinson's disease) [34].

After multiple rejections and reviews we finally achieved our first publication, where our primary objective was to demonstrate the presence of proteinopathy on the skin and secondly to quantify its presence and compare it among a population with Parkinson's disease, another with atypical Parkinson's and a control population. We found a clear difference with moderately high expression in Parkinson's disease, low in Atypical Parkinson's, and scarce in controls [35].

At the meeting of the Movement Disorders Society in Australia in 2013 and that of the American Academy of Neurology (AAN) with a more significant number of cases, we presented a comparative study between the expression of α-synuclein in patients with Parkinson's disease and PSP, finding that it could be a method to differentiate a Parkinsonism due to synucleinopathy from one due to tauopathy [36].

At the 2014 AAN Annual Meeting, we showed how proteinopathies were expressed in the skin and how the α-synuclein, phosphorylated Tau, beta-amyloid protein, could be seen similarly in the brain, in the nerves (PNS) and the skin, demonstrating for the first time in our knowledge the expression of the phosphorylated Tau protein in the skin of patients with Alzheimer's disease [37] (Fig. 7.1).

We were convinced that the expression of aggregated proteins found in the brain characterizing neurodegeneration was not exclusive to this organ. We set about the task of demonstrating its presence in the skin and presented our results again at the annual meeting of the AAN of 2015, concerning the presence of the natural proteins of neurodegeneration, demonstrating their presence on the skin of patients with Alzheimer's disease and Parkinson's disease, with high significance for both pathologies compared to controls [38]. This work was very importantly seized by the AAN and multiple times mentioned in the media, among others Scientific American [39], Medscape [40], Mdedge Neurology [41]. The fact that our work appeared in many media around the world was very stimulating, but there were also multiple criticisms and rejections of this article that was finally published [42].

Next, we demonstrated the presence of α-synuclein in skin cells derived from the neural crest. By comparing its expression in the skin of patients with Parkinson's disease, melanomas, nevi, skin tags and normal skin. This work is fascinating and important, because it clearly shows how melanocytes express this protein and how its expression is notably increased in melanomas, followed by nevi and Parkinson's disease [43]. This work led us to propose that neurons and melanocytes, derived from neuroectoderm cells, share the synthesis and regulatory pathways of α-synuclein,

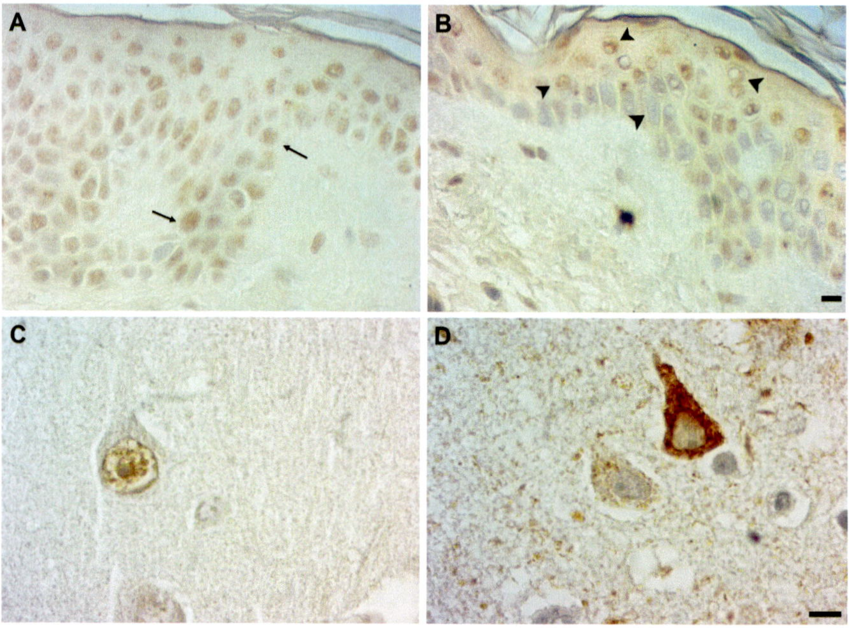

Fig. 7.1 Human epidermis (**a**, **b**) and human CA1 pyramidal hippocampal cells (**c**, **d**) immunopositive to anti-Tau antibody (pSer202/pThr205) (AH36, StressMarq Biosciences Inc, Victoria, CAN). Phosphorylated Tau at Ser202/Thr205 is located inside nuclei of epidermal cells in a healthy 65-year-old control (arrows in **a**) as well as in the nucleus of CA1 pyramidal cells (**c**). In a skin biopsy of a patient with Alzheimer disease immunopositivity is located in the cytoplasm and extracellular space (arrow heads, **b**), and nuclei do not contain this phosphorylated form anymore (arrowhead, **b**) Notice that extranuclear Tau does not form tangles in the skin. In neurons, neurofibrillary tangles of cytoplasmic Tau and neurites with aggregated protein are evident in a section of hippocampus belonging to a deceased Alzheimer´s disease patient at Braak stage III–IV (**d**)

involved both in PD and melanoma, which explains their relationship and increased comorbidity [44–46].

In an exciting proposal, our group began to work on the expression of proteinopathies in the oral mucosa, demonstrating the presence of p-Tau in subjects with cognitive impairment at a significantly higher level than control subjects with normal cognition, proposing that this site may also be a fully accessible means of sampling a population at risk of tauopathy [47].

Since α -synuclein has been related to neuroinflammatory processes and could play an important role in conditions such as multiple sclerosis, we decided to study its presence in peripheral blood cells and skin, comparing 34 controls against 23 patients with recurrent remitting multiple sclerosis (RRMS). Protein was measured by immunohistochemistry and by flow cytometry. We found no difference in their presence in lymphocytes and monocytes between the two groups. But a significantly lower level of skin's alpha-synuclein of patients in relapse than in those in remission and controls. This makes us think of a modulating role of synuclein in the acute inflammatory response [48].

7.6 Conclusions

The work carried out along ten years shows that it is possible to find and to quantify the presence of α-synuclein in recognized synucleinopathies (Parkinson's disease, multiple system atrophy, Lewy body dementia) and tau protein in the skin of subjects with tauopathies (Alzheimer's disease, cortico-basal degeneration, progressive supranuclear palsy, frontotemporal dementia). Although skin cells do not present the characteristic aggregates of neurodegenerative proteinopathies, namely Lewy bodies or tangles, due to their different cytoskeleton and cell cycle, there are clear difference in the distribution of these proteins among disease states. Furthermore, synuclein is expressed in a very significant way in nevi and melanoma and it plays a regulatory role in neuroinflammatory processes such as relapsing multiple sclerosis.

Since neurodegenerative diseases are currently a diagnostic and therapeutic challenge, all these facts allow us to state that skin biopsy is a minimally invasive, safe, low-cost method that enables approaching the diagnosis and would possibly allow to see the response to the therapy and to get closer to the diagnosis of a patient who is at risk or suffering a neurodegenerative process. Moreover, this initial approach underlies the recent measurement of the ability of synuclein to aggregate in the skin of patients with Parkinson´s disease by means of more efficient techniques [49, 50].

References

1. Golde TE, Borchelt DR, Giasson BI, Lewis J. Thinking laterally about neurodegenerative proteinopathies. J Clin Invest. 2013;123(5):1847–55. https://doi.org/10.1172/JCI66029.
2. Association A. 2019 Alzheimer's disease facts and figures. Alzheimer's Dementia. 2019;15(3):321–87. https://doi.org/10.1016/j.jalz.2019.01.010.
3. Grady CL. Brain imaging and age-related changes in cognition. Exp Gerontol. 1998;33(7–8):661–73. https://doi.org/10.1016/s0531-5565(98)00022-9.
4. Ganguly G, Chakrabarti S, Chatterjee U, Saso L. Proteinopathy, oxidative stress and mitochondrial dysfunction: cross talk in Alzheimer's disease and Parkinson's disease. Drug Des Devel Ther. 2017;11:797. https://doi.org/10.2147/DDDT.S130514.
5. Maruszak A, Gaweda-Walerych K, Sołtyszewski I, Zekanowski C. Mitochondrial DNA in pathogenesis of Alzheimer's and Parkinson's diseases. Acta Neurobiol Exp. 2006;66(2):153.
6. Biomarkers Definitions Working Group. Biomarkers and surrogate endpoints: preferred definitions and conceptual framework. Clin Pharmacol Ther. 2001;69(3):89–95.
7. Morgan JC, Mehta SH, Sethi K. Biomarkers in Parkinson's disease. Curr Neurol Neurosci Rep. 2010;10(6):423–30. https://doi.org/10.1007/s11910-010-0144-0.
8. Poblador-Plou B, Calderón-Larrañaga A, Marta-Moreno J, Hancco-Saavedra J, Sicras-Mainar A, Soljak M, Prados-Torres A. Comorbidity of dementia: a cross-sectional study of primary care older patients. BMC Psychiatry. 2014;14(1):84. https://doi.org/10.1186/1471-244X-14-84.
9. Turner RS. Biomarkers of Alzheimer's disease and mild cognitive impairment: are we there yet? Exp Neurol. 2003;183(1):7–10. https://doi.org/10.1016/s0014-4886(03)00203-6.

10. Consensus report of the Working Group on molecular and biochemical markers of Alzheimer's disease. The Ronald and Nancy Reagan Research Institute of the Alzheimer's Association and the National Institute on Aging Working Group. Neurobiol Aging. 1998;19(2):109–16.
11. Clos AL, Kayed R, Lasagna Reeves CA. Association of skin with the pathogenesis and treatment of neurodegenerative amyloidosis. Front Neurol. 2012;3:5. https://doi.org/10.3389/fneur.2012.00005.
12. Sharma N, McLean PJ, Kawamata H, Irizarry MC, Hyman BT. Alpha-synuclein has an altered conformation and shows a tight intermolecular interaction with ubiquitin in Lewy bodies. Acta Neuropathol. 2001;102(4):329–34.
13. Clayton DF, George JM. Synucleins in synaptic plasticity and neurodegenerative disorders. J Neurosci Res. 1999;58(1):12012–9.
14. Parihar MS, Parihar A, Fujita M, Hashimoto M, Ghafourifar P. Mitochondrial association of alpha-synuclein causes oxidative stress. Cell Mol Life Sci. 2008;65(7–8):1272–84. https://doi.org/10.1007/s00018-008-7589-1.
15. Wennström M, Surova Y, Hall S, Nilsson C, Minthon L, Boström F, Hansson O, Nielsen HM. Low CSF levels of both α-synuclein and the α-synuclein cleaving enzyme neurosin in patients with synucleinopathy. PLoS ONE. 2013;8(1): e53250. https://doi.org/10.1371/journal.pone.0053250.
16. Beyer K, Domingo-Sábat M, Lao JI, Carrato C, Ferrer I, Ariza A. Identification and characterization of a new alpha-synuclein isoform and its role in Lewy body diseases. Neurogenetics. 2008;9(1):15–23. https://doi.org/10.1007/s10048-007-0106-0.
17. Bisaglia M, Trolio A, Bellanda M, Bergantino E, Bubacco L, Mammi S. Structure and topology of the non-amyloid-β component fragment of human α-synuclein bound to micelles: implications for the aggregation process. Protein Sci. 2006;15(6):1408–16. https://doi.org/10.1110/ps.052048706.
18. Fonseca-Ornelas L, Eisbach SE, Paulat M, Giller K, Fernández CO, Outeiro TF, Becker S, Zweckstetter M. Small molecule-mediated stabilization of vesicleassociated helical α-synuclein inhibits pathogenic misfolding and aggregation. Nat Commun. 2014;5:5857. https://doi.org/10.1038/ncomms6857.
19. Freeman D, Cedillos R, Choyke S, Lukic Z, McGuire K, Marvin S, Burrage AM, Sudholt S, Rana A, O'Connor C, Wiethoff CM, Campbell EM. Alpha-synuclein induces lysosomal rupture and cathepsin dependent reactive oxygen species following endocytosis. PLoS ONE. 2013;8(4): e62143. https://doi.org/10.1371/journal.pone.0062143.
20. Frost B, Diamond MI. Prion-like mechanisms in neurodegenerative diseases. Nat Rev Neurosci. 2010;11(3):155–9. https://doi.org/10.1038/nrn2786.
21. Schaser AJ, Osterberg VR, Dent SE, Stackhouse TL, Wakeham CM, Boutros SW, Weston LJ, Owen N, Weissman TA, Luna E, Raber J, Luk KC, McCullough AK, Woltjer RL, Unni VK. Alpha-synuclein is a DNA binding protein that modulates DNA repair with implications for Lewy body disorders. Sci Rep. 2019;9(1):10919. https://doi.org/10.1038/s41598-019-47227-z.
22. Meles SK, Teune LK, de Jong BM, Dierckx RA, Leenders KL. Metabolic imaging in Parkinson disease. J Nucl Med. 2017;58(1):23–8. https://doi.org/10.2967/jnumed.116.183152.
23. Kassubek J. MRI-based neuroimaging: atypical parkinsonisms and other movement disorders. Curr Opinion Neurol. 2018;31(4):425–30. https://doi.org/10.1097/WCO.0000000000000578.
24. Seifan A, Schelke M, Obeng-Aduasare Y, Isaacson R. Early life epidemiology of Alzheimer's disease—a critical review. Neuroepidemiology. 2015;45(4):237–54. https://doi.org/10.1159/000439568.
25. Garre-Olmo J. Epidemiology of Alzheimer's disease and other dementias. Rev Neurol. 2018;66(11):377–86.
26. Mudher A, Colin M, Dujardin S, Medina M, Dewachter I, Alavi Naini SM, Mandelkow EM, Mandelkow E, Buée L, Goedert M, Brion JP. What is the evidence that tau pathology spreads through prion-like propagation? Acta Neuropathol Commun. 2017;5(1):99. https://doi.org/10.1186/s40478-017-0488-7.
27. Selkoe DJ. Cell biology of protein misfolding: the examples of Alzheimer's and Parkinson's diseases. Nat Cell Biol. 2004;6(11):1054–61. https://doi.org/10.1038/ncb1104-1054.

28. Sergeant N, et al. Biochemistry of Tau in Alzheimer's disease and related neurological disorders. Expert Rev Proteomics. 2008;5(2):207–24.
29. Braak H, Braak E. Neuropathological stageing of Alzheimer-related changes. Acta Neuropathol. 1991;82(4):239–59. https://doi.org/10.1007/BF00308809.
30. Braak H, Braak E. Staging of Alzheimer's disease-related neurofibrillary changes. Neurobiol Aging. 1995;16(3):271–8. https://doi.org/10.1016/0197-4580(95)00021-6.
31. Miki Y, Tomiyama M, Ueno T, Haga R, Nishijima H, Suzuki C, Mori F, Kaimori M, Baba M, Wakabayashi K. Clinical availability of skin biopsy in the diagnosis of Parkinson's disease. Neurosci Lett. 2010;469(3):357–9. https://doi.org/10.1016/j.neulet.2009.12.027.
32. Rentería-Palomo AA, Rodriguez-Leyva I, Valdes-Rodríguez R, Fuentes-Ahumada C, Calderon-Garciduenas AL, Moncada B, Castanedo Cazares JP. Expression of alpha-synuclein in skin patients with Parkinson's disease. J Invest Dermatol. 2011;131(75):10013–1917.
33. Rodríguez-Leyva I, Rentería-Palomo AA, Calderón-Garcidueñas A, Fuentes-Ahumada C, Hernández HE, Mendoza-Esquivel F, Castanedo-Cázares JP. Usefulness of α-synuclein as a marker for early diagnosis of Parkinson's disease in skin biopsy (S22.005). Neurology; 2012:78 (1 Supplement).
34. Donadio V, Incensi A, Leta V, Giannoccaro MP, Scaglione C, Martinelli P, Capellari S, Avoni P, Baruzzi A, Liguori R. Skin nerve α-synuclein deposits: a biomarker for idiopathic Parkinson disease. Neurology. 2014;82(15):1362–9. https://doi.org/10.1212/WNL.0000000000000316.
35. Rodríguez-Leyva I, Calderón-Garcidueñas AL, Jiménez-Capdeville ME, Rentería-Palomo AA, Hernández-Rodríguez HG, Valdés-Rodríguez R, Fuentes-Ahumada C, Torres-Álvarez B, Sepúlveda-Saavedra J, Soto-Domínguez A, Santoyo ME, Rodríguez-Moreno JI, Castanedo-Cázares JP. α-Synuclein inclusions in the skin of Parkinson's disease and parkinsonism. Ann Clin Transl Neurol. 2014;1(7):471–8. https://doi.org/10.1002/acn3.78.
36. Rodríguez-Leyva I, Calderón-Garcidueñas A, Santoyo M, Chi E, Medina-Mier V, Jiménez-Capdeville M. Progressive supranuclear palsy (PSP): diagnosis through skin biopsy (P1.014). Neurology. 2014;82.
37. Rodríguez-Leyva I, Calderón-Garcidueñas A, Santoyo M, Chi E, Medina-Mier V, Jiménez-Capdeville M. Presence of phosphorylated tau, alpha-synuclein and amyloid protein in the skin of patients with clinical diagnosis of Alzheimer disease (S38.003). Neurology. 2014;82.
38. Rodríguez-Leyva I, Chi-Ahumada E, Calderón-Garcidueñas A, Medina-Mier V, Martel-Gallegos G, Zarazúa S, Jiménez-Capdeville M. Skin cells express altered proteins that characterize the most common neurodegenerative diseases (S33.006). Neurology. 2015;84 (14 Supplement).
39. British Broadcasting Corporation. Científicos en México proponen prueba cutánea para detectar Alzheimer. https://www.bbc.com/mundo/ultimas_noticias/2015/02/150225_ultnot_alzheimer_piel_prueba_wbm. https://www.scientificamerican.com/espanol/noticias/elalzheimer-y-el-parkinson-podrian-detectarse-en-la-piel/. Accessed 18 June 2021.
40. Anderson P. Skin test may aid Alzheimer's, Parkinson's diagnosis. 2015. https://www.medscape.com/viewarticle/840387. Accessed 18 June 2021.
41. American Academy of Neurology. Skin test may shed new light on Alzheimer's and Parkinson's diseases. 2015. https://www.mdedge.com/neurology/article/99000/movementdisorders/skin-test-may-shed-new-light-alzheimers-and-parkinsons. Accesed 18 June 2021.
42. Rodríguez-Leyva I, Chi-Ahumada E, Calderón-Garcidueñas A, Medina-Mier V, Santoyo M, Martel-Gallegos G, Zarazúa S, Carrizales-Rodríguez J, Jiménez-Capdeville M. Presence of phosphorylated tau protein in the skin of Alzheimer's disease patients. J Mol Biomark Diagn. 2015;S6:005–10. https://doi.org/10.4172/2155-9929.S6-005.
43. Rodriguez-Leyva I, Jimenez-Capdeville M, Chi-Ahumada E, Eng W, Saikaly S, Carrizalez-Rodriguez J, Castanedo-Cazares J, Norman R. Expression of proteinopathies in the skin: alpha-synuclein in cells derived from the neural crest and in Parkinson disease. Neurology. 2016;86(16 Suppl):P6.238.
44. Rodríguez-Leyva I, Chi-Ahumada E, Mejía M, Castanedo-Cazares JP, Eng W, Saikaly SK, Carrizales J, Levine TD, Norman RA, Jiménez-Capdeville ME. The presence of alpha-synuclein in skin from Melanoma and patients with Parkinson's disease. Mov Disord Clin Pract. 2017;4(5):724–32. https://doi.org/10.1002/mdc3.12494.

45. Dean DN, Lee JC. Linking Parkinson's disease and Melanoma: interplay between α-synuclein and Pmel17 amyloid formation. Mov Disord. 2021. https://doi.org/10.1002/mds.28655. Epub ahead of print. PMID: 34021920.
46. Dexter DN, Lee JC. Linking Parkinson's disease and melanoma: interplay between α-synuclein and Pmel17 amyloid formation. Mov Disord. 2021. https://doi.org/10.1002/mds.28655.
47. Arredondo LF, Aranda-Romo S, Rodríguez-Leyva I, Chi-Ahumada E, Saikaly SK, Portales-Pérez DP, González-Amaro R, Salgado-Bustamante M, Enriquez-Macias L, Eng W, Norman RA, Jimenez-Capdeville ME. Tau protein in oral Mucosa and cognitive state: a cross-sectional study. Front Neurol. 2017;8:554. https://doi.org/10.3389/fneur.2017.00554.
48. Mejía M, Rodríguez-Leyva I, Cortés-Enríquez F, Chi-Ahumada E, Portales-Pérez DP, Macías-Islas MA, Jiménez-Capdeville ME. Low levels of alpha-synuclein in peripheral tissues are related to clinical relapse in relapsing-remitting multiple sclerosis: a pilot cross-sectional study. J Neurol Sci. 2019;396:87–93. https://doi.org/10.1016/j.jns.2018.11.003.
49. Wang Z, Becker K, Donadio V, Siedlak S, Yuan J, Rezaee M, Incensi A, Kuzkina A, Orrú CD, Tatsuoka C, Liguori R, Gunzler SA, Caughey B, Jimenez-Capdeville ME, Zhu X, Doppler K, Cui L, Chen SG, Ma J, Zou WQ. Skin α-synuclein aggregation seeding activity as a novel biomarker for Parkinson disease. JAMA Neurol. 2010;78:1–11. https://doi.org/10.1001/jamaneurol.2020.3311.
50. Donadio V, Wang Z, Incensi A, Rizzo G, Fileccia E, Vacchiano V, Capellari S, Magnani M, Scaglione C, Stanzani Maserati M, Avoni P, Liguori R, Zou W. In vivo diagnosis of synucleinopathies: a comparative study of skin biopsy and RT-QuIC. Neurology. 2021;96(20):e2513–24. https://doi.org/10.1212/WNL.0000000000011935.

Chapter 8
Skin Biomarker in Parkinson Disease

Donadio Vincenzo

Abstract Parkinson's disease (PD) is the second most common neurodegenerative disease. The majority of PD patients presented an idiopathic disease (IPD), whereas a small subgroup showed a genetic form. At present, the IPD diagnosis is largely based on clinical criteria. Due to the imperfect sensitivity and specificity, a combination of diagnostic tests has been proposed to achieve an acceptable sensitivity and specificity for the PD diagnosis. This chapter is focused on analyzing skin biopsy as new biomarker for PD. Skin biopsy represents a promising diagnostic tool for PD and other synucleinopathies also suitable for the in vivo study of pathogenetic mechanisms correlated to misfolded α-syn deposition in neurons.

Keywords PD · Skin · Diagnostic criteria · Tissues biomarkers · Skin biopsy

8.1 Parkinson's Disease

Parkinson's disease (PD) is the second most common neurodegenerative disease, estimated to occur in approximately 1% of individuals > 60 years of age, a number predicted to more than double by 2030, because of the aging population [24]. The majority of PD patients presented an idiopathic disease (IPD), whereas a small subgroup showed a genetic form of this disease (GPD) associated with dominant or recessive mutations mainly involving α-synuclein, LRRK2, PINK1, parkin or DJ-1 genes [45].

Clinical features of IPD include four cardinal signs that can be grouped under the acronym TRAP: Tremor at rest, Rigidity, Akinesia (or bradykinesia) and Postural instability. In addition, flexed posture and freezing (motor blocks) have been included among classic features of parkinsonism, with PD as the most common form. In

D. Vincenzo (✉)
IRCCS Istituto Delle Scienze Neurologiche, UOC Clinica Neurologica, Via Altura 3, 40139 Bologna, Italy
e-mail: vincenzo.donadio@unibo.it

Dipartimento di Scienze Biomediche e Neuromotorie, Università di Bologna, Bologna, Italy

R. Norman (ed.), *Biomarkers in Dermatology*,
https://doi.org/10.1007/978-3-031-66513-4_8

addition, several non-motor symptoms are a common and underappreciated feature of IPD [79]. These include autonomic dysfunction, cognitive/neurobehavioral disorders and sensory and sleep abnormalities and sometimes could also be the early symptoms of IPD anticipating motor dysfunctions. Because of the diverse profiles and lifestyles of patients affected by IPD, motor and non-motor impairments should be evaluated in the context of each patient's needs and goals [37].

A number of rating scales are used for the evaluation of motor impairment and disability in patients with IPD. The Hoehn and Yahr scale is commonly used to compare groups of patients and to provide gross assessment of disease progression, ranging from stage 0 (no signs of disease) to stage 5 (wheelchair bound or bedridden unless assisted). The Unified Parkinson's Disease Rating scale (UPDRS) revised by the Movement Disorder Society (MDS) is the most well established scale for assessing disability and impairment [32]. Studies making use of MDS-UPDRS to track the progression of PD suggest that the course of PD is not linear and that the rate of deterioration is variable and more rapid in the early phase of the disease and in patients with the postural instability gait difficulty (PIGD) of PD [36, 43, 57]. In a large study prospectively followed-up 297 patients (181 men, 116 women) with clinically diagnosed PD for at least 3 years the total MDS-UPDRS scores increased of 1.34 points when assessed during ON and 1.58 points when assessed during OFF [37]. Patients who were older and had the postural instability gait difficulty form of PD at onset experienced more rapid disease progression than did those who were younger at onset and had the tremor dominant form of PD. On the other hand, many studies have shown that younger patients are at a higher risk for levodopa induced dyskinesias than older patients [38]. In a prospective study of 145 clinic-based patients followed-up for 1 year and of 124 community-based patients followed-up for 4 years, the annual mean rate of deterioration in motor and disability scores ranged from 2.4 to 7.4% [64]. Other types of rating scales include those that assess psychiatric manifestations (e.g., depression) [62] and quality of life [27, 62].

8.2 The Diagnosis of Parkinson's Disease

At present, the IPD diagnosis is largely based on clinical criteria. Several sets of clinical diagnostic criteria have been proposed, based mainly on the presence of the classical motor signs of the disease, combined with the absence of incompatible or atypical signs (the so-called red flags suggestive of atypical parkinsonism). The most widely used clinical criteria for the diagnosis of PD are those introduced by the Queen Square Brain Bank (QSBB) [30]. These criteria provide a three-step method:

1. Signs that must be present
2. Signs that should not be present
3. Supportive criteria

The first diagnostic step requires the presence of bradykinesia which is not just slowness of movements but rather a progressive fatiguing and decrement of repetitive alternating movements during finger or foot tapping [2]. In addition, important signs to be considered included muscular rigidity, 4- to 6-Hz rest tremor and/or postural instability not caused by primary visual, vestibular, cerebellar or proprioceptive dysfunctions. The second step involves a checklist of symptoms and signs that argue against a diagnosis of PD such as history of repeated strokes with stepwise progression of parkinsonian features or neuroleptic treatment at onset of symptoms or cerebellar or Babinski signs. Finally, the diagnosis of PD requires the presence of three or more supportive criteria as unilateral onset, rest tremor present, progressive disorder, excellent response to L-dopa for at least 5 years or hyposmia.

However, the clinical accuracy of PD diagnosis is low ranging close to 50% in the early disease stage [3]. This leads to a frequent misdiagnosis as underlined by autopsy studies reporting that 20% of patients with a clinical diagnosis of MSA showed instead PD or DLB [41] or alternatively MSA patients presenting with parkinsonism may be misdiagnosed as PD [56]. Misdiagnosis could be responsible for delayed treatment or increased risk of drug-related adverse events and can lead to wrong eligibility for clinical trials preventing to develop a disease-modifying treatment. Thus, although the QSBB clinical diagnostic criteria are widely used in clinical practice, a number of pitfalls have been recognized:

1. Having more than one affected relative cannot be considered an exclusion criterion of PD anymore;
2. Some of the supportive criteria such as persistent asymmetry, prolonged disease course or continuous levodopa response may occur in atypical parkinsonian disorders as well. A critical revision of the QSBB criteria will be required to address these drawbacks.

In addition, clinical expertise of the neurologist assessing PD diagnosis has been shown to predict the diagnostic effectiveness of the QSBB clinical diagnostic criteria in two independent studies [47]. In the first study, the QSBB clinical diagnostic criteria were applied by movement disorder specialists to 402 cases previously diagnosed as PD from general practitioners in North Wales [47]. A definite diagnosis of PD could be reached in only 53% of cases, suggesting an error rate of 47% outside of specialized centers. The most common misdiagnoses were essential tremor, Alzheimer's disease and vascular parkinsonism. The second study compared the diagnostic accuracy of PD clinical diagnosis, as made by movement disorder experts, in comparison with non-expert physicians in the community [63]. In this study, 126 patients with a pre-existing clinical diagnosis of probable or possible PD underwent diagnostic reassessment by movement disorder specialists using the QSBB clinical diagnostic criteria. The results showed that experts reached a greater sensitivity (93.5% for experts versus 73.5% for non-experts) and positive predictive value (88.7% for experts versus 73.5% for non-experts), whereas the negative predictive value was similar (76.9% for experts vs. 79.1% for non-experts) [63]. These results underscored a relatively high diagnostic inaccuracy by non-experts.

Even if made by a movement disorder expert, PD diagnosis may change at follow-up, for several reasons: development of atypical signs (red flags), insufficient response to dopaminergic treatment or neuroimaging clues for an alternative diagnosis. This makes important to support the clinical diagnosis by means of reliable biomarkers obtained by using standardized tests.

8.3 Diagnostic Markers for Parkinson's Disease Diagnosis

Due to the imperfect sensitivity and specificity, a combination of diagnostic tests has been proposed to achieve an acceptable sensitivity and specificity for the PD diagnosis [65, 67]. They mainly included olfactory function testing, cardiovascular autonomic testing, biological fluids (including CSF and blood) testing and imaging.

8.3.1 Olfactory Function Testing

It has been extensively studied as a diagnostic marker for Parkinson's disease even in the premotor and preclinical disease phase. Standardized tests of olfactory function include the University of Pennsylvania Smell Identification Test (UPSIT) [26] and Sniffin' Sticks [35, 40]. Olfactory dysfunction is present in more than 90% of Parkinson's disease patients [25], with deficits present in odor identification, discrimination, and threshold [51, 70]. In addition, in early Parkinson's disease, olfactory dysfunction correlates with the extent of striatal dopaminergic loss as assessed by radiolabeled tracer imaging [68], but it does not otherwise correlate with disease duration or severity [68].

8.3.2 Cardiovascular Autonomic Testing

Uptake of I-123-metaiodobenzylguanidine (MIBG) on cardiac SPECT imaging reflects cardiac postganglionic sympathetic innervation. A reducted MIBG SPECT signal has been reported in patients with Parkinson's disease [52]. Nevertheless MIBG SPECT has low specificity, in distinguishing PD from different parkinos-misms syndromes [76]. However, most MIBG scintigraphy studies demonstrated that myocardial sympathetic innervation was normal in Multiple System Atrophy (MSA) patients although a mildly reduced sympathetic innervation has been reported in some cases [55, 71]. In contrast, multiple imaging studies with MIBG in PD patients have shown decreased cardiac uptake, indicating myocardial postganglionic sympathetic dysfunction, even when cardiovascular reflexes remain intact [55, 71]. However, in early stages of PD, MIBG uptake can be normal [61]. Overall, recent meta-analyses suggest that MIBG imaging is useful to discriminate PD from MSA in moderate to advanced disease stages, but unreliable in early stages since early stage PD patients may have a normal cardiac sympathetic innervation [55, 71]. In addition, MSA cannot be discriminated from neurodegenerative disorders of different origin (i.e., tauopathies as progressive supranuclear palsy-PSP) based on MIBG scintigraphy alone [42].

8.3.3 Magnetic Resonance Imaging

Conventional magnetic resonance imaging (MRI) and magnetic resonance spectroscopy are of little utility for the diagnosis of PD, although conventional MRI is important for the exclusion of secondary causes of parkinsonism [69]. Diffusion weighted imaging may be useful in distinguishing MSA-P [54] and tauopathies (as PSP and corticobasal disorder-CBD) [59] from PD. Other promising MRI techniques in the PD diagnosis included measurement of midbrain proton transverse relaxation time (as an estimate of iron content) using high field strength MRI [46] and assessment of fractional anisotropy using diffusion tensor imaging [72].

8.3.4 CSF and Blood

A decrease of total alpha-synuclein levels has been reported in the CSF of PD patients [34, 50]. However, the diagnostic utility of alpha-synuclein is poor [9] and the detection of specific target such as DJ-1 levels [34] or neurofilament light chain [1] holds more promising. In addition, low CSF tau form ratio is useful in distinguishing PSP from PD [10] and CSF amyloid-b peptides in distinguishing dementia with Lewy body disease from PD with dementia [7]. Taking into consideration, all available data probably a combination of CSF tests will be of greatest utility for PD diagnosis [1].

As for CSF, even plasma alpha-synuclein has not been useful as a diagnostic tool [44, 66].

8.3.5 Transcranial Doppler Ultrasonography

PD patients showed an increased echogenicity of the substantia nigra on transcranial Doppler ultrasonography [6, 74] that likely reflect an increased iron content and ferritin together with reduced neuromelanin [74, 78]. Hyperechogenicity of the substantia nigra is useful in distinguishing PD from healthy controls [58] and PD from parkinsonisms [5, 73]. However, the specificity of this technique is relatively low which precludes its use in isolation as a diagnostic test, and the difficulty to achieve enough bone windows, particularly in older adults, can interfere with testing in up to 15% of patients [6].

8.3.6 *Positron Emission Tomography (PET) or SPECT Imaging*

The use of radiolabeled tracer using is important to ascertain a nigro-striatal terminals damage. This test is promising for the early detection of PD or for disease severity and progression [11]. Radiolabeled tracers used in PD mainly include molecules that bind to the presynaptic markers such as vesicular monoamine transporter type 2 (VMAT2), 18F-DOPA, a cocaine analogs such as 11C-WIN, 123Ib-FP-CIT or 99mTc-TRODAT binding to the presynaptic dopamine transporter [28, 29]. Technical differences exist between these tracers and the use of PET and SPECT [29]. This test is useful in distinguishing PD from psychogenic parkinsonism or essential tremor [8, 39] but may not be as useful in distinguishing PD from other parkinsonisms such as MSA and PSP [12].

8.4 Skin Biopsy in Parkinson's Disease

The skin biopsy allows to study the skin innervation contained in a small sample. Skin biopsy is an easily performed, inexpensive and minimally invasive technique with minor discomfort for the patient.

The skin innervation includes a more superficial epidermal innervation belonging to somatic fibers and a deeper autonomic innervation in the dermis.

The epidermal innervation encompasses nociceptors as free-ending fibers in the epidermal layer originating from the subepidermal plexus.

Autonomic fibers are included deeper in the dermis. The autonomic innervation of hairy skin encompasses different subsets of adrenergic and cholinergic fibers both in humans and animals but the chemical code of autonomic nerve terminals is complex and not well known. This is unfortunate since the neuropeptide content of a fiber subpopulation is likely to define important aspects of its functional characteristics. The hairy skin autonomic innervation contains sympathetic (both adrenergic and cholinergic) and parasympathetic fibers co-expressing specific neuropeptides. They are differentially distributed in skin structures. NPY is co-expressed in adrenergic fibers of skin vessels and sweat glands but absent in adrenergic fibers of arrector pili muscles, whereas CGRP, VIP and SP are co-expressed in cholinergic fibers both of sympathetic and parasympathetic types [16].

8.4.1 Skin Deposition of Misfolded α-synuclein as Biomarker for PD

The autonomic skin innervation is a useful site for the search of abnormal α-syn aggregates since peripheral sympathetic nerves could be the earliest affected neural region and autonomic symptoms may precede the classical symptoms of synucleinopathy, such as motor dysfunction in PD [13]. The Table reported the main in vivo study of skin innervation in PD.

Primary antibody	Authors	Reference test	Features of patients (age, H&Y, disease duration)	Sampling site	Sample number	Sampling technique	Technique	Fixation	Embedding	Section thickness	Section number	Neuronal marker
Syn: N4 pSyn: P2, P5	Donadio et al. [16]	Gelb's criteria UKBBC	66 (+-9), 2,4 (± 1) 8(± 10) Wurzburg/ Marborg 68 (± 7), 2,6 (± 1) 6 (± 2) Bologna,	C7 paravertebral area, thigh, distal leg	6	3-mm punch biopsy	Dual-label immunofluorescence	Cold Zamboni, overnight	Frozen	10 μ	50	PGP 9.5
Syn: N4 pSyn: P2, P5	Donadio et al. [15]	UKBBC	70(± 3), 6(± 4)	C7 paravertebral area, thigh, distal leg	6	3-mm punch biopsy	Dual-label immunofluorescence	Cold Zamboni, overnight	Frozen	10 micron	24	PGP 9.5
Syn: N4 pSyn: P2, P5	Donadio et al. [18]	Gelb's criteria	68 (± 7), 1.9 (± 0.5), 8 (± 5)	C7 paravertebral area, thigh, distal leg	6	3-mm punch biopsy	Dual-label immunofluorescence	Cold Zamboni, overnight	Frozen	10 μ	24	PGP 9.5, DBH, VIP
pSyn: P1	Donadio et al. [17]	Gelb's criteria	71 (± 8), 2.7 (± 0.9), 13 (± 6)	C7 paravertebral area, thigh, distal leg	6	3-mm punch biopsy	Dual-label immunofluorescence	Cold Zamboni, overnight	Frozen	10 μ	24	PGP 9.5, DBH, VIP
pSyn: P5	Doppler [21]	UKBBC	65 (34–88), 3 (1–5), 9 (0–27)	Th12 paravertebral area, proximal leg, distal leg, index finger	4	5 or 3-mm punch biopsy	Dual-label immunofluorescence	4% PFA	Frozen	20 μ	3	PGP 9.5, VIP, TH, CGRP, SP, S100, MBP

(continued)

(continued)

Primary antibody	Authors	Reference test	Features of patients (age, H&Y, disease duration)	Sampling site	Sample number	Sampling technique	Technique	Fixation	Embedding	Section thickness	Section number	Neuronal marker
pSyn: P6	Doppler [22]	UKBBC	67, N.S, 12	Th12 paravertebral area, proximal leg, distal leg	3	5-mm punch biopsy	Dual-label immunofluorescence	4% PFA, 30 min	Frozen	20 μ	5	PGP 9.5, VIP, TH, CGRP, SP, S100, MBP
pSyn: P7	Doppler [23]	UKBBC	63 [59-67] 1.5 (± 0.5) N.S	Th12 paravertebral area, proximal leg, distal leg	3	5-mm punch biopsy	Dual-label immunofluorescence	4% PFA, 30 min	Frozen	20 μ	5	PGP 9.5
pSyn: P1	Navarro-Otano et al. [53]	UKBBC	67 (± 8) 2.1 (± 0.7) 10 (± 6)	Distal leg	1	3-mm punch biopsy	Conventional immunohistochemistry	10% formaldehyde	Paraffin	5 μ	N.S	PGP 9.5, TH
pSyn: P1	Zange [77]	UKBBC	70 (± 9), NS, 6 (± 4)	Ventral forearm	1	3-mm punch biopsy	Conventional immunohistochemistry	4% formaldehyde (24 h-2 weeks)	Paraffin	3 μ	N.S	PGP 9.5, TH
nSyn: N12, N13	Rodríguez-Leyva [60]	UKBBC	68 (± 9), 3,5 (± 0,8) 6,1 (± 3,8)	3 cm behind the ear insertion	N.S	4-mm punch biopsy	Conventional immunohistochemistry Dual-label immunofluorescence	4% formaldehyde, 24 h	Paraffin	5 μ	N.S	*
pSyn: P1	Haga [33]	UKBBC	64,1(± 5,7), 2,5(± 0,7,) 4,8 (± 3,2)	Chest wall, lower limb	N.S	6-mm punch biopsy	Dual-label immunofluorescence	Cold Zamboni, overnight	Frozen	60 μ	N.S	PGP 9.5
nSyn: N4	Wang [75]	N.S	61(± 10), 2,6(± 1) 4 (± 4)	Proximal thigh, distal thigh, distal leg	3	3-mm punch biopsy	Dual-label immunofluorescence	Cold Zamboni, 18 h	Frozen	50 μ	N.S	PGP 9.5, DBH, VIP, TH

(continued)

(continued)

Primary antibody	Authors	Reference test	Features of patients (age, H&Y, disease duration)	Sampling site	Sample number	Sampling technique	Technique	Fixation	Embedding	Section thickness	Section number	Neuronal marker
nSyn: N2 pSyn: P1	Melli [48]	UKBBC	66 (57–73), N.S, 5 (3–8)	C8 paravertebral area, thigh, distal leg	6	3-mm punch biopsy	Dual-label immunofluorescence	2% PLP, N.S	Frozen	50 μ	8	PGP 9.5
nSyn	Gibbons [31]	UKBBC	NAF: 2.0 (± 0.3) AF: 2.2 (± 0.4) N.S, NAF: 4 (± 5) AF: 9 (± 7)	Ventral forearm, proximal thigh, distal thigh, distal leg	4	3-mm punch biopsy	Dual-label immunofluorescence	Cold Zamboni, 18 h	Frozen	50 μ	20	PGP 9.5
	Nolano	UKBBC	62,7 (± 8), 2,6 (± 1), 7,6 (± 5)	Fingertip, thigh and distal leg	N.S	3-mm punch biopsy	Dual-label immunofluorescence	N:S	N:S	50 μ	N:S	PGP 9.5
pSyn	Miki [49]	UKBBC	65,4 (± 7,3), 2,8 (± 0,9), 5,7 (± 4)	Chest wall (central precordium) and lower limb (10 cm above the lateral malleolus)	6	3-mm punch biopsy	Conventional immunohistochemistry	10% buffered formalin for 48 h	Paraffin	30 μ	3	*

NAF not autonomic failure
AF with autonomic failure
*Localization in neuronal structures was confirmed in adjacent sections stained with neuronal markers using conventional immunohistochemistry
Primary antibodies against native α-synuclein (n-syn):
N1 = mouse anti-α-synuclein monoclonal antibody (Santa Cruz Biotechnology, catalog number unknown)
N2 = mouse anti-α-synuclein monoclonal antibody (Analytik Jena AG or Roboscreen, clone 5G4)
N3 = mouse anti-α-synuclein monoclonal antibody (Novocastra or Leica Biosystems, clone KM51)

N4 = rabbit anti-α-synuclein polyclonal antibody (Millipore or Chemicon, catalog number ab5038)
N5 = mouse anti-α-synuclein monoclonal antibody (Cell Signaling, clone Syn 204)
N6 = mouse anti-α-synuclein monoclonal antibody (Abcam, clone MJFR1)
N7 = rat anti-α-synuclein monoclonal antibody (Enzo Life Sciences, clone 15G7)
N8 = mouse anti-α-synuclein monoclonal antibody (Abcam or Zymed or Invitrogen, clone LB509)
N9 = mouse anti-α-synuclein monoclonal antibody (custom-made, clone 3G5)
N10 = rabbit anti-α-synuclein polyclonal antibody (Gene Way Biotech, catalog number GWB-F102F6)
N11 = mouse anti-α-synuclein monoclonal antibody (BD Biosciences, clone 42)
N12 = anti-α-synuclein polyclonal antibody (Thermo Scientific, Rockford, IL)
N13 = anti-α-synuclein monoclonal antibody (Becton, Dickinson and Co. Franklin Lakes NJ, USA)
Primary antibodies against phosphorylated α-synuclein (p-syn):
P1 = mouse anti-α-synuclein phosphorylated at serine-129 monoclonal antibody (WAKO, clone pSyn#64)
P2 = rabbit anti-α-synuclein phosphorylated at serine-129 monoclonal antibody (Abcam, clone EP1536Y)
P3 = rabbit anti-α-synuclein phosphorylated at serine-129 monoclonal antibody (Abcam, clone MJF-R13 (8–8))
P4 = rabbit anti-α-synuclein phosphorylated at serine-129 polyclonal antibody (Abcam, catalog number ab59264)
P5 = mouse anti-α-synuclein phosphorylated at serine-129 monoclonal antibody (BioLegend or Covance, clone P-Syn/81A)
P6 = rabbit anti-α-synuclein phosphorylated at serine-129 polyclonal antibody (custom-made)

Skin biopsy was able to differentiate IPD from healthy controls and different forms of parkinsonism by searching for proximal peripheral nerve deposits of phosphorylated α-synuclein, considered the pathological form of α-synuclein. In addition, Doppler et al. [19] reported that this approach was able to identify abnormal α-synuclein deposits in skin nerves as found in post-mortem brain tissue of PD patients supporting this approach as in vivo diagnostic tool for synucleinopathies. Reported data showed that neuritic Lewy body inclusions account for > 90% of sporadic PD [53]. Subsequent studies disclosed a highest sensitivity (100%) by studying two cervical skin samples, whereas the analysis of only one sample may disclose a lower positivity rate [13]. This is due to a likely patchy deposition of misfolded α-synuclein in skin nerves and to the higher positivity in proximal (i.e., cervical) skin sites as suggested by a lower rate of positive staining in peripheral skin nerves of chest, abdominal or leg (ranging from 10 to 70%). The higher positivity in the proximal (i.e., cervical) sites is interesting since these sites included the skin around the spine, i.e., close to autonomic ganglia, and the possibility of detecting p-syn with higher incidence in this site may suggest that misfolded α-syn comes from ganglia and spread up firstly to the closest autonomic skin terminals. In line with this explication, abnormal α-syn deposits may reach the longest autonomic terminals in the distal leg later and to a lesser extent. By contrast, it is possible to speculate that the widespread p-syn distribution in skin autonomic nerves in PD with OH [15] may support a different pathogenetic mechanism with misfolded α-syn arising in autonomic nerve terminals or the higher α-syn aggregates in these disorders could be due to more favorable predisposing conditions.

Another important aspect that should be underlined is that studies reaching the highest rate of pathological α-synuclein positivity were based on a new, advanced immunohistochemistry technique. This technique was settled up in the skin biopsy laboratory of Bologna and it is based on an indirect immunofluorescence method [13]. Shortly, this technique is based on the correspondence between two different staining in the same image by using different fluorescent filter: the first staining allows to disclose the skin innervation by using a pan-neuronal marker (i.e., PGP), while the second staining may allow to disclose the pathological form of α-synuclein phosphorylated at Ser 129 that can be found inside a nerve fiber. The correspondence between the two staining may help to verify the intraneuronal deposits of misfolded α-synuclein (Fig. 8.1), excluding possible non-specific staining arising from the background.

The analysis was usually made at high magnification (×40) using a fluorescent microscopy usually confocal (see Donadio [13] for details) in a blinded fashion to the clinical diagnosis. The inter- and intra-laboratory analyses of this technique revealed an excellent reproducibility supporting its use as diagnostic tool in clinical practice [14]. By using this technique, additional interesting findings have been collected in PD or prodromal PD. Data from the Bologna laboratory indicated the higher incidence of misfolded α-synuclein in skin nerves of paravertebral cervical C7 area compared to the thoracic Th12 area supporting a spine gradient [13]. Importantly, the analysis of C7 distribution of p-syn in patients with unilateral PD showed that abnormal deposits were evenly distributed between affected and non-affected motor

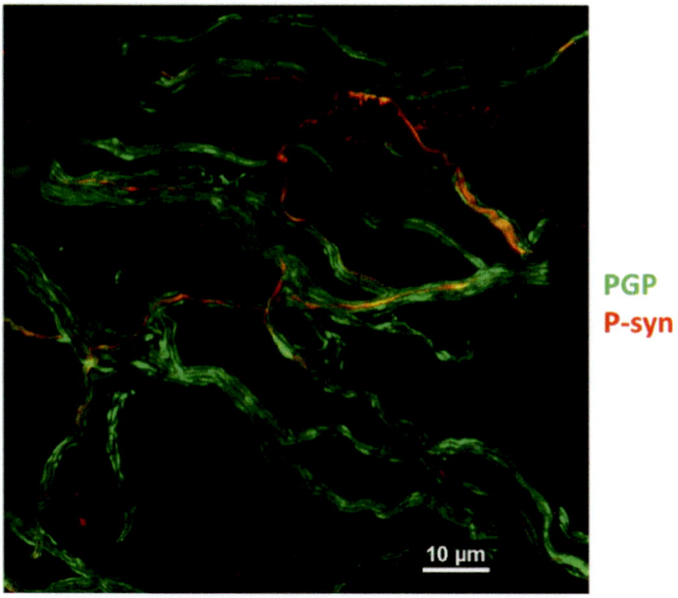

Fig. 8.1 Phosphorylated α-synuclein deposition around a skin arterioles of a PD patient. Confocal microscope (×400) study of phosphorylated α-synuclein deposits in skin nerves of a patient with PD. Nerve fibers around an arteriole in the deep derma are identified by a PGP 9.5 staining (green). Most of these fibers showed positive phosphorylated α-synuclein (stained by a p-syn antibody in red) as neuritic inclusions demonstrated by the merged image

side suggesting that skin nerves p-syn could be independent of the motor and nigrostriatal damage, whereas PD patients with bilateral motor symptoms presented with a widespread spine diffusion of p-syn. These findings point to the need to perform skin biopsy on both cervical sides when searching for p-syn in PD patients with prevalent unilateral motor dysfunctions [13].

Interestingly, the same distribution with the highest incidence of p-syn in proximal sites has been described in idiopathic REM sleep behavior disorder (iRBD), a clinical condition often preceding PD [4, 20]. These data come from the experience of few skin laboratories and need confirmation on a larger scale.

However, taking into account the several important results achieved by skin biopsy as diagnostic tool for PD, it should be underlined that skin biopsy represent a promising diagnostic tool for PD and other synucleinopathies also suitable for the in vivo study of pathogenetic mechanisms correlated to misfolded α-syn deposition in neurons.

References

1. Abdo WF, Bloem BR, Van Geel WJ, et al. CSF neurofilament light chain and tau differentiate multiple system atrophy from Parkinson's disease. Neurobiol Aging. 2007;28:742–7.
2. Abdo WF, van de Warrenburg BP, Burn DJ, Quinn NP, Bloem BR. The clinical approach to movement disorders. Nat Rev Neurol. 2010;6:29–37.
3. Adler CH, Beach TG, Hentz JG, et al. Low clinical diagnostic accuracy of early vs advanced Parkinson disease: clinicopathologic study. Neurology. 2014;83:406–12.
4. Antelmi E, Donadio V, Incensi A, Plazzi G, Liguori R. Skin nerve phosphorylated α-synuclein deposits in idiopathic REM sleep behavior disorder. Neurology. 2017;88(22):2128–31.
5. Behnke S, Berg D, Naumann M, Becker G. Differentiation of Parkinson's disease and atypical parkinsonian syndromes by transcranial ultrasound. J Neurol Neurosurg Psychiatry. 2005;76:423–5.
6. Berg D, Siefker C, Ruprecht-Dorfler P, Becker G. Relationship of substantia nigra echogenicity and motor function in elderly subjects. Neurology. 2001;56:13–7.
7. Bibl M, Mollenhauer B, Esselmann H, et al. CSF amyloid-beta-peptides in Alzheimer's disease, dementia with Lewy bodies and Parkinson's disease dementia. Brain. 2006;129:1177–87.
8. Booij J, Speelman JD, Horstink MW, Wolters EC. The clinical benefit of imaging striatal dopamine transporters with [123I]FP-CIT SPET in differentiating patients with presynaptic parkinsonism from those with other forms of parkinsonism. Eur J Nucl Med. 2001;28:266–72.
9. Borghi R, Marchese R, Negro A, et al. Full length alpha-synuclein is present in cerebrospinal fluid from Parkinson's disease and normal subjects. Neurosci Lett. 2000;287:65–7.
10. Borroni B, Malinverno M, Gardoni F, et al. Tau forms in CSF as a reliable biomarker for progressive supranuclear palsy. Neurology. 2008;71:1796–803.
11. Brucke T, Asenbaum S, Pirker W, et al. Measurement of the dopaminergic degeneration in Parkinson's disease with [123I] beta-CIT and SPECT. Correlation with clinical findings and comparison with multiple system atrophy and progressive supranuclear palsy. J Neural Transm Suppl 1997;50:9–24.
12. Deeb J, Shah M, Muhammed N, et al. A basic smell test is as sensitive as a dopamine transporter scan: comparison of olfaction, taste and DaTSCAN in the diagnosis of Parkinson's disease. QJM. 2010;103:941–52.
13. Donadio V. Skin nerve α-synuclein deposits in Parkinson's disease and other synucleinopathies: a review. Clin Auton Res. 2019;29(6):577–85.
14. Donadio V, Doppler K, Incensi A, Kuzkina A, Janzen A, Mayer G, Volkmann J, Rizzo G, Antelmi E, Plazzi G, Sommer C, Liguori R, Oertel WH. Abnormal α-synuclein deposits in skin nerves: intra- and inter-laboratory reproducibility. Eur J Neurol. 2019b;26(10):1245–51.
15. Donadio V, Incensi A, Del Sorbo F, Rizzo G, Infante R, Scaglione C, Modugno N, Fileccia N, Elia AE, Cencini F, Liguori R. Skin nerve phosphorylated α-synuclein deposits in Parkinson's disease with orthostatic hypotension. J Neuropathol Exp Neurol. 2018;77(10):942–9.
16. Donadio V, Incensi A, Vacchiano V, Infante R, Magnani M, Liguori. The autonomic innervation of hairy skin in humans: an in vivo confocal study. R Sci Rep 2019a;9(1):16982.
17. Donadio V, Incensi A, Leta V, Giannoccaro MP, Scaglione C, Martinelli P, et al. Skin nerve α-synuclein deposits: a biomarker for idiopathic Parkinson disease. Neurology. 2014;82(15):1362–9.
18. Donadio V, Incensi A, Piccinini C, Cortelli P, Giannoccaro MP, Baruzzi A, Liguori R. Skin nerve misfolded α-synuclein in pure autonomic failure and Parkinson disease. Ann Neurol. 2016;79(2):306–16.
19. Doppler K, Ebert S, Uçeyler N, Trenkwalder C, Ebentheuer J, Volkmann J, Sommer C. Cutaneous neuropathy in Parkinson's disease: a window into brain pathology. Acta Neuropathol. 2014;128(1):99–109.
20. Doppler K, Jentschke HM, Schulmeyer L, Vadasz D, Janzen A, Luster M, Höffken H, Mayer G, Brumberg J, Booij J, Musacchio T, Klebe S, Sittig-Wiegand E, Volkmann J, Sommer C, Oertel WH. Dermal phospho-alpha-synuclein deposits confirm REM sleep behaviour disorder as prodromal Parkinson's disease. Acta Neuropathol. 2017;133(4):535–45.

21. Doppler K, Ebert S, Uçeyler N, Trenkwalder C, Ebentheuer J, Volkmann J, Sommer C. Cutaneous neuropathy in Parkinson's disease: a window into brain pathology. Acta Neuropathol. 2014;128(1):99–109.
22. Doppler K, Weis J, Karl K, Ebert S, Ebentheuer J, Trenkwalder C, Klebe S, Volkmann J, Sommer C. Distinctive distrubution of phospho-alpha-synuclein in dermal nerves in multiple system atrophy. Mov Disord. 2015;30(12):1688–92.
23. Doppler K, Jentschke HM, Schulmeyer L, Vadasz D, Janzen A, Luster M, Höffken H, Mayer G, Brumberg J, Booij J, Musacchio T, Klebe S, Sittig-Wiegand E, Volkmann J, Sommer C, Oertel WH. Dermal phospho-alpha-synuclein deposits confirm REM sleep behaviour disorder as prodromal Parkinson's disease. Acta Neuropathol. 2017;133(4):535–45
24. Dorsey ER, Constantinescu R, Thompson JP, et al. Projected number of 408. people with Parkinson disease in the most populous nations, 2005 through 2030. Neurology 2007;68:384–6.
25. Doty RL, Deems DA, Stellar S. Olfactory dysfunction in parkinsonism: a general deficit unrelated to neurologic signs, disease stage, or disease duration. Neurology. 1988;38:1237–44.
26. Doty RL, Shaman P, Dann M. Development of the university of Pennsylvania smell identification test: a standardized microencapsulated test of olfactory function. Physiol Behav. 1984;32:489–502.
27. Ebersbach G, Baas H, Csoti I, et al. Scales in Parkinson's disease. J Neurol 2006;253:iv32–5.
28. Frey KA, Koeppe RA, Kilbourn MR, et al. Presynaptic monoaminergic vesicles in Parkinson's disease and normal aging. Ann Neurol. 1996;40:873–84.
29. Frost JJ, Rosier AJ, Reich SG, et al. Positron emission tomographic imaging of the dopamine transporter with 11C-WIN 35,428 reveals marked declines in mild Parkinson's disease. Ann Neurol. 1993;34:423–31.
30. Gibb WR, Lees AJ. The relevance of the Lewy body to the pathogenesis of idiopathic Parkinson's disease. J Neurol Neurosurg Psychiatry. 1988;51:745–52.
31. Gibbons CH, Garcia J, Wang N, Shih LC, Freeman R. The diagnostic discrimination of cutaneous α-synuclein deposition in Parkinson disease. Neurology. 2016;87(5):505–12.
32. Goetz CG, Fahn S, Martinez-Martin P, et al. Movement disorder society-sponsored revision of the unified Parkinson's disease rating scale (MDS-UPDRS): process, format, and clinimetric testing plan. Mov Disord. 2007;22:41–7.
33. Haga R, Sugimoto K, Nishijima H, Miki Y, Suzuki C, Wakabayashi K, Baba M, Yagihashi S, Tomiyama M. Clinical utility of skin biopsy in differentiating between Parkinson's disease and multiple system atrophy. Parkinsons Dis. 2015;2015:167038.
34. Hong Z, Shi M, Chung KA, et al. DJ-1 and alpha-synuclein in human cerebrospinal fluid as biomarkers of Parkinson's disease. Brain. 2010;133:713–26.
35. Hummel T, Sekinger B, Wolf SR, et al. 'Sniffin' sticks': olfactory performance assessed by the combined testing of odor identification, odor discrimination and olfactory threshold. Chem Senses. 1997;22:39–52.
36. Jankovic J, Kapadia AS. Functional decline in Parkinson disease. Arch Neurol. 2001;58:1611–5.
37. Jankovic J. Pathophysiology and assessment of parkinsonian symptoms and signs. In: Pahwa R, Lyons K, Koller WC, editors. Handbook of Parkinson's disease. New York: Taylor and Francis Group, LLC; 2007. p. 79–104.
38. Jankovic J, Stacy M. Medical management of levodopa-associated motor complications in patients with Parkinson's disease. CNS Drugs. 2007;21:677–92.
39. Jennings DL, Seibyl JP, Oakes D, et al. (123I) beta-CIT and single-photon emission computed tomographic imaging vs clinical evaluation in Parkinsonian syndrome: unmasking an early diagnosis. Arch Neurol. 2004;61:1224–9.
40. Kobal G, Hummel T, Sekinger B, et al. Sniffin' sticks': screening of olfactory performance. Rhinology. 1996;34:222–6.
41. Koga S, Aoki N, Uitti RJ, van Gerpen JA, Cheshire WP, Josephs KA, Wszolek ZK, Langston JW, Dickson DW. When DLB, PD, and PSP masquerade as MSA: an autopsy study of 134 patients. Neurology. 2015;85(5):404–12.

42. Kurata T, Kametaka S, Ohta Y, et al. PSP as distinguished from CBD, MSA-P and PD by clinical and imaging differences at an early stage. Intern Med 2011;50(22):2775–81.
43. Lang AE. The progression of Parkinson disease: a hypothesis. Neurology. 2007;68:948–52.
44. Maita C, Tsuji S, Yabe I, et al. Secretion of DJ-1 into the serum of patients with Parkinson's disease. Neurosci Lett. 2008;431:86–9.
45. Martin I, Dawson VL, Dawson TM. Recent advances in the genetics of Parkinson's disease. Annu Rev Genomics Hum Genet. 2011;12:301–25.
46. Martin WR, Wieler M, Gee M. Midbrain iron content in early Parkinson disease: a potential biomarker of disease status. Neurology. 2008;70:1411–7.
47. Meara J, Bhowmick BK, Hobson P. Accuracy of diagnosis in patients with presumed Parkinson's disease. Age Ageing. 1999;28:99–102.
48. Melli G, Vacchi E, Biemmi V, Galati S, Staedler C, Ambrosini R, Kaelin-Lang A. Cervical skin denervation associates with alpha-synuclein aggregates in Parkinson disease. Ann Clin Transl Neurol. 2018;5(11):1394–407.
49. Miki Y, Tomiyama M, Ueno T, Haga R, Nishijima H, Suzuki C, Mori F, Kaimori M, Baba M, Wakabayashi K. Clinical availability of skin biopsy in the diagnosis of Parkinson's disease. Neurosci Lett. 2010;469(3):57–9.
50. Mollenhauer B, Cullen V, Kahn I, et al. Direct quantification of CSF alpha-synuclein by ELISA and first cross-sectional study in patients with neuro-degeneration. Exp Neurol. 2008;213:315–25.
51. Muller A, Mungersdorf M, Reichmann H, et al. Olfactory function in Parkin-sonian syndromes. J Clin Neurosci. 2002;9:521–4.
52. Nagayama H, Hamamoto M, Ueda M, et al. Reliability of MIBG myocardial scintigraphy in the diagnosis of Parkinson's disease. J Neurol Neurosurg Psychiatry. 2005;76:249–51.
53. Navarro-Otano J, Casanova-Mollà J, Morales M, Valls-Solé J, Tolosa E. Cutaneous autonomic denervation in Parkinson's disease. J Neural Transm (Vienna). 2015;122(8):1149–55.
54. Nicoletti G, Lodi R, Condino F, et al. Apparent diffusion coefficient measurements of the middle cerebellar peduncle differentiate the Parkinson variant of MSA from Parkinson's disease and progressive supranuclear palsy. Brain. 2006;129:2679–87.
55. Orimo S, Suzuki M, Inaba A, Mizusawa H. 123I-MIBG myocardial scintigraphy for differentiating Parkinson's disease from other neurodegenerative parkinsonism: a systematic review and meta-analysis. Parkinsonism Relat Disord 2012;18(5):494–500.
56. Palma JA, Norcliffe-Kaufmann L, Kaufmann H. Diagnosis of multiple system atrophy. Auton Neurosci. 2018;211:15–25.
57. Post B, Merkus MP, Haan RJ, et al. Prognostic factors for the progression of Parkinson's disease: a systematic review. Mov Disord. 2007;22:1839–51.
58. Prestel J, Schweitzer KJ, Hofer A, et al. Predictive value of transcranial sonography in the diagnosis of Parkinson's disease. Mov Disord. 2006;21:1763–5.
59. Rizzo G, Martinelli P, Manners D, et al. Diffusion-weighted brain imaging study of patients with clinical diagnosis of corticobasal degeneration, progressive supranuclear palsy and Parkinson's disease. Brain. 2008;131:2690–700.
60. Rodríguez-Leyva I, Chi-Ahumada EG, Carrizales J, Rodríguez-Violante M, Velázquez-Osuna S, Medina-Mier V, Martel-Gallegos MG, Zarazúa S, Enríquez-Macías L, Castro A, Calderón-Garcidueñas AL, Jiménez-Capdeville ME. Parkinson disease and progressive supranuclear palsy: protein expression in skin. Ann Clin Transl Neurol. 2016;3(3):191–9.
61. Satoh A, Serita T, Seto M, et al. Loss of 123I-MIBG uptake by the heart in Parkinson's disease: assessment of cardiac sympathetic denervation and diagnostic value. J Nucl Med 1999;40(3):371–5.
62. Schrag A, Barone P, Brown RG, et al. Depression rating scales in Parkinson's disease: critique and recommendations. Mov Disord. 2007;22:1077–92.
63. Schrag A, Ben-Shlomo Y, Quinn N. How valid is the clinical diagnosis of Parkinson's disease in the community? J Neurol Neurosurg Psychiatry. 2002;73:529–34.
64. Schrag A, Dodel R, Spottke A, et al. Rate of clinical progression in Parkinson's disease. A prospective study. Mov Disord. 2007;22:938–45.

65. Shapira AH. Recent developments in biomarkers in Parkinson disease. Curr Opin Neurol. 2013;26(4):395–400.
66. Shi M, Zabetian CP, Hancock AM, et al. Significance and confounders of peripheral DJ-1 and alpha-synuclein in Parkinson's disease. Neurosci Lett. 2010;480:78–82.
67. Shtilbans A, Henchcliffe C. Biomarkers in Parkinson's disease: an update. Curr Opin Neurol. 2012;25(4):460–5.
68. Siderowf A, Newberg A, Chou KL, et al. [99mTc]TRODAT-1 SPECT imaging correlates with odor identification in early Parkinson disease. Neurology. 2005;64:1716–20.
69. Siderowf A, Stern MB. Premotor Parkinson's disease: clinical features, detection, and prospects for treatment. Ann Neurol. 2008;64(Suppl 2):S139–47.
70. Tissingh G, Berendse HW, Bergmans P, et al. Loss of olfaction in de novo and treated Parkinson's disease: possible implications for early diagnosis. Mov Disord. 2001;16:41–6.
71. Treglia G, Stefanelli A, Cason E, Cocciolillo F, Di Giuda D, Giordano A. Diagnostic performance of iodine-123-metaiodobenzylguanidine scintigraphy in differential diagnosis between Parkinson's disease and multiple-system atrophy: a systematic review and a meta-analysis. Clin Neurol Neurosurg 2011;113(10):823–9.
72. Vaillancourt DE, Spraker MB, Prodoehl J, et al. High-resolution diffusion tensor imaging in the substantia nigra of de novo Parkinson disease. Neurology. 2009;72:1378–84.
73. Walter U, Dressler D, Probst T, et al. Transcranial brain sonography findings in discriminating between Parkinsonism and idiopathic Parkinson disease. Arch Neurol. 2007;64:1635–40.
74. Walter U, Niehaus L, Probst T, et al. Brain parenchyma sonography discriminates Parkinson's disease and atypical parkinsonian syndromes. Neurology. 2003;60:74–7.
75. Wang N, Gibbons CH, Lafo J, Freeman R. α-Synuclein in cutaneous autonomic nerves. Neurology. 2013;81(18):1604–10.
76. Yoshita M. Differentiation of idiopathic Parkinson's disease from striatonigral degeneration and progressive supranuclear palsy using iodine-123 meta- iodobenzylguanidine myocardial scintigraphy. J Neurol Sci. 1998;155:60–7.
77. Zange L, Noack C, Hahn K, Stenzel W, Lipp A. Phosphorylated α-synuclein in skin nerve fibres differentiates Parkinson's disease from multiple system atrophy. Brain. 2015;138(Pt 8):2310–21.
78. Zecca L, Berg D, Arzberger T, Ruprecht P, et al. In vivo detection of iron and neuromelanin by transcranial sonography: a new approach for early detection of substantia nigra damage. Mov Disord. 2005;20:1278–85.
79. Zesiewicz TA, Sullivan KL, Hauser RA. Nonmotor symptoms of Parkinson's disease. Exp Rev Neurother. 2006;6:1811–22.

Chapter 9
Merkel Cell Carcinoma Biomarkers

Diem-Phuong D. Dao, Zachary H. Rollins, Jessica N. Pixley, Christine Ahn, and Steven R. Feldman

Abstract Merkel cell carcinoma (MCC) is an aggressive malignant neuroendocrine tumor of the skin. While considerable advances in the management of MCC have been made, the clinical utility of potential biomarkers remains unclear. Biomarkers play a crucial role in assessing prognosis, diagnosis, and therapeutic interventions in many chronic diseases and may be similarly beneficial in MCC. This chapter focuses on examining potential biomarkers in MCC. Through conducting a literature search, 22 biomarkers were identified and classified based on the classification standards provided by the World Health Organization (WHO). These biomarkers have the potential to aid in screening, diagnosis, prognosis, monitoring, and pharmacodynamic properties of MCC.

Keywords Merkel cell carcinoma · Merkel cell polyomavirus · Biomarkers · Skin cancer · Survival · Pathophysiology · Cytokeratin-20 · MCPyV-positive · Neuron-specific enolase · Phosphatidylinositol-3-kinase · Programmed death ligand-1 · Tertiary lymphoid structures · P63 · p14ARF methylation · γδ T-cells · Stathmin · Vasculogenic mimicry · A disintegrin and metalloproteinase 10 and 17 · Major capsid protein antibodies and T antigen · MiRNAs · Pan-immune-inflammation value · Circulating tumor cells · $CD8^+$ lymphocytes · High neutrophil-to-CD8-lymphocyte ratio · Anaplastic lymphoma kinase · Phosphohistone-H3

D.-P. D. Dao · Z. H. Rollins · C. Ahn
Wake Forest School of Medicine, 4618 Country Club Road, Winston-Salem, NC 27104, USA

J. N. Pixley (✉)
Virginia Commonwealth University, Richmond, USA
e-mail: pixleyjn@vcu.edu

S. R. Feldman
Professor of Dermatology, Pathology and Social Sciences & Health Policy, Wake Forest School of Medicine, 4618 Country Club Road, Winston-Salem, NC 27104, USA
e-mail: sfeldman@wakehealth.edu

R. Norman (ed.), *Biomarkers in Dermatology*,
https://doi.org/10.1007/978-3-031-66513-4_9

9.1 Introduction

Merkel cell carcinoma (MCC) is a malignant neuroendocrine tumor that arises from Merkel cells, a type 1 mechanoreceptor in the skin. Relative to other skin cancers, MCCs are uncommon, with an incidence of approximately 2000 cases in the USA [1]. The primary population affected is older individuals between 60 and 85 years of age with lighter skin types. MCC is associated with high rates of recurrence, metastasis, and mortality.

MCC classically presents as a single asymptomatic, skin-colored to red papule or nodule on sun-exposed areas of the head and neck [2, 3]. The pathogenesis of MCC is believed to be multifactorial, related to the presence of Merkel cell polyomavirus (MCPyV) and ultraviolet (UV) exposure [3, 4]. MCC may resemble other more common skin lesions such as a cysts or pyogenic granulomas, which can lead to a delay in diagnosis [5]. Skin biopsy is diagnostic; subsequent workup should include a thorough skin examination, evaluation of regional lymph node basins, and additional imaging to evaluate for distant disease [6].

Initial treatment for non-metastatic MCC is wide local excision with 1–2 cm margins, whenever possible. Excision should be performed in coordination with evaluation of regional lymph nodes. For clinically evident lymph nodes, patients may undergo fine needle aspiration (FNA) or core needle biopsy. In other cases, patients undergo sentinel lymph node biopsy (SNLB) [7]. Patients with clear margins and without any evidence of nodal spread can be managed with observation alone, though some providers may additionally recommend adjuvant radiotherapy in patients with increased risk factors. If negative margins are not achieved on initial excision, patients can either undergo re-excision or adjuvant radiotherapy. Positive SLNB can be managed with radiotherapy to the nodal basin, complete nodal dissection, or adjuvant therapy [8]. If nodal spread or metastasis is noted before the primary excision, then neoadjuvant immunotherapy may also be considered [9].

The utility of biomarkers is still poorly understood [10]. In some tumor processes, biomarkers serve as valuable tools in diagnosis as they can help to distinguish MCC from other tumors with similar or overlapping histologic features. Due to the aggressive clinical course of most MCC, prognostic biomarkers may be helpful in tumor progression and response to treatment.

In this chapter, we discuss biomarkers that have a potential role in the diagnosis, prognosis, and management of MCC. The selected MCC biomarkers were classified based on characteristics assigned by the World Health Organization. These subtypes included the following: screening, biomarkers that facilitate identifying patients at risk of developing the disease; monitoring, biomarkers that indicate a higher disease severity; prognosis, biomarkers that have indicative serum or tissue levels; pharmacodynamic, biomarkers that inform pharmacologic approaches or treatment; diagnostic, and biomarkers that aid in diagnosis of the disease.

9.2 Methods

A literature search was conducted through the PubMed database including key words: "*Merkel cell carcinoma*", "*pathophysiology*", "*Merkel cell polyomavirus*", "*MCPyV-positive*", "*biomarkers*", "*survival*", and "*CK-20*". There were 128 articles identified of which 46 relevant articles were identified to be relevant from reviewing abstracts and relevant sections. The references of identified articles were reviewed for further relevant articles. The National Comprehensive Cancer Network guidelines were also reviewed. Articles included were published between 2002 and 2022, were written in English, and were relevant to the objectives of this chapter. Guided by the WHO classification guidelines, biomarkers were categorized into one of five categories including screening, prognostic, monitoring, pharmacodynamic, and diagnostic.

9.3 Pathogenesis of Merkel Cell Carcinoma

9.3.1 Merkel Cell Polyomavirus

MCPyV is a circular, non-enveloped, double-stranded DNA virus and is considered to be one of seven known human oncoviruses [11]. The virus is ubiquitous and can be found on the skin of healthy individuals. Infection is typically asymptomatic and is thought to infect most people during early childhood [12]. A small subset of these infections will go on to cause MCC, which suggests a multifactorial component to the tumor development. In most studies, integrated MCPyV DNA has been found in approximately 80% of MCC tumors [13]. There are two proteins encoded in the MCPyV genome that are primarily responsible for oncogenesis, the large tumor antigen (LT) and small tumor antigen (ST). For both of these antigens, MCC is thought to progress through incorporation of MCPyV genome into host cell DNA, resulting in inactivation of tumor suppressor genes such as retinoblastoma 1 (RB1) [4, 12].

9.3.2 UV Radiation Exposure

The majority of MCCs that are negative for MCPyV are associated with a high burden of tumor mutations, many consistent with a UV mutational signature [4]. Mutations include single nucleotide variants, translocations, and copy number alterations, which are not seen in MCPyV associated tumors [14]. Loss of function mutations has been noted in TP53, RB1, and NOTCH1. In addition, a subset of tumors is also noted to have increased amplification of the MYC proto-oncogene family. This pathway is further supported by the predilection of MCC to arise in skin-exposed areas.

9.4 Diagnostic Biomarkers

9.4.1 Cytokeratin-20 (CK-20)

CK-20 is a low-molecular-weight keratin expressed normally in the gastrointestinal epithelium and in some gastrointestinal and transitional cell carcinomas [15]. Through immunohistochemical markers such as CK-20, diagnostic accuracy for MCC has increased. Perinuclear staining with CK-20 has 95% sensitivity and 60% specificity for MCC. CK-20 staining in lymph nodes is also specific for MCC; however, some tumors may have low or absent CK-20 expression, which limits sensitivity [16]. Classically seen as a paranuclear dot-like pattern, CK-20 is a crucial diagnostic biomarker for MCC. CK-20 has been used to differentiate MCC from small cell lung cancers, small neuroendocrine carcinomas, and other cutaneous cancers. About 5–10% of cases of MCC completely lack CK-20 expression, and as a result, other diagnostic biomarkers are needed for confirmation of MCC [16].

9.4.2 Neuron-Specific Enolase (NSE)

Neuron-specific enolase (NSE) is an isozyme of the glycolytic enzyme enolase and has three isozymes, which are expressed by different genes, and are found in their respective locations: enolase α is found everywhere in the body; enolase β is muscle specific; enolase γ gene is neuron specific. The expression of NSE, which presents as $\gamma\gamma$- and $\alpha\gamma$-dimers, occurs later in neural differentiation, indicating its role in neural maturation. Because NSE is a highly specific marker for neurons and neuroendocrine cells, increased levels of NSE may be identified in malignancies of these tissue types and may serve as a useful biomarker for diagnosis, staging, and treatment response [17].

To date, NSE has been used as a biomarker for small cell carcinomas. NSE has been identified in cases of MCC using immunohistochemistry, although its clinical use has not been well established. In one study with 84 patients, blood sampling to measure NSE levels was obtained. There were 565 NSE blood samples that correlated with disease extension ($p = 0.01$). A NSE level of 18.2 ng/ml was proposed to the level best for clinical use, with a sensitivity of 91%, specificity of 78%, PPV of 48%, and NPV of 98%. The study also examined the response of NSE levels to immunotherapy in 23 patients, in which all complete responders had normalized NSE (< 18.2 ng/ml), all incomplete responders had decreasing NSE and all non-responders continued to have NSE levels that were elevated [18]. Therefore, NSE may be used to trend immunotherapy responses during treatment and serve as a pharmacodynamic biomarker, as well as a diagnostic biomarker.

9.4.3 *Phosphatidylinositol-3-Kinase (PI3K)*

Phosphatidylinositol-3-kinase (PI3K)/protein kinase B (AKT) pathway activation has been described in many human malignancies such as those of the lung, breast, and brain. Mutation frequencies in this pathway are high. Activating mutations in *PIK3CA*, a gene encoding for PI3K, have been observed in MCC. As a result of these mutations, PIK3CA proteins have increased kinase activity and may play a role in tumor pathogenesis. Examining PIK3CA activating mutations in MCC may provide valuable insight into the role of the PI3K/pAKT pathway in MCC oncogenesis [19].

In 60 MCC samples, mutations were identified in 9 MCC primary tumors, including 6 activating *PIK3CA* gene mutations. MCPyV-positive tumors and *PIK3CA* activating mutations seemed to be mutually exclusive, with the exception of one case. However, the presence of this mutation was associated with sensitivity to treatment with a PI3K inhibitor and dual PI3K-mTOR inhibitor [19]. Though the association of *PIK3CA* mutations in the PI3K/AKT pathway for MCC oncogenesis has limited research, identifying mutations in these oncogenes may serve as a future screening and diagnostic indicator. In addition, the sensitivity of MCC with *PIK3CA* mutations to PI3K inhibitor and dual PI3K-mTOR inhibitor treatment offers potential therapeutic interventions and may additionally be classified as a pharmacodynamic biomarker.

9.5 Prognostic Biomarkers

9.5.1 *Merkel Cell Polyomavirus (MCPyV)*

MCC can present with MCPyV-positive tumors or MCPyV-negative tumors. MCPyV integrates into the host genome. Through subsequent coding of viral oncoproteins, p53 and Tb tumor suppressor proteins are inactivated. These viral oncoproteins are sufficient to maintain tumor burden as cellular gene mutations are not usually detected in virus-positive MCC [20].

Virus-positive or negative status plays a critical role in MCC overall survival and MCC-specific survival. Virus-positive MCC cases have better outcomes with greater overall survival and MCC-specific survival [20]. MCPyV status serves as an independent prognostic biomarker for MCC.

9.5.2 *Programmed Death Ligand-1 (PD-L1)*

Programmed death ligand-1 (PD-L1) is an immune-inhibitory ligand that down modulates the immune response and inhibits damage to normal cells. Programmed death-1 (PD-1) is the main receptor for PD-L1 and is expressed by T lymphocytes.

Many tumor cells overexpress PD-L1 and are able to evade a host immune anti-tumor response. As a result, immunotherapy aimed against PD-1, such as nivolumab, has been demonstrated to be efficacious in eliciting an anti-tumor response in other malignancies such as melanoma by blockading the PD-1/PD-L1 pathway and mediating tumor regression [21]. Due to the role of PD-L1 in modulating the immune system's reaction to tumor cells, tumor cell expression of PD-L1 may be an independent positive prognostic factor.

In a study examining if PD-1/PD-L1 blockade may be a plausible treatment for MCC, 67 specimens from 49 patients were examined for PD-L1 tumor cell and tumor-infiltrating lymphocyte expression. Cells that were Merkel cell polyomavirus negative were also PD-L1 negative. Improved overall survival was associated with tumor cell PD-L1 expression ($p = 0.046$). MCC that did not express PD-L1 had worse patient survival overall ($p = 0.012$) [21]. In another study regarding MCC tumor cell PD-1 expression, 78 patient tissue samples were examined and patients who were not treated with immune checkpoint inhibitors did not have different median survival rates based on their expression of PD-L1 ($p = 0.60$) [22]. As a result, expression of PD-L1 did not affect prognosis. Therefore, MCC expression of PD-L1 may be a prognostic and pharmacodynamic biomarker; however, more studies are needed to elucidate this association.

9.5.3 Tertiary Lymphoid Structures (TLSs)

Involvement of tertiary lymphoid structures (TLSs) in malignancies indicates better prognosis and response to immune checkpoint inhibitors. Ectopic lymphoid tissues, TLSs, are found in tumor or infected tissues. In solid tumors, TLSs play a role in creating a favorable immune environment against the tumor [23].

Previous studies have examined the presence of TLS in MCC and have concluded that the presence of TLS indicates a better prognosis in patients with MCPyV-positive MCC. Similarly, in a study examining 61 patients with both MCPyV-positive and MCPyV-negative MCC cases, samples with TLS had a better prognosis than those without TLS. The same results were found regardless of MCPyV status. Samples that were MCPyV-negative and TLS-negative were associated with a poor prognosis. Samples that exhibited spontaneous regression were MCPyV-positive and TLS-positive [23]. As a result, TLS presence, regardless of MCPyV status, may be a useful prognostic biomarker in MCC.

9.5.4 p63

P63 is a transcription factor in the p53 family that is found in stem cells and basal cells of the epidermis and other locations [24]. Multiple isoforms of this protein encompass many functions such as proliferation, differentiation, cell death, cell survival, and DNA response and metabolism. P63 is associated with many carcinomas [25].

Expression of p63 may correlate with MCC disease course. In one study identifying 70 cases of MCC, p63 expression was determined by immunohistochemistry, reverse-transcription-PCR, and fluorescence in situ hybridization (FISH). Expression of p63 was correlated with decreased overall survival ($p < 0.0001$) and decreased disease-free survival ($p < 0.0001$). In addition, p63 expression was associated with evolution of MCC as well ($p < 0.0001$) [24]. This indicates that the expression of p63 in patients with MCC may confer a worse prognosis and may be used to predict survival. In addition, p63 expression may predict clinical progression of disease.

9.5.5 Delta-Like Protein 3 (DLL3)

MCC typically has dysregulated NOTCH expression. The Notch signaling pathway regulates epithelial or neuroendocrine cell fate in developing lungs. Delta-like protein 3 (DLL3) is an important protein in the Notch signaling pathway and acts as an inhibitory ligand of NOTCH receptors. Small cell lung cancers have increased expression of DLL3. Due to the neuroendocrine features of small cell lung cancer and the predisposition of MCC and MCC for dysregulated NOTCH expression, DLL3 expression in MCC has been evaluated for a role in prognosis [26].

Sixty-five patients with MCC were examined for DLL3 expression. DLL3 expression in patients with MCC did not correlate with overall survival ($p = 0.15$) and DLL3 expression was not associated with prognostic value in this study, despite MCC cells overexpressing DLL3 [26]. There is no current evidence to suggest the use of DLL3 as a prognostic biomarker.

9.5.6 Kit Receptor Tyrosine Kinase (CD117)

KIT receptor tyrosine kinase (CD117) is a transmembrane receptor that regulates germ cell development, hematopoiesis, melanocytes, and interstitial cells of Cajal with its ligand, stem cell factor. Many tissues, both normal and malignant, express CD117. Tumors that express CD117 include small cell lung cancer, melanoma, germ cell tumors, and acute myeloid leukemia, among others [27].

In one study of CD117 expression in MCC, the intensity of CD117 did not impact rate of metastasis. Many MCCs do express CD117; however, the function of CD117 in MCC remains ambiguous and its role as a prognostic biomarker requires further investigation [27].

9.5.7 Phosphohistone-H3 (PHH3 or Ser10)

Phosphohistone-H3 (PHH3 or Ser10) is a mitotic count biomarker that examines mitotic activity in various cancers such as melanoma and breast cancer. Histone-H3 is phosphorylated during the late G2 and mitosis (M) phases of the cell cycle and therefore is a biomarker specific for mitotic activity [28].

In a study evaluating the prognostic indication of PHH3 index in 19 MCPyV-positive MCC and 9 MCPyV-negative MCC samples, PHH3-positive cell counts had some prognostic utility for overall survival when combined with MCPyV status. When combining MCPyV status and PHH3 counts, MCPyV-negative MCC samples with high PHH3-positive cells counts had worse overall survival ($p = 0.035$) and increased MCC-specific death ($p < 0.001$). As a result, the combined analysis yielded prognostic value [28]. Though MCPyV status in MCC patients remains a more reliable prognostic indicator, combining the MCPyV status with PHH3-positivity may provide more insight into overall survival and MCC-specific death rates.

9.5.8 Anaplastic Lymphoma Kinase (ALK)

Anaplastic lymphoma kinase (ALK), a tyrosine kinase receptor, regulates nervous system development. This receptor possesses oncogenic properties. ALK is activated through phosphorylation and, once phosphorylated, activates other signaling cascades such as the extracellular signal regulated kinase pathway, mitogen-activated protein kinase pathway, protein kinase B pathway, and phosphoinositide 3-kinase pathway. Several cancers have targeted ALK for treatment, and increased expression of ALK in MCC has been reported. Regardless of MCPyV status, ALK is expressed in MCC at the RNA level [29].

In a case–control study of 136 patients with MCC, ALK immunohistochemistry was positive in 74% of MCC patients. Phosphorylated APK (p-ALK) was observed in 48% of MCC. Lower median age at diagnosis was associated with high and intermediate p-ALK positive cases, compared to low and negative p-ALK cases ($p = 0.005$). Presence of p-ALK at the time of diagnosis was associated with no metastatic disease ($p = 0.012$). Higher overall survival and MCC-specific survival were seen in ALK and p-ALK positivity. In addition, MCPyV positivity, younger age, and lack of metastasis at the time of diagnosis were associated with p-ALK presence as well [29]. Therefore, ALK has promising utility as a prognostic biomarker.

9.5.9 High Neutrophil-to-CD8-Lymphocyte Ratio

The presence of infiltrating immune cells such as neutrophils and $CD8^+$ lymphocytes plays a major role in the creation of either a pro- or anti-tumor microenvironment. The type of microenvironment affects the migratory ability of tumor cells and response to immune checkpoint inhibitors. In other skin malignancies such as melanoma, ulceration is a leading prognostic factor that indicates a pro-tumor microenvironment. Examining ulceration and presence of infiltrating immune cells may provide better insight into the prognosis of MCC [30].

In a study examining the association of ulceration, MCPyV status, and microenvironment in MCC, increased infiltration of neutrophils and decreased infiltration of $CD8^+$ lymphocytes were observed in MCCs with ulceration. Ulceration was associated with MCPyV-negative tumors, which correlate to worse outcomes in MCC-specific survival [30]. High neutrophil-to-$CD8^+$ lymphocyte ratios, ulceration, virus-negative status, and absence of $CD8^+$ lymphocytes were negative prognostic markers in MCC-specific survival which therefore serve as prognostic biomarkers.

9.5.9.1 $CD8^+$ Lymphocytes

Cellular immune responses may play a critical role in controlling the progression of MCC. Improved outcomes in cohorts with MCC have been linked to brisk $CD8^+$ lymphoid infiltrates. These tumor-infiltrating myeloid cells are believed to be involved in MCC immune regulation. Myeloid-derived suppressor cells are due to tumor-secreted factors that block myeloid progenitor differentiation. $CD33^+$ cells are suspected to be tumor-infiltrating myeloid-derived suppressor cells, and $CD33^+$ macrophage densities were associated with $CD8^+$ T-cell infiltrates [31].

Among 242 MCC patients, 103 FFPE samples were examined. MCC tumors with the most $CD8^+$ T-cell infiltrates were associated with greater $CD33^+$ myeloid-cell infiltration ($p = 0.001$). These $CD33^+$ infiltrates were associated with PD-L1 expression. MCC with $CD8^+$ T-cell and $CD33^+$ myeloid-cell infiltrates had improved overall survival and recurrence-free rates. $CD33^+$ cells were not found to be myeloid-derived suppressor cells, and instead, brisk $CD33^+CD8^+$ cells were associated with improved prognosis and may be targeted by PD-1/PD-L1 therapy [31]. As a result, $CD8^+$ lymphocytes, associated with $CD33^+$ cells, may be used as both prognostic and pharmacodynamic biomarkers.

9.6 Monitoring Biomarkers

9.6.1 Circulating Tumor Cells (CTCs)

Circulating tumor cells (CTCs) are useful biomarkers in several carcinomas such as prostate, colon, breast, pancreatic, and neuroendocrine tumors. These blood-based biomarkers correlate with disease progression and relapse prediction [32].

In 52 specimens from 34 patients with MCC, patients without CTC had 80% disease-specific survival 2 years after testing, while patients with CTC had 29%

disease-specific survival 2 years after testing ($p = 0.015$). Patients without CTC had 72% MCC-specific survival versus patients with CTC had 25% survival [32]. As a result, CTC detection in patients with MCC may provide valuable insight as monitoring biomarkers.

9.6.2 Pan-Immune-Inflammation Value (PIV)

The pan-immune-inflammation value (PIV) is a biomarker of inflammation based on a complex complete blood count (CBC). It is a proposed scoring system including neutrophil, platelet, monocyte, and lymphocyte counts. As the PIV was recently developed, a formal assessment regarding its utility and efficacy as an inflammatory biomarker has yet to be determined. PIV has been associated with disease progression-free survival and overall survival [33].

Compared to the cutaneous melanoma patient control group and healthy patient control group, median PIV in patients with MCC was increased. Additionally, PIV was much higher in stage II and stage III MCC patients than in MCC stage I patients. PIVs greater than 372 were associated with MCC disease recurrence ($p < 0.0001$). Higher MCC stage correlated with disease recurrence as well [33]. Though a systematic assessment of the PIV scale's utility is needed, PIV has a promising prognostic potential in MCC patients and may serve as a monitoring biomarker. PIV independently predicted MCC disease recurrence; however, PIV scoring was still dependent on disease stage.

9.6.3 Circulating MicroRNAs (MiRNAs)

Circulating microRNAs (miRNAs) may regulate neoplastic processes such as proliferation, invasion, and metastasis [34]. Specific miRNA levels in serum and plasma may act as prognostic biomarkers or therapy predictors. MiRNAs may be released from active cancer cells and remain resistant to degradation. The role of miRNA as a biomarker for other cancers has been recognized [35].

Expression of miRNA was higher in MCC patients when compared to non-MCC or healthy patient controls ($p < 0.0005$). In patients with tumors, miRNA serum levels correlated with tumor stage ($p = 0.037$) and had high accuracy differentiating between tumor-positive and tumor-negative MCC patients regarding diagnosis. Many biomarkers rely on the presence of polyomavirus positivity to be useful; however, miRNA serum levels gave insight into MCC tumor burden without the need for polyomavirus positivity [35]. This biomarker, best classified as a monitoring biomarker, would be useful in assessing treatment efficacy in patients with MCC.

9.6.4 Major Capsid Protein Antibodies and T Antigen

Merkel cell polyomavirus is a naked DNA virus that possesses oncogenic properties. It includes the following structural proteins: VP1, which is the major capsid protein, and two minor capsid proteins (VP2 and VP3). T antigens of the MCPyV possess oncogenic properties as well. In approximately 80% of MCCs, MCPyV DNA and T antigen expression are detected. VP1 antibodies have been observed in healthy adults; however, patients with MCC have higher levels of VP1 antibodies [36].

In patients with MCC, VP1 antibodies at low titers have been associated with an elevated recurrence risk ($p = 0.026$) and mortality ($p = 0.004$). T antigen antibodies did not affect outcome in patients with MCC, but were more likely to be detected in patients with relapse or progression at 12 months ($p = 0.20$) and 24 months ($p = 0.016$) after initial diagnosis. VP1 antibodies did not give insight in the above-mentioned factors during follow-up [36]. Therefore, baseline prognostic biomarkers should focus on VP1 antibodies, while follow-up biomarkers should examine T antigen at least 12 months after diagnosis. VP1 antibodies and T antigens may serve as monitoring biomarkers.

9.7 Pharmacodynamic Biomarkers

9.7.1 A Disintegrin and Metalloproteinase (ADAM) 10 and 17

A disintegrin and metalloproteinase (ADAM) is zinc-dependent transmembrane proteins that facilitate shedding of various proteins. Thirteen of the 21 ADAMs regulate membrane cytokines, growth factors, cell adhesion molecules, and their receptors through proteolytic sheddase activities. These sheddase activities play a role in inflammation, tumor progression, and tumor metastasis. Levels of specific ADAMs correlate to tumor progression and as a result may facilitate cancer development and metastasis. ADAM 10 and 17 are upregulated in MCPyV-positive MCC [37].

Inhibiting ADAM 10 and 17 activity impaired MCPyV-induced metastases as a result of reduced cell motility and dissociation [37]. As a result, ADAM protein expression may be used as a pharmacodynamic biomarker. Inhibiting ADAM 10 and 17 remains a potential therapeutic target for MCPyV-positive MCC.

9.7.2 Vasculogenic Mimicry

Vasculogenic mimicry (VM) is the ability of cancer cells to drive tumor proliferation and form patterned networks that mimic vasculogenesis. VM may be associated with tumor aggressiveness, where tumors develop anastomosing laminin-like networks. These tumor cells express genes that encode for vascular endothelial growth factor receptor (VEGFR-1) and vascular endothelial-cadherin (CD144) are identified in VM networks [38].

Two human MCC lines were used in a xenograft model where induced tumor histologically resembled MCC. These lines contained the laminin networks associated with VEGFR-1 and CD144. Etoposide and carboplatin, chemotherapeutic agents established for treatment of MCC, did induce necrosis in the xenografts. However, resistance tumor regions in laminin networks persisted, indicating that MCC regions with high levels of VM may not respond to conventional chemotherapeutic agents [38]. Therefore, VM-like laminin biomarkers may serve pharmacodynamic purposes.

9.7.3 Stathmin

Stathmin is a microtubule-associated protein that binds tubulin dimers and reduces the substrate for growing microtubule polymers when unphosphorylated. However, phosphorylated stathmin has a weakened tubulin-binding ability and increases free tubulin concentration for microtubule assembly. Overexpression of stathmin is observed in many malignancies. Increased stathmin expression is associated with poorer outcomes and increased metastatic potential [39].

Stathmin facilitated MCPyV small tumor-mediated microtubule destabilization and cell motility through the cellular phosphatase catalytic subunit protein phosphatase 4C (PP4C). Due to this microtubule destabilization leading to increased cell mobility and migration, tumors with phosphorylated stathmin may exhibit a propensity for metastasis [39]. The role of stathmin as a biomarker for MCC has not yet been defined; however, stathmin is a possible pharmacodynamic biomarker as stathmin-targeted therapeutic interventions may curb MCC metastasis.

9.7.4 Γδ T-Cells

Γδ T-cells are a subset of MHC-restriction lacking, unconventional T-cells. They are defined by expression of a γδ T-cell receptor, encoded by T-cell receptor-γ and T-cell receptor-δ genes that differentiate these cells from αβ T–cell lineage. γδ T-cells rapidly proliferate and produce pro-inflammatory cytokines upon activation, primed to create a rapid immune response. As a result, these cells may have some value in tumor surveillance. γδ T-cells have been observed in skin, colon, breast, and pancreatic tumors, but do not currently have a known role in MCC [40].

In a study examining 58 MCC lesions from 39 patients, CD4/CD8 double-negative T-cells were characterized as unconventional γδ T-cells through flow cytometry. γδ T-cells predicted better survival in patients with MCC. These cells elicit a pro-inflammatory and response, likely antigen-driven. T-cell infiltration in MCC tumors correlated with improved patient survival. In addition, disease-specific survival was increased in patients with high enrichment scores. There was a positive correlation between double-negative T-cell infiltrates and enrichment scores, and complete response to immune checkpoint inhibitor therapy (anti-PD-1/PD-L1) was observed in three out of four cases with high enrichment scores [40]. Therefore, examining γδ T-cell infiltration may serve as a future pharmacodynamic biomarker.

9.7.5 *p14ARF Methylation*

Epigenetic mechanisms such as gene methylation status or histone modifications influence MCC tumorigenesis. Thought to be one of the most common molecular alterations, aberrant DNA methylation is common in many cancer cells. Human promoter *p14ARF* is aberrantly methylated in many cancers such as gliomas, esophageal carcinomas, and cutaneous squamous cell carcinoma [41].

From 19 MCC tumor samples, methylation of *p14ARF* occurred in 8 samples. Methylation-specific PCR was used to determine methylation of the *p14ARF* promoter [41]. There is limited evidence supporting the use of *p14ARF* methylation as a prognostic or pharmacodynamic biomarker. Therefore, though *p14ARF* hypermethylation and subsequent, silencing, may be a potential therapeutic target in MCC intervention, its clinical utility has yet to be determined.

9.8 Discussion

Biomarkers play an important role in screening, prognosis, diagnosis, monitoring, and therapeutic interventions for many diseases. Merkel cell carcinoma has a paucity of established biomarkers. Advances in diagnosis and management of MCC have improved greatly over the years; however, identifying clear biomarkers and establishing their utility in MCC have yet to be done, likely due in part to the rarity of the disease. In addition to elucidating prognosis and diagnosis, MCC biomarkers would also provide insight into metastasis and guide new therapeutic interventions.

In this chapter, 22 potential biomarkers were identified to have a possible role in MCC. CK-20 is the most sensitive and specific MCC biomarker that is able to differentiate MCC from other neuroendocrine and cutaneous cancers [16]. In addition, MCPyV-positive status in MCC tumors has been correlated with improved overall survival and MCC-specific survival several times [19, 23, 28, 30, 42]. These two biomarkers are effective and useful in the prognosis and diagnosis of MCC.

The other biomarkers mentioned in this chapter have had clinical efficacy in limited studies and sample sizes. Therefore, additional studies are needed to determine if these biomarkers can translate to clinical use. Many biomarkers, such as CD8 lymphocytes or double-negative/γδ T-cells, intersect with the potential prognostic and pharmacodynamic biomarker, PD-L1 [21, 30, 31, 33, 40]. These biomarkers combined may determine future response to immune checkpoint inhibitors and therapeutic interventions that target blockading the PD-1/PD-L1 pathway. Other potential biomarkers that may play an important role in MCC tumorigenesis rely on immune system response and immune system infiltration.

Although biomarkers have the potential to facilitate screening and diagnostic purposes, there are several limitations to the use of biomarkers in MCC. Not all MCC cells exhibit the biomarkers listed and some of the biomarkers identified in this chapter are not mutually exclusive with MCPyV-presence [19, 20]. As a result, these biomarkers are not able to serve as independent prognostic biomarkers and depend on MCPyV positivity. This poses a limitation as some forms of MCC are MCPyV-negative. MCPyV-negative MCC has poorer outcomes in general, and thus, ascertaining their prognosis and monitoring recurrence of the disease is important to patients who already do not have a favorable disease course.

Other risk factors of MCC include immunosuppression due to organ transplantation, HIV infection, or other malignancies. Hematologic malignancies are strongly linked to MCC development with the strongest correlation in multiple myeloma, and chronic lymphocytic leukemia [43]. Identifying biomarkers that overlap between MCC and these malignancies may have future value.

9.9 Conclusion

Merkel cell carcinoma is an aggressive neuroendocrine tumor that arises from Merkel cells, a type 1 mechanoreceptor in the skin. MCC is less common than other cutaneous cancers, and comparatively less is known about this type of skin cancer. MCC has high rates of recurrence, metastasis, and mortality. Diagnosis is typically through skin biopsy and favored pathogenesis mechanisms center around MCPyV DNA into the tumor's genome and UV exposure. Many potential biomarkers have been identified for MCC; however, their clinical utility must be further explored. Other than CK-20 and MCPyV status, there is limited evidence to determine the value of the other biomarkers listed in this chapter. More studies are needed to elucidate their value.

References

1. American Cancer Society: Key Statistics for Merkel Cell Carcinoma. https://www.cancer.org/cancer/merkel-cell-skin-cancer/about/key-statistics.html. 2022. Accessed 10 Oct 2022.
2. Zwijnenburg EM, Lubeek SFK, Werner JEM, Amir AL, Weijs WLJ, Takes RP, Pegge SAH, van Herpen CML, Adema GJ, Kaanders JHAM. Merkel cell carcinoma: new trends. Cancers (Basel). 2021;13(7):1614. https://doi.org/10.3390/cancers13071614.
3. Popp S, Waltering S, Herbst C, Moll I, Boukamp P. UV-B-type mutations and chromosomal imbalances indicate common pathways for the development of merkel and skin squamous cell carcinomas. Int J Cancer. 2002;99(3):352–60. https://doi.org/10.1002/ijc.10321.

4. DeCaprio JA. Molecular pathogenesis of merkel cell carcinoma. Annu Rev Pathol. 2021;16:69–91. https://doi.org/10.1146/annurev-pathmechdis-012419-032817.
5. Heath M, Jaimes N, Lemos B, Mostaghimi A, Wang LC, Peñas PF, Nghiem P. Clinical characteristics of merkel cell carcinoma at diagnosis in 195 patients: the AEIOU features. J Am Acad Dermatol. 2008;58(3):375–81. https://doi.org/10.1016/j.jaad.2007.11.020.
6. Singh N, Alexander NA, Lachance K, Lewis CW, McEvoy A, Akaike G, Byrd D, Behnia S, Bhatia S, Paulson KG, Nghiem P. Clinical benefit of baseline imaging in merkel cell carcinoma: analysis of 584 patients. J Am Acad Dermatol. 2021;84(2):330–9.
7. Cornejo C, Miller CJ. Merkel cell carcinoma: updates on staging and management. Dermatol Clin. 2019;37(3):269–77. https://doi.org/10.1016/j.det.2019.03.001.
8. Cramer JD, Suresh K, Sridharan S. Completion lymph node dissection for merkel cell carcinoma. Am J Surg. 2020;220(4):982–6. https://doi.org/10.1016/j.amjsurg.2020.02.018.
9. National Comprehensive Cancer Network: Merkel Cell Carcinoma. https://merkelcell.org/wp-content/uploads/2021/11/2022-NCCN-Guidelines-for-Non-Melanoma-Skin-Cancer-v1.2022.pdf. 2021. Accessed 10 Oct 2022.
10. Schadendorf D, Lebbé C, Zur Hausen A, Avril MF, Hariharan S, Bharmal M, Becker JC. Merkel cell carcinoma: Epidemiology, prognosis, therapy and unmet medical needs. Eur J Cancer 2017;71:53–69.https://doi.org/10.1016/j.ejca.2016.10.022
11. Mui UN, Haley CT, Tyring SK. Viral oncology: molecular biology and pathogenesis. J Clin Med. 2017;6(12):111. https://doi.org/10.3390/jcm6120111.
12. Krump NA, You J. From merkel cell polyomavirus infection to merkel cell carcinoma oncogenesis. Front Microbiol. 2021;12: 739695. https://doi.org/10.3389/fmicb.2021.739695.
13. Pietropaolo V, Prezioso C, Moens U. Merkel cell polyomavirus and merkel cell carcinoma. Cancers (Basel). 2020;12(7):1774. https://doi.org/10.3390/cancers12071774.
14. Ahmed MM, Cushman CH, DeCaprio JA. Merkel cell polyomavirus: oncogenesis in a stable genome. Viruses. 2021;14(1):58. https://doi.org/10.3390/v14010058.
15. Mistry K, Levell NJ, Craig P, Steven NM, Venables ZC. Merkel cell carcinoma. Skin Health Dis. 2021;1(4): e55. https://doi.org/10.1002/ski2.55.
16. Stanoszek LM, Chan MP, Palanisamy N, Carskadon S, Siddiqui J, Patel RM, Harms KL, Lowe L, Fullen DR, Harms PW. Neurofilament is superior to cytokeratin 20 in supporting cutaneous origin for neuroendocrine carcinoma. Histopathology. 2019;74(3):504–13. https://doi.org/10.1111/his.13758.
17. Isgrò MA, Bottoni P, Scatena R. Neuron-specific enolase as a biomarker: biochemical and clinical aspects. Adv Exp Med Biol. 2015;867:125–43. https://doi.org/10.1007/978-94-017-7215-0_9.
18. van Veenendaal LM, Bertolli E, Korse CM, Klop WMC, Tesselaar MET, van Akkooi ACJ. The clinical utility of neuron-specific enolase (NSE) serum levels as a biomarker for merkel cell carcinoma (MCC). Ann Surg Oncol. 2021;28(2):1019–28. https://doi.org/10.1245/s10434-020-08656-7.
19. Nardi V, Song Y, Santamaria-Barria JA, et al. Activation of pI3K signaling in merkel cell carcinoma. Clin Cancer Res. 2012;18(5):1227–36. https://doi.org/10.1158/1078-0432.CCR-11-2308.
20. Harms KL, Zhao L, Johnson B, et al. Virus-positive merkel cell carcinoma is an independent prognostic group with distinct predictive biomarkers. Clin Cancer Res. 2021;27(9):2494–504. https://doi.org/10.1158/1078-0432.CCR-20-0864.
21. Lipson EJ, Vincent JG, Loyo M, et al. PD-L1 expression in the merkel cell carcinoma microenvironment: association with inflammation, merkel cell polyomavirus and overall survival. Cancer Immunol Res. 2013;1(1):54–63. https://doi.org/10.1158/2326-6066.CIR-13-0034.
22. Hanna GJ, Kacew AJ, Tanguturi AR, et al. Association of programmed death 1 protein ligand (PD-L1) expression with prognosis in merkel cell carcinoma. Front Med (Lausanne). 2020;7:98. https://doi.org/10.3389/fmed.2020.00198.
23. Nakamura M, Magara T, Kano S, Matsubara A, Kato H, Morita A. Tertiary lymphoid structures and chemokine landscape in virus-positive and virus-negative merkel cell carcinoma. Front Oncol. 2022;12: 811586. https://doi.org/10.3389/fonc.2022.811586.

24. Asioli S, Righi A, de Biase D, et al. Expression of p63 is the sole independent marker of aggressiveness in localised (stage I-II) merkel cell carcinomas. Mod Pathol. 2011;24(11):1451–61. https://doi.org/10.1038/modpathol.2011.100.
25. Fisher ML, Balinth S, Mills AA. p63-related signaling at a glance. J Cell Sci. 2020;133(17):jcs228015. https://doi.org/10.1242/jcs.228015
26. Xie H, Kaye FJ, Isse K, et al. Delta-like protein 3 expression and targeting in merkel cell carcinoma. Oncologist. 2020;25(9):810–7. https://doi.org/10.1634/theoncologist.2019-0877.
27. Su LD, Fullen DR, Lowe L, Uherova P, Schnitzer B, Valdez R. CD117 (KIT receptor) expression in merkel cell carcinoma. Am J Dermatopathol. 2002;24(4):289–93. https://doi.org/10.1097/00000372-200208000-00001.
28. Iwasaki T, Matsushita M, Nonaka D, et al. Phosphohistone-H3 (PHH3) is prognostic relevant in merkel cell carcinomas but merkel cell polyomavirus is a more powerful prognostic factor than AJCC clinical stage, PHH3, Ki-67 or mitotic indices. Pathol Int. 2015;65(8):404–9. https://doi.org/10.1111/pin.12305.
29. Jaatinen J, Veija T, Salmikangas M, Böhling T, Sihto H, Koljonen V. ALK is frequently phosphorylated in merkel cell carcinoma and associates with longer survival. PLoS ONE. 2021;16(5): e0252099. https://doi.org/10.1371/journal.pone.0252099.
30. Naseri S, Steiniche T, Georgsen JB, et al. Tumor ulceration, reduced infiltration of CD8-lymphocytes, high neutrophil-to-CD8-lymphocyte ratio and absence of MC virus are negative prognostic markers for patients with merkel cell carcinoma. Cancers (Basel). 2020;12(4):888. https://doi.org/10.3390/cancers12040888.
31. Kervarrec T, Gaboriaud P, Berthon P, et al. Merkel cell carcinomas infiltrated with $CD33^+$ myeloid cells and $CD8^+$ T cells are associated with improved outcome. J Am Acad Dermatol. 2018;78(5):973-982.e8. https://doi.org/10.1016/j.jaad.2017.12.029.
32. Blom A, Bhatia S, Pietromonaco S, et al. Clinical utility of a circulating tumor cell assay in Merkel cell carcinoma. J Am Acad Dermatol. 2014;70(3):449–55. https://doi.org/10.1016/j.jaad.2013.10.051.
33. Gambichler T, Said S, Abu Rached N, et al. Pan-immune-inflammation value independently predicts disease recurrence in patients with Merkel cell carcinoma. J Cancer Res Clin Oncol. 2022. https://doi.org/10.1007/s00432-022-03929-y.
34. Durante G, Broseghini E, Comito F, et al. Circulating microRNA biomarkers in melanoma and non-melanoma skin cancer. Expert Rev Mol Diagn. 2022;22(3):305–18. https://doi.org/10.1080/14737159.2022.2049243.
35. Fan K, Ritter C, Nghiem P, et al. Circulating cell-free miR-375 as surrogate marker of tumor burden in merkel cell carcinoma. Clin Cancer Res. 2018;24(23):5873–82. https://doi.org/10.1158/1078-0432.CCR-18-1184.
36. Samimi M, Molet L, Fleury M, Laude H, Carlotti A, Gardair C, Baudin M, Gouguet L, Maubec E, Avenel-Audran M, Esteve E, Wierzbicka-Hainaut E, Beneton N, Aubin F, Rozenberg F, Dupin N, Avril MF, Lorette G, Guyetant S, Coursaget P, Touzé A. Prognostic value of antibodies to Merkel cell polyomavirus T antigens and VP1 protein in patients with Merkel cell carcinoma. Br J Dermatol. 2016;174(4):813–22. https://doi.org/10.1111/bjd.14313.
37. Nwogu N, Boyne JR, Dobson SJ, et al. Cellular sheddases are induced by Merkel cell polyomavirus small tumour antigen to mediate cell dissociation and invasiveness. PLoS Pathog. 2018;14(9): e1007276. https://doi.org/10.1371/journal.ppat.1007276.
38. Lezcano C, Kleffel S, Lee N, et al. Merkel cell carcinoma expresses vasculogenic mimicry: demonstration in patients and experimental manipulation in xenografts. Lab Invest. 2014;94(10):1092–102. https://doi.org/10.1038/labinvest.2014.99.
39. Knight LM, Stakaityte G, Wood JJ, et al. Merkel cell polyomavirus small T antigen mediates microtubule destabilization to promote cell motility and migration. J Virol. 2015;89(1):35–47. https://doi.org/10.1128/JVI.02317-14.
40. Gherardin NA, Waldeck K, Caneborg A, et al. $\gamma\delta$ T Cells in merkel cell carcinomas have a proinflammatory profile prognostic of patient survival. Cancer Immunol Res. 2021;9(6):612–23. https://doi.org/10.1158/2326-6066.CIR-20-0817.

41. Lassacher A, Heitzer E, Kerl H, Wolf P. P14ARF hypermethylation is common but INK4a-ARF locus or p53 mutations are rare in Merkel cell carcinoma. J Invest Dermatol. 2008;128(7):1788–96. https://doi.org/10.1038/sj.jid.5701256.
42. Boyer M, Cayrefourcq L, Dereure O, Meunier L, Becquart O, Alix-Panabières C. Clinical relevance of liquid biopsy in melanoma and merkel cell carcinoma. Cancers (Basel). 2020;12(4):960. https://doi.org/10.3390/cancers12040960.
43. Howard RA, Dores GM, Curtis RE, Anderson WF, Travis LB. Merkel cell carcinoma and multiple primary cancers. Cancer Epidemiol Biomarkers Prev. 2006;15(8):1545–9. https://doi.org/10.1158/1055-9965.EPI-05-0895.

Chapter 10
Melanoma Biomarkers

Rachel E. Tao, Jessica N. Pixley, Christine Ahn, and Steven R. Feldman

Abstract Melanoma is a skin cancer that originates from melanocytes, cells that sit in the basal layer of the epidermis and synthesize melanin. The gold standard for the diagnosis is histopathologic evaluation; however, melanoma can show a wide range of histopathologic features, including subtle histologic atypia, which can pose diagnostic challenges. Additionally, there are other melanocytic tumors that remain incompletely understood, designated as melanocytic tumors of uncertain malignant potential (MELTUMP). Biomarkers could potentially address limitations in disease screening, diagnosis, prognosis, and management of melanoma. This chapter focuses on analyzing the biomarkers most closely associated with clinical outcomes in melanoma patients. We conducted a literature review of 14 biomarkers and used classification standards provided by the World Health Organization (WHO). In this review, we discuss the measurable levels of antigens, proteins, and antibodies associated with melanoma diagnosis, prognosis, and response to treatment. The presence and extent of immunohistochemical staining, the serum levels of biomarkers, and the presence of inflammatory cell infiltrates can be analyzed to identify patients who qualify for further testing for melanoma, to distinguish malignant melanoma from benign nevi, to differentiate melanoma from other tumor types, to predict patient outcomes, to monitor the progression of melanoma, and to predict response to therapies.

Keywords Melanoma · Ki-67 · PTEN · P16 · S100B · MCAM · HMB-45 · MITF · LDH · Tyrosinase · PHH3 · T-lymphocytes · Inflammatory cells · VISTA · BRAF · PRAME

R. E. Tao · C. Ahn
Wake Forest School of Medicine, 4618 Country Club Road, Winston-Salem, NC 27104, USA

J. N. Pixley (✉)
Virginia Commonwealth University, Richmond, VA 23284, USA
e-mail: pixleyjn@vcu.edu

S. R. Feldman
Professor of Dermatology, Pathology and Social Sciences & Health Policy, Wake Forest School of Medicine, 4618 Country Club Road, Winston-Salem, NC 27104, USA

R. Norman (ed.), *Biomarkers in Dermatology*,
https://doi.org/10.1007/978-3-031-66513-4_10

10.1 Introduction

Melanoma is a malignant skin cancer that originates from melanocytes, cells that sit in the basal layer of the epidermis and synthesize melanin [1]. In the American Cancer Society's estimates of cancers that will have the most new cases in 2022, melanoma ranked fifth [2]. Melanomas can arise de novo or as the result of malignant transformation of a pre-existing nevus [1]. Definitive diagnosis of melanoma requires biopsy and histopathological evaluation, using criteria that include cytologic atypia and pleomorphism, architectural disorder, and mitotic activity [3]. Poor prognostic indicators used in the TNM staging system include increased tumor thickness, presence of ulceration, and sentinel lymph node involvement [4].

There are limitations to the histopathologic criteria used to diagnose melanoma. Melanoma variants can be devoid of distinctive diagnostic histopathologic features [5]. The histologic interpretation of challenging melanocytic lesions can also pose challenges, with studies showing variability in interrater interpretation of melanocytic lesions among board-certified dermatopathologists [6, 7]. Therefore, the use of biomarkers may be used as an adjunctive tool for diagnosing challenging or borderline melanocytic tumors [5]. Biomarkers can also assist in screening patients for melanoma by identifying patients who may benefit from further testing, distinguishing melanoma from MELTUMP or other borderline melanocytic tumors, differentiating melanomas from other tumor types, predicting prognosis, monitoring for progression or regression of melanoma, and predicting melanoma response to specific therapies. A biomarker is a measurable molecular change in the cancer cell including DNA or chromosomal, epigenetic, mRNA, or protein that can be used prognostically or therapeutically to identify and treat melanoma and address the limitations of our current set of histopathologic assessment tools [8, 9].

This chapter presents a summary of biomarkers that are used in the diagnosis, prognosis, and treatment of melanoma. The selected melanoma biomarkers have been classified as screening (detecting the presence of melanoma), diagnostic (facilitating the diagnosis of melanoma), prognostic (predicting the outcome of melanoma), monitoring (determining the progression of disease), and pharmacodynamic (indicating the effect of a drug on melanoma).

10.2 Methods

A literature search was performed using the PubMed search engine from June to July 2022. Keywords used included *biomarkers, melanoma, diagnostic, prognostic, immunotherapy, role of biomarkers in melanoma, and pathophysiology of melanoma.* Articles included were published between 1979 and 2022, written in English, and relevant to this chapter. The "similar results" feature on PubMed was used to find additional articles. The search resulted in 85 articles that were prescreened by reviewing the abstracts and conclusions. References of these articles were further reviewed to find additional relevant articles. Information regarding each biomarker was classified into the following categories: screening, prognostic, monitoring, pharmacodynamic, and diagnostic.

10.3 Ki-67

10.3.1 Ki-67 Function

Ki-67 is a human protein that is closely associated with cell proliferation and is detected in all cell cycle active phases including G1, S1, G2, and mitosis [10]. Ki-67 is absent from resting phase, G0 [10]. Ki-67 has several important roles in dividing cells [11]. Ki-67 assists in the synthesis of the peri-chromosomal compartment [11]. It assists in spatially organizing heterochromatin to control gene expression [12]. Ki-67 forms a component of the mitotic chromosome periphery and prevents chromosomes from collapsing after the nuclear envelope disassembles to allow for independent chromosomal motility and interaction with the mitotic spindle [13].

10.3.2 Ki-67 Role as Diagnostic Biomarker

Analysis of Ki-67 in benign nevi and melanoma lesions indicates that elevated levels of Ki-67 correlate with the classification of the lesion as a melanoma, while lower quantities of Ki-67 correlate with the classification of the lesion as benign. Ki-67 therefore has the potential to serve as a diagnostic biomarker for melanoma. In a study that stained 23 compound nevi, 17 dysplastic nevi, 8 Spitz nevi, and 24 malignant melanomas with Ki-67 antibody, the average number of Ki-67 positive nuclei was greater in malignant melanomas compared to the other groups of benign nevi [14]. A study examined the use of a combined triple p16-Ki-67-HMB-45 immunohistochemistry scoring system in a set of 44 melanomas and 57 nevi. In this study, the strength of agreement between the final diagnosis and the triple immunohistochemistry score had a k value of 1.00 [15]. This study included six "challenging" tumors that were initially diagnosed as nevi but definitively diagnosed as melanomas either because of metastatic evolution or after review by experts in melanocytic pathology [15]. Further studies are needed to test the reproducibility of the combined triple p16-Ki-67-HMB-45 immunohistochemistry scoring system in additional ambiguous melanocytic lesions [15].

10.3.3 Ki-67 Role as Prognostic Biomarker

Elevated levels of Ki-67 correlate with an increased risk of metastatic dissemination [16, 17]. Ki-67 therefore also has the potential to serve as a prognostic biomarker for melanoma. In a study that assessed Ki-67 reactivity in 55 specimens, there was a positive correlation between Ki-67 reactivity and metastatic dissemination in primary melanomas less than 1.5 mm thick [18]. In a study that analyzed the clinical course of 167 thin melanomas, the tumors that metastasized had no statistically significant difference compared with the others in terms of patient age, Clark level, tumor thickness, or mitotic count. Metastases of the tumors were closely associated with increased Ki-67 immunohistochemical proliferative activity [19]. In a prospective cohort study of 396 patients with thin invasive primary melanomas, the vertical growth phase was closely associated with increased dermal Ki-67 expression compared to the radial growth phase. In addition, dermal Ki-67 expression was associated with metastasis at 10 years and was classified as an independent prognostic factor [16].

The role of Ki-67 as a prognostic biomarker includes predicting survival. A study compared 12 patients with thick Stage I nodular melanomas who were without signs of progression after 5 years of follow-up to 12 patients who did not survive the first 5 years after removal of the tumor. Patients without progression had decreased Ki-67 antigen expression with a mean staining index of 159 compared to 282 in non-survivors with a two-tailed p value of 0.02. Immunostaining for the Ki-67-antigen could help identify individuals with thick nodular melanomas who are at risk of metastatic disease [20]. In another study, elevated Ki-67 expression was superior to mitotic count as a prognostic factor in thick cutaneous melanoma. In the cases with high Ki-67 expression, 5-year survival was 57% and the 10-year survival was 47%. In the group with low Ki-67 positivity, the 5- and 10-year survival rates were 89% and 86%, respectively [17]. In oral mucosal melanoma, patients with lower Ki-67 scores had a survival advantage over those with higher Ki-67 [21]. Ki-67's independent prognostic capabilities are present in Stage I/II melanomas [22].

10.4 PTEN

10.4.1 PTEN Function

Phosphatase and tensin homologue (PTEN) is a tumor suppressor that is frequently lost from a region of chromosome 10q23 in a variety of human tumors. PTEN has distinct functions in the cytoplasm and nucleus of the cell whereby it serves as a tumor suppressor. In the cytoplasm, PTEN acts as a tumor suppressor by blocking phosphatidylinositol 3 kinase (PI3K) signaling to inhibit cell survival, growth, proliferation, angiogenesis, and metabolism [23]. In the nucleus, PTEN exhibits protein phosphatase activity that allows it to inhibit cell migration or induce cell cycle arrest in a manner independent of the PI3K pathway [24].

Melanocytes express the melanocortin-1 receptor (MC1R) which binds to PTEN and can prevent PTEN degradation to suppress PI3K signaling and protect against UV damage. Mutations in MC1R have been identified that are unable to bind to PTEN, causing increased activation of the PI3K pathway upon exposure to UV rays. In primary MC1R variant melanocytes without a BRAF V600E mutation, this hyperactivation of the PI3K signaling results in premature senescence. However, in MC1R variant melanocytes with an activated BRAF V600E mutation, the elevated PI3K signaling allows for oncogenic transformation [25].

10.4.2 PTEN Role as a Diagnostic Biomarker

PTEN has different levels of cytoplasmic staining in melanoma versus benign nevi. In a study that observed cytoplasmic PTEN staining in 41 nevi, 162 primary melanomas, and 71 melanoma metastases, 88% of primary tumors had positive PTEN cytoplasmic staining, 90% of the metastases had detectable PTEN cytoplasmic staining, and no PTEN immunoreactivity was observed in benign nevi [26]. Further studies are needed to analyze PTEN expression in ambiguous melanocytic lesions to conclude if it can function as a diagnostic biomarker to distinguish between melanoma and benign melanocytic lesions.

10.4.3 PTEN Role as a Prognostic Biomarker

Loss of PTEN expression is associated with worse melanoma outcomes. In an analysis of PTEN in 112 primary cutaneous melanomas, loss of cytoplasmic PTEN expression is closely associated with higher stage of melanoma and a lower disease-free survival [27]. In a study that examined PTEN expression in patients with Stage IIIB or III melanoma, complete loss of PTEN expression was associated with shorter overall survival but not shorter distant disease-free survival. The loss of PTEN was closely associated with shorter time to melanoma brain metastasis. In patients with BRAF V600E mutations, loss of PTEN was associated with shorter overall survival and time to melanoma brain metastasis [28]. In patients with melanoma, loss of PTEN was associated with decreased T-lymphocyte infiltration at tumor sites, reduced likelihood of successful T-cell expansion from resected tumors, and inferior outcomes with PD-1 inhibitor therapy. PTEN loss in tumor cells increased the expression of immunosuppressive cytokines, resulting in decreased T-cell infiltration into tumors and inhibited autophagy, which decreased T-cell-mediated cell death [29].

10.5 P16

10.5.1 P16 Function

P16 is a tumor-suppressor protein encoded by the CKDN2A gene on chromosome 9p21. P16 has a well-established role in both hereditary and sporadic melanoma [30]. P16 functions as a tumor suppressor by inhibiting the binding of cyclin-dependent kinase (CDK)-4 and CDK-6 to cyclin D, which activates substances necessary for progression from the G1 to S phase of the cell cycle [31, 32]. When p16 is mutated or lost, it is unable to oppose the CDK4/6-cyclin D complex at the transition from the G1 to S phase. This allows the mitotic rate to increase which plays a role in the development of a melanoma [33].

Loss of function mutations at the CDKN2A locus that encodes p16 creates susceptibility to melanoma. P16 gene germline mutations occur in 25% of families with inheritable melanoma [31]. Familial melanoma syndrome is associated with a homozygous loss of CDKN2A and the development of multiple melanomas [33].

In sporadic melanomas, promoter methylation and loss of heterozygosity are common mechanisms of silencing p16 gene activity. Benign melanocytic nevi uniformly express the p16 protein and increasing loss of p16 expression occurs with melanoma progression [31]. Melanoma in situ has either no alterations or only a decrease in p16. Thus, the loss of p16 is a late rather than initiating event in melanoma [31]. In 60–70% of sporadic melanomas, there is a heterozygous or homozygous loss of the CDKN2A gene. In 10–15% of sporadic melanomas, there is a mutation of the CDKN2A gene [33].

10.5.2 P16 Role as a Diagnostic Biomarker

P16 may function as a diagnostic biomarker, with high specificity but limited sensitivity.

P16 has different levels of expression in childhood nodular spitzoid malignant melanoma and a benign Spitz nevus [34]. In a study that examined the expression of p16 in 6 spitzoid malignant melanomas, 18 Spitz nevi, and 12 compound melanocytic nevi in children younger than 18 years, 100% of the childhood melanoma cases were associated with loss of P16 while 100% of the Spitz nevi and benign melanocytic nevi had strong positive nuclear and cytoplasmic p16 staining [34]. Further studies are needed to analyze P16 expression in ambiguous melanocytic lesions to conclude if it can function as a diagnostic biomarker to distinguish between childhood nodular spitzoid malignant melanoma and a benign Spitz nevus. It would be helpful to have a diagnostic biomarker for this situation because Spitz nevi and spitzoid nodular melanoma in childhood overlap clinically and histopathologically and can be difficult to differentiate [34].

P16 expression can also help distinguish desmoplastic Spitz nevi from desmoplastic melanomas. In a study that compared 15 desmoplastic Spitz nevi and 11 desmoplastic melanomas, only 18% of desmoplastic melanomas reacted with the antibody to p16 and less than 30% of the cells were immunoreactive for p16. All desmoplastic Spitz nevi stained positive for p16, and in 93% of the nevi, over 80% of the cells were immunoreactive for p16 [33].

Loss of p16 expression is far more specific for borderline and malignant spitzoid neoplasms than Spitz nevi. In a study of immunohistochemical p16 protein expression in 24 benign, 27 borderline, and 19 malignant spitzoid lesions, loss of p16 expression was not observed in Spitz nevi but occurred in atypical spitzoid tumors with uncertain malignant potential and spitzoid melanomas. Spitz nevi were associated with higher levels of p16 expression compared to atypical spitzoid tumors and spitzoid melanomas [35].

P16 immunohistochemical staining can be used to confirm the benign nature of blue nevi tumors. A study evaluated p16 immunohistochemical staining in 14 atypical cellular blue nevi, 8 conventional and atypical melanocytic nevi, and 16 melanomas, including 4 malignant cellular blue nevi. P16 staining was far higher in all cellular blue nevi when compared to melanomas and malignant cellular blue nevi. Increased p16 expression was also seen in mildly and moderately atypical cellular blue nevi, but not severely atypical cellular blue nevi compared to melanomas. When used together with additional markers and histology, p16 staining may confirm the benign nature of these blue nevi tumors, but cannot distinguish severely atypical cellular blue nevi from malignant cases [36].

P16 can distinguish benign nevi from melanoma. In a study analyzing 15 skin nevi, 18 nodal nevi, 26 sentinel lymph node melanoma metastases, 10 non-sentinel lymph node melanoma metastases, and 13 melanoma organ metastases, 100% of skin and nodal nevus cells had extensive nuclear and cytoplasmic staining for p16. However, p16 nuclear staining was absent in all cells of melanoma metastasis, except for one skin metastasis. Thus, lack of p16 nuclear staining is a reliable biomarker to distinguish lymph node nevi, nevi located in lymph nodes, from melanoma metastasis [37].

The pattern of p16 expression in a lesion can also be helpful in establishing the diagnosis of melanoma. A study evaluated p16 staining pattern as well as p16 expression. It defined two major categories of p16 staining pattern: simple/homogenous and multiple/heterogeneous. The single/homogenous pattern of expression was defined as a uniform distribution of p16 staining across the lesion and included homogenously strong, diffuse, completely negative, patchy, or rare staining. Multiple/heterogeneous pattern expression was characterized by distinct changes in staining pattern in a zonal distribution within the same lesion. The presence of multiple patterns of p16 expression in a single lesion, in the absence of a region of total loss, should raise concern for melanoma. Multiple patterns of p16 expression occur in 50% of nevoid melanomas and 100% of melanomas arising in precursor nevi. Other nevi categories, besides epithelioid nevi, had only 0–25% of cases with multiple patterns. All lesions that included total pattern loss, both single and multiple pattern lesions, were malignant. However, the total pattern loss of expression was not seen in some cases of nevoid melanoma, some cases of melanoma arising in a precursor nevus, and in most cases of non-nevoid melanoma. Thus, loss of p16 expression is a specific but not sensitive marker for melanocytic malignancy [30].

10.5.3 P16 Role as a Prognostic Biomarker

P16 may also function as a prognostic biomarker.

Absent p16 expression can serve as an independent prognostic factor for overall relapse-free and distant metastasis-free survival, independent of Breslow thickness, ulceration, and tumor stage [38]. Melanoma subtypes associated with deep vertical growth have consistently had loss of p16, and p16 loss has been linked to decreased 5-year survival [33]. Melanomas with the p16/ARF + BRAF/RAS mutational profile are closely associated with longer survival than melanoma cases with more complex mutational profiles. In contrast, melanomas with loss of p16 protein expression are associated with increased cell proliferation as measured by the Ki-67 index, more advanced stage, and metastases. In cases of invasive vertical growth phase melanomas, loss of nuclear p16 immunoreactivity is associated with poor 10-year survival, while the presence of p16 gene polymorphisms is associated with improved 10-year survival [31].

Absent p16 expression is associated with other criteria used for advanced staging. In a study that analyzed p16 expression and cell proliferation in 79 primary cutaneous malignant melanomas and 10 benign melanocytic nevi, 58% of melanomas and 100% of benign melanocytic nevi were p16 positive, while 42% of melanomas were p16 negative. The p16-negative melanomas were closely associated with higher extent of invasion and higher rates of cell proliferation [32]. Loss of the p16 tumor-suppressor gene is associated with increased Breslow thickness, melanoma ulceration, vascular invasion, increased mitotic index, advanced tumor stage, decreased recurrence-free survival, lymph node metastasis, and decreased 5-year survival [33, 38].

10.6 S100B

10.6.1 S100B Function

S100B is an immunohistochemical protein that was first discovered in melanoma cell cultures [39]. It is overexpressed in most cells of neuroectodermal origin [39]. The S100 proteins are members of a multigene family of low-molecular-weight calcium-modulated proteins [40]. S100B is a cytoplasmic protein with many cellular functions including cytoskeleton integrity, calcium homeostasis, and regulation of enzyme activity [39, 40]. S100B also has a role in signal transduction, cell cycle regulation, and apoptosis through its interaction with p53 [39, 40]. It can inhibit calcium-dependent phosphorylation of p53 by protein kinase C which leads to suppression of the p53 tumor-suppressor mechanism and uncontrolled tumor growth [40]. S100B could potentially have a functional role in melanogenesis due to its ability to interact with p53 and to activate STK38/NDR1, a protein kinase involved in cell survival and proliferation [41]. S100B is expressed in elevated levels in melanocyte cytoplasm, and elevated serum S100B levels occur in melanoma due to loss of melanoma cell integrity [40, 42]. It is not fully understood how S100B enters the blood, but it is likely related to cell damage and death. Therefore, the elevation of S100B in patients with melanoma is interpreted as evidence of subclinical microscopic metastatic disease [42]. The elevated S100B level in patients with melanoma is not a result of over expression or increased release [43].

10.6.2 S100B Role as a Prognostic Biomarker

S100B may serve as a prognostic factor for melanoma as elevated levels correlate with disease progression and poor outcome.

Elevated levels of S100B are associated with a higher stage and worse prognosis of melanoma. The mean concentration of S100B protein is closely associated with clinical melanoma stage with increasing levels associated with progressively higher stages [43]. In a study examining 40 patients with Stage IIa and IIb primary melanoma (tumor thickness between 2.0–4.0 mm) and 40 high-risk patients with Stage IIc primary melanoma (tumor thickness over 4.0 mm), patients with Stage IIa and IIb primary melanomas had lower levels of S100B compared to patients with Stage IIc melanoma. Increased levels of S100B were associated with shorter disease-free survival in patients with Stage IIa, IIb, and IIc melanomas. In patients with Stage IIc melanoma, having an S100B level above 0.106 correlated with decreased overall survival and disease-free survival rate [44]. In a study that examined 22 patients with melanoma of unknown origin, serum S100B was elevated in 7 patients. The PET scan detected metastases in 6 of 7 patients with elevated serum S100B protein. Patients with metastases had higher S100B levels than the ones without. Serum S100B protein is discriminative between patients with and without metastases with 75% sensitivity and 92% specificity. Overall, serum S100B protein is a sensitive as well as specific marker for detection of metastases [45]. In patients with distant metastases, the serum concentration of S100B protein is closely associated with the number of affected organs [46]. An increased mean concentration of S100B protein is correlated with increased clinical melanoma stage with the highest S100B concentrations in patients with liver or bone metastases [43].

In a study of 82 healthy subjects and 84 patients with biopsy-proven malignant melanoma, clinical staging was performed according to the TMN system. In 100% of the healthy volunteers, the S100B value was < 0.3 ug/L. In 100% of the patients with clinical Stage II melanoma without metastases, none of the patients had elevated

S100B serum concentrations. In clinical Stage III melanoma with metastases, S100B values > 0.3 ug/L were present in 31% of patients. In clinical Stage IV melanoma with metastases, 69% of patients had elevated serum levels of S100B. Progressive disease was associated with rising S100B values. Even in patients with partial remission or stable disease under chemoimmunotherapy, no decline in S100B serum levels could be observed [46].

Baseline S100B levels can be used as prognostic biomarkers. Elevated pre-operative S100B in patients with clinical Stage III melanoma is associated with decreased disease-free survival. A study analyzed the potential prognostic value of pre-operative S100B concentrations in patients who underwent a therapeutic lymph node dissection after pre-operative staging with FDG-PET and CT. The proportion of patients with pre-operative elevated S100B concentrations was 0–9% in Stage I/II, 5–98% in Stage III, and 40–100% in Stage IV melanoma. Pre-operative elevated concentrations of S100B were associated with a decreased disease-free survival [42]. In another study that analyzed serum S100B level measurements pre-operatively and on post-operative days 1 and 2 of 119 patients who underwent therapeutic lymph node dissection for nodal macrometastases, pre-operative S100B and S100B measured on day 2 were most closely associated with disease-free survival. For disease-specific survival, the pre-operative S100B level was the strongest independent predictor of melanoma prognosis in patients undergoing therapeutic lymph node dissection for nodal macrometastases [47].

10.6.3 S100B Role as a Monitoring Biomarker

Levels of S100B can also be used to monitor melanoma for progression and response to treatment. A rising level of serum S100B is a specific and sensitive marker of melanoma progression. In a study that analyzed patients with melanoma recurrence after a disease-free interval, serum S100B was elevated in 37% of patients at the time of relapse. In cases of progression to Stage III melanoma, 32% of the patients had elevated S100B levels. In cases of progression to Stage IV melanoma, 48% of patients presented with increased S100B. In 5.5% of patients, S100B was the first indicator of disease progression [48]. Another study analyzed 64 different patients during chemotherapy and/or immunotherapy for advanced Stage IV metastatic melanoma. Rising S100B levels were present in 84% of patients with tumor progression during treatment, while 95% of patients with stable or regressing metastatic disease had constant or declining S100B levels [49]. Baseline S100 can help predict metastatic spread because patients with greater than or equal to 3 metastatic sites had higher S100 baseline levels compared to patients with 1 metastatic site [40].

S100B levels can be used as a tumor marker during melanoma treatment. Effective therapy through methods including lymph node dissection, systemic therapy, or immunotherapy is associated with declining S100B levels. Disease progression is associated with elevated S100B levels. S100B serves as a biomarker of disease progression in addition to inducing disease progression itself. It interacts with p53 to down-regulate its function as a tumor-suppressor protein and prevent induction of apoptosis of potential melanoma cells [43].

A study evaluated 137 malignant melanoma patients both retrospectively and prospectively. Serum levels of S100B were far higher in all patients before immunotherapies including anti-BRAF and ipilimumab anti-PD-1 therapies were applied, and the levels decreased thereafter. After therapy, lower S100B levels remained while response lasted. Increases in S100B were associated with recurrence and unresponsiveness. Higher levels of S100B are associated with active disease, higher stage, and metastases [50].

In a study that analyzed 116 patients with metastatic melanoma, changes in S100 from baseline were associated with progression of disease. Patients with progressive disease had an increase from baseline S100 of 143.8% compared to patients with response to treatment who had a decrease from baseline S100 of 60.8%. Patients with a greater than 50% increase from baseline S100 in 12 weeks had lower overall survival than patients with a greater than 50% decrease from baseline S100 [40].

10.7 MCAM

10.7.1 MCAM Function

Melanoma cell adhesion molecule (MCAM) is the main melanoma–melanoma cell adhesion molecule linked with melanoma progression and metastasis. It mediates the aggregation of melanoma cells by binding to an unidentified ligand and may mediate melanoma cell interactions that allow new foci of growth to form in other tissues [51]. In melanoma, MCAM establishes close cell–cell communication for growth, survival, invasion, and metastases [52]. Thus, MCAM expression is closely associated with tumor progression. Approximately 70% of melanoma metastases express this molecule. In primary melanoma tumors, MCAM expression increases with increasing vertical thickness, a predictor of metastatic disease [53].

The production of tumorigenic variants from a non-tumorigenic melanoma cell line is associated with MCAM upregulation. Transfection of MCAM-negative melanoma cells with MCAM-encoding cDNA led to an increase in homotypic adhesion between the cells and increased tumor growth in vivo. While MCAM is strongly expressed by the majority of advanced primary and metastatic cutaneous melanomas, it cannot be detected on normal epidermal melanocytes in situ and is expressed weakly on a fraction of benign nevi [53].

10.7.2 MCAM Role as a Prognostic Biomarker

The expression and intensity of MCAM are closely associated with patient outcome, supporting the use of MCAM as a prognostic biomarker for melanoma [52]. A study investigated expression of MCAM in melanoma and compared this with patient outcome [52]. MCAM expression was negatively associated with survival [52]. Patients with MCAM-positive tumors had a 46% 5-year survival rate and higher risk of dying compared to a 94% 5-year survival rate for patients whose tumors were MCAM negative [52]. Patients whose melanomas expressed MCAM had a 16-fold greater risk of poor outcome in terms of disease survival compared to patients whose melanomas did not express MCAM [52]. MCAM intensity was also negatively associated with survival [52]. Increasing MCAM staining intensity was associated with worsening survival [52]. The 5-year survival rates of mildly positive, moderately positive, and strongly positive MCAM staining melanoma patients were 33%, 48%, and 19%, respectively [52].

Increased immunohistochemical staining of MCAM in primary melanomas that meet the criteria for sentinel lymph node biopsy is predictive of developing regional lymph node disease and worse survival [51]. A study compared MCAM expression in primary and metastatic melanomas and related MCAM expression to regional lymph node disease and patient survival [51]. MCAM positivity was increased in cases of lymph node metastases with 68% of primary melanomas and 89% of lymph node metastases staining positive for the cell adhesion molecule MCAM [51]. MCAM staining intensity was also increased in cases of lymph node metastases with 61% of lymph node metastases exhibiting moderate or strong staining compared to 38% of primary tumors [51]. Patients with primary melanomas that were MCAM positive had poorer outcomes compared with those where MCAM expression was not detectable [51]. The 5-year survival for the MCAM-negative patients with melanoma was 92% compared with 40% for the MCAM-positive patients with melanoma [51]. Patients with primary melanomas that were MCAM-positive were more likely to develop lymph node metastases compared to primary lesions that were negative [51]. Within 5 years of primary excision, 38% of MCAM-positive patients developed lymph node metastases [51]. MCAM expression was more predictive of patients at risk for sentinel node metastasis compared to Breslow thickness, with MCAM-positive patients having a risk of lymph node disease 14-fold greater compared to patients who did not express this adhesion molecule [51]. In the future, MCAM expression and staining intensity could be used to identify patients with melanoma that are candidates for further treatment including lymphadenectomy [51].

10.8 HMB-45

10.8.1 HMB-45 Function

HMB-45 is a monoclonal antibody to a glycoprotein present in pre-melanosomes [54]. The specific cellular structures and antigens recognized are still being determined [55]. Previous immunofluorescence data suggest that the antigen is cytoplasmic [55].

10.8.2 HMB-45 Role as a Screening Biomarker

HMB-45 may be used as a screening biomarker for melanoma because it can be used as an immunohistochemical stain to detect primary and metastatic melanoma [54]. This antibody reacts with melanoma cells, junctional nevus cells, and fetal melanocytes but not with completely melanized normal adult melanocytes or intradermal nevus cells [54]. HMB-45 also does not react with most non-melanoma human malignancies, except for rare tumors with evidence of melanogenesis and tumors associated with tuberous sclerosis [54]. When HMB-45 was assayed on 62 melanomas and 168 non-melanomas, HMB-45 recognized 97% of the melanomas tested and none of the non-melanomas [55]. Based on these data, the predictive value of a positive HMB-45 staining test on a given malignant tumor would be 100% for melanoma [55]. The predictive value of a negative HMB-45 staining test to "rule out" melanoma would be 98% [55]. HMB-45 is specific for melanocytic lesions and does not create false-positive reactions with undifferentiated tumors [55]. Therefore, HMB-45 could be used in cases of undifferentiated malignant tumors where it is difficult to distinguish between melanoma, sarcoma, carcinoma, and lymphoma [55]. Undifferentiated neoplasms that react with HMB-45 can be identified as melanomas [55].

In lymph node dissections, HMB-45 is also useful in identifying microscopic clusters of metastatic melanoma cells [55]. HMB-45 staining in sentinel lymph nodes has low false-positive results because of good resolution and low background staining [54]. Therefore, it can identify small foci of melanoma cells within nodes that were thought to be negative [55].

A disadvantage is that HMB-45 is not useful in distinguishing benign and malignant melanocytic proliferations because it recognizes junctional nevi, Spitz tumors, and atypical melanocytic hyperplasia [55].

10.9 MITF

10.9.1 MITF Function

Microphthalmia-associated transcription factor (MITF) is a nuclear protein that is the master regulator of melanocyte differentiation, development, and melanin synthesis [56]. MITF is involved in melanocyte specification, differentiation, and transformation [56]. It modulates extracellular signals including alpha-MSH, c-Kit ligand, and pro-survival signals from two the ERK and PI3-kinase anti-apoptotic pathways [56, 57]. The protein encoded by the microphthalmia gene is a transcription factor important for development and survival of melanocytes [57]. Melanocyte stimulating hormone (alpha-MSH) upregulates pigment enzyme expression through a signaling cascade that stimulates expression of MITF followed by MITF-mediated activation of pigment enzyme expression [57].

10.9.2 MITF Role as a Diagnostic Biomarker

The essential role of MITF in melanocyte development allows it to serve as a diagnostic biomarker for melanoma. The antibody D5 is an anti-human MITF antibody used to detect MITF in melanocytes [56]. MITF expression is present in both primary and metastatic malignant melanomas as well as benign nevi [58]. In a series of 76 histologically confirmed melanomas, the MITF antibody detected 100% of cases. S100 and HMB-45 failed to detect 5 and 7 cases [57]. The MITF antibody was able to identify an area of deep dermal staining on a specimen that was difficult to visualize with H&E and negative with HMB-45 staining [57]. MITF's sensitivity for identifying melanocytic lesions makes it useful for melanomas, which are more difficult to diagnose, including melanomas that lack a primary site, arise from an internal site, or are diagnosed at the metastatic stage [57]. The deep staining altered the measured thickness of the tumor and thus treatment decisions about optimal surgical margins and adjuvant therapy [57]. Because MITF is a nuclear protein, MITF staining in melanomas produces a nuclear pattern which poses some advantages over cytoplasmic immunostains [57]. It can be difficult to distinguish cytoplasmic staining from background staining [57]. Nuclear staining does not obscure cellular architecture [57]. In a study that evaluated MITF immunostaining in 62 benign nevi, 58 primary cutaneous melanomas, and 53 non-melanocytic tumors, all primary cutaneous melanomas were immunopositive, with the exception of desmoplastic melanomas [58]. MITF immunostaining was conserved in all benign nevi [58]. Immunolabeling with anti-MITF antibodies increases the lymphovascular invasion detection rate in primary cutaneous melanoma compared to detection with hematoxylin and eosin (H&E) staining alone [59].

A disadvantage to using MITF as a diagnostic biomarker is that in addition to immunoreactivity in both benign and malignant melanoma lesions, MITF is also immunoreactive in macrophages, lymphocytes, fibroblasts, Schwann cells, and smooth muscle cells at various sites and tumors derived from these cell types [56]. Thus, the use of antibody D5 may lack sufficient sensitivity and specificity for widespread diagnostic use [56].

10.10 LDH

10.10.1 LDH Function

Lactate dehydrogenase's (LDH) role in normal cellular homeostasis is to convert pyruvate to lactate to produce ATP in anaerobic glycolysis. While this process is less efficient at producing ATP compared to oxidative phosphorylation through the Krebs cycle in aerobic glycolysis, it is the major mechanism of ATP production in most melanomas due to changes in glucose metabolism [60]. Rapidly growing melanomas are poorly vascularized, which causes them to rely on anaerobic glycolysis mediated by LDH as an alternative energy source [61].

10.10.2 LHD Role as a Prognostic Biomarker

LDH is a prognostic biomarker for melanoma. In the 7th revision of the American Joint Committee on Cancer (AJCC) for melanoma staging and classification published in 2009, serum LDH was incorporated as a biomarker used for staging [62]. Under the new AJCC guidelines, serum LDH is measured at the time Stage IV disease is documented [63]. If LDH level is elevated, these patients are classified as M1c: more than one area of cancer in several organs, regardless of the site of their distant metastases [63]. Elevated serum LDH is a predictor of survival even after accounting for site and number of metastases [62]. In the 2008 AJCC Melanoma Staging Database, elevated serum LDH was associated with worse survival in patients with Stage IV melanoma [63]. The 1- and 2-year overall survival rates for patients with Stage IV melanoma were 65 and 40% compared to 32 and 18% in patients with elevated serum LDH at the time of staging [63].

Elevated baseline LDH twice the upper limit of normal is also associated with a decreased likelihood of benefitting from ipilimumab therapy in Netherland and United Kingdom cohorts [61]. Treatment benefit from ipilimumab is likely increased in the LDH-low group because lactate accumulation decreases extracellular pH, which negatively affects the function of lymphocytes present in the melanoma environment [61]. Thus, the median overall survival in the LDH-high group was lower than in the LDH-low group [61]. The 1- and 2-year survival rates for the LDH-low patients were 51.2 and 34.6% compared to 4.7 and 0% in the LDH-high patients [61]. Ipilimumab treatment benefits were exclusively in the LDH-low group [61]. In the future, LDH may be used to guide treatment when selecting patients for ipilimumab therapy [61].

10.11 Tyrosinase

10.11.1 Tyrosinase Function

Tyrosinase is a cytoplasmic protein in melanoma cells and normal melanocytes that serves as a key enzyme in melanin synthesis and belongs to a group of melanocyte differentiation antigens. Peptide epitopes derived from tyrosinase serve as targets for cytotoxic T-lymphocytes and tumor-infiltrating lymphocytes in the context of HLA Class I and Class II molecules. The specific monoclonal antibody T311 targets tyrosinase [64].

10.11.2 Tyrosinase Role as a Diagnostic Biomarker

T311 monoclonal antibody is able to stain melanoma for tyrosinase with a sensitivity of 94% [64]. Anti-tyrosinase antibodies exhibit positivity in all melanocytes, whether resting or in an activated state, and label all compartments of all lesions (intraepidermal, junctional, and dermal) [65]. Benign and malignant melanocytic cells are immunoreactive, but non-melanocytic cells are immunonegative. Detection of tyrosinase protein in a melanoma series ranges from 86 to 100% according to clinical stage. Tyrosinase immunoreactivity decreases with progression from clinical Stage I to Stage IV. Since tyrosinase is a melanocyte differentiation marker, it is lost in dysplastic and metastatic melanocytic tumors [64].

A disadvantage of using tyrosinase as a diagnostic biomarker is that it cannot distinguish between benign and malignant melanoma. In addition to staining melanoma, nevi of all types, lentigo maligna, nevus Spitz, and nevus Reed stain homogeneously positive for tyrosinase [64].

10.11.3 Tyrosinase Role as a Prognostic Biomarker

The detection of tyrosinase mRNA by reverse transcriptase-polymerase chain reaction (RT-PCR) can also be a negative prognostic biomarker for melanoma [66].

From January 2000 to February 2003, blood samples were drawn from 114 melanoma patients following surgery and were tested with RT-PCR reaction for tyrosinase mRNA. Overall, 79.1% of patients tested negative for tyrosinase mRNA and 20.9% tested positive for tyrosinase mRNA. The percent of patients who tested positive for tyrosinase mRNA was closely associated with stage. The number of patients who tested positive was 7.9% for Stage I, 13.6% for Stage II, 16.7% for Stage III, and 54.2% for Stage IV. After median follow-up of 372 days or until death, median progression-free survival has not been reached for tyrosinase-negative patients and was 265 days for tyrosinase-positive patients. Median overall survival was 344 days for tyrosinase-negative patients and has not been reached for tyrosinase-negative patients. Detection of circulating melanoma cells by RT-PCR for tyrosinase mRNA is an adverse prognostic factor for disease-free survival in patients with malignant melanoma [66].

10.11.4 Tyrosinase Role as a Monitoring Biomarker

The detection of tyrosinase mRNA by reverse transcriptase-polymerase chain reaction (RT-PCR) can also be a monitoring biomarker for melanoma [67].

A total of 200 patients with Stage IV metastatic melanoma were analyzed including 149 with active metastatic disease undergoing systemic therapies and 51 who were disease free after surgery. A baseline sample was obtained within 3 weeks of either the clinical/radiological demonstration of metastatic disease or the surgical treatment for each patient. Then, tyrosinase determinations were performed at day 1 of each therapy course before chemotherapy administration or at each follow-up visit for a total of three determinations. Standard RT-PCR techniques were used to determine tyrosinase expression. A baseline positive tyrosinase determination was obtained in 72.5% of the patients with active metastatic disease, but not in any of the patients who were disease free after surgery. In the patients undergoing systemic therapy, an early clearance of circulating melanoma cells was expressed as a decline in tyrosinase from 72.5 at the first determination to 44.9% at the second determination to 29.5% at the third determination. The level of tyrosinase expression before the third cycle was associated with the clinical response: 69.1% of patients with a negative tyrosinase determination obtained a response or a stable disease, while 85.3% patients with a positive tyrosinase determination developed a progressive disease. All patients who had a negative tyrosinase at the first three determinations had a clinical response. All patients who had a positive tyrosinase at the first three determinations developed progressive disease. The presence of a constant positive tyrosinase expression during follow-up was associated with the development of new metastatic sites in 95.6%of patients with active metastatic disease. Tyrosinase expression in the peripheral blood both at baseline and during follow-up is a monitoring biomarker associated with the response to treatment, development of new metastatic sites, time to progression, and survival [67].

10.12 PHH3

10.12.1 PHH3 Function

The proliferation marker phosphohistone 3 (PHH3) marks cells in the four phases of mitosis and late G2 [22]. Therefore, it can be combined with a melanocytic marker in an immunohistochemical double stain to facilitate counting of mitosis and serve as a prognostic biomarker for melanoma [68].

10.12.2 PHH3 Role as a Prognostic Biomarker

Mitosis in melanoma lesions has traditionally been assessed using H&E stains. The proliferation index of H&E-stained thin melanomas is included in the American Joint Committee on Cancer staging system [22]. However, using the proliferation index on H&E stains has presumed inaccuracy and low reproducibility and causes excessive time-consumption [22]. In a study that examined 153 consecutive Stage I/II melanoma patients, the prognostic impact of primary cutaneous melanoma proliferation using immunohistochemical dual labeling with PHH3/MART-1 to detect mitoses was superior to H&E staining [22]. PHH3 was a more reliable marker of mitosis in melanoma than H&E stains, and time spent to determine the proliferation index was reduced by at least 50% [22]. In another study that examined 457 cases of nodular cutaneous melanoma, increased mitotic count and PHH3 value were both associated with increased tumor thickness and presence of ulceration [69]. Per univariate survival analysis, there is a prognostic impact of mitotic count and PHH3 [69]. Per multivariate analysis, PHH3 is a stronger prognostic indicator than mitotic count [69]. The detection rate of mitoses in melanocytic cells using immunohistochemical dual labeling with PHH3/Melan-A was compared to H&E staining [69]. PHH3 improved the accuracy of mitotic counts [69]. The combined immunohistochemical stain for PHH3/Melan-A yielded similar results as the H&E-stained sections and was more time efficient [69].

10.13 Inflammatory Cells

10.13.1 Inflammatory Cells' Function

One of the skin's primary defenses against melanoma is the lymphocytes and inflammatory cells that extravasate from the circulation into the skin to fight the cancer. These various cells can serve as prognostic factors to predict the outcome of melanoma patients.

10.13.2 *Inflammatory Cells' Role as a Prognostic Biomarker*

Cells in the lymphocytic infiltrate include T-lymphocytes and dendritic cells that perform tumor-cell apoptosis and regression [70]. The presence of a dense peri-tumoral and intratumoral lymphocytic infiltrate is strongly associated with a better melanoma prognosis [70]. The inflammatory infiltrate tends to diminish as the tumor grows in size [70]. Activated CD4+ T-cells express OX40, a cell surface glycoprotein that belongs to the TNF receptor family and has the potential to be a prognostic marker for melanoma [70]. Having higher peri-tumoral OX40+ and CD25+ lymphocytic infiltration is strongly associated with having a longer melanoma survival rate [70]. Dendritic cells can express a maturation marker called DC lysosomal-associated membrane protein (DC-LAMP) [70]. The presence of DC-LAMP-positive dendritic cells has been strongly associated with decreased thickness of melanomas [70]. In addition, having a high peri-tumoral concentration of mature dendritic cells has been strongly associated with increased survival. Increased density of dendritic cells in the tumor has been associated with an increased number of activated CD25+ or OX40+ T-lymphocytes [70]. The combination of high peri-tumoral DC-LAMP-positive dendritic cells with high numbers of CD25+ or OX40+ lymphocytes is strongly associated with a favorable survival prognosis [70].

Clark's tumor-infiltrating lymphocyte scoring system further supports tumor-infiltrating lymphocytes as a prognostic factor in melanoma [71]. Clark defined tumor-infiltrating lymphocytes as lymphocytes that infiltrate and disrupt the tumor-cell nests [71]. He classified tumor-infiltrating lymphocytes as brisk (present throughout the substance of the vertical growth phase or present and infiltrating across the entire base of the vertical growth phase), non-brisk (noted in one or more foci of the vertical growth phase), or absent (entirely absent from the tumor or present but not infiltrating the melanoma cell nests) [71]. Brisk is associated with a better prognosis and has been validated in multiple studies involving over 5000 patients [71].

Tumor-infiltrating B cells can also serve as a prognostic factor in melanoma [72]. A low number of CD20-positive B cells has been associated with greater melanoma progression [72]. The presence of less than or equal to 15% of CD20-positive tumor-infiltrating lymphocytes was associated with a worse prognosis in terms of increased tumor recurrence, decreased disease-free interval, increased development of lymph node metastasis, and shorter overall survival [72].

In a study that analyzed sentinel lymph nodes containing metastatic melanoma from 60 treatment naive patients, the number of CD3+, CD4+, and CD8+ tumor-infiltrating lymphocytes was associated with increased recurrence-free and overall survival [73]. Therefore, T-cell subsets in sentinel lymph node metastases could serve as a prognostic factor for melanoma patient outcome [73].

10.13.3 Inflammatory Cells Role as a Pharmacodynamic Biomarker

Assessing the presence of pre-existing CD8+ T-cells also has potential to be a pharmacodynamic marker for selecting melanoma patients that could respond to PD-L1 therapy. A mechanism that cancer cells use to limit the host immune response is upregulation of the programmed cell death ligand (PD-L1) [74]. PD-L1 binds to programmed cell death (PD-1), an immune checkpoint receptor expressed by activated T-cells. When PD-L1 on cancer cells binds to PD-1 on T-cells, this downregulates T-cell activation to create T-cell exhaustion and immune tolerance to the cancer [74]. Administration of anti-PD-1 antibodies including pembrolizumab and nivolumab allows for long-term survival of patients with metastatic melanoma [75]. The use of nivolumab compared to chemotherapy to treat metastatic melanoma is associated with increased progression-free survival and overall survival [76]. The use of pembrolizumab compared to the CTLA-4 inhibitor, ipilimumab, to treat metastatic melanoma is also associated with increased progression-free survival and overall survival [76]. Response to therapies that target PD-1 can be predicted by the presence of pre-existing CD8 T-cells [77]. In a study that analyzed 46 metastatic melanoma samples obtained from patients before and during pembrolizumab therapy, proliferation of intratumoral CD8+ T-cells correlated with reduction in tumor size [77]. Tumor regression following PD-1 blockade therapy was associated with the presence of pre-existing CD8+ T-cells at the margin of the tumor and inside the tumor that could be negatively regulated by PD-1/PD-L1 mediated immune resistance [77]. In another study that analyzed metastatic melanoma samples from 20 patients prior to anti-PD-1 treatment, the presence of increased PD-1 CD8+ T-cells was strongly associated with increased response to anti-PD-1 therapy and progression-free survival [78]. When the metastatic lesions were analyzed during anti-PD-1 therapy, there was an accumulation of highly activated CD8+ T-cells in the tumors, suggesting a release of T-cell exhaustion [78]. This association between presence of CD8+ T-cells and response to anti-PD-1 therapy could be used to select melanoma patients with a high likelihood of achieving a clinical response to PD-1 pathway inhibition [78].

10.14 VISTA

10.14.1 VISTA Function

V-domain Ig suppressor of T-cell activation (VISTA) is a recently identified negative regulator of T-cell-mediated immune responses expressed in melanoma patient samples [79]. VISTA is primarily expressed on hematopoietic cells and myeloid cells including neutrophils, monocytes, macrophages, and dendritic cells [79]. When overexpressed, VISTA suppresses T-cell proliferation and production of T-cell cytokines such as interleukin (IL)-2 and interferon (IFN)-gamma, impairing the immune response to cancer [79].

10.14.2 VISTA Role as Prognostic Biomarker

In a study that analyzed 136 cases of melanoma for VISTA expression via immunohistochemistry, VISTA expression is associated with negative prognostic factors, including increased Breslow thickness and advanced stage of disease [79]. VISTA expression is an independent prognostic factor in cutaneous melanoma, and high expression of VISTA is associated with worse survival [79]. VISTA expression correlated with the expression of the myeloid-derived suppressor cell marker CD33 in cutaneous melanoma; thus, VISTA is mainly expressed on hematopoietic cells and myeloid cells [79]. A study that performed survival analysis on The Cancer Genome Atlas cutaneous melanoma dataset of non-recurrent Stage III patients with a regional lymph, cutaneous, or subcutaneous tumor sample supported that VISTA suppresses T-cell function [80]. In patients with low levels of VISTA, there was decreased survival in patients with lower cytotoxic T-lymphocytes compared to patients with higher cytotoxic T-lymphocytes [80]. In patients with high levels of VISTA, there was no difference in survival between patients with lower versus higher cytotoxic T-lymphocytes, likely because VISTA suppressed the cytotoxic T-lymphocytes [80]. High VISTA expression is associated with decreased cytotoxic T-lymphocyte function, and in melanoma patients with low VISTA expression, high cytotoxic T-lymphocytes is associated with improved survival [80].

In a study that selected 85 primary melanoma specimens from pathology tissue archives and immunohistochemically stained for CD3, PD-1, PD-L1, and VISTA, the presence of VISTA was associated with worse disease-specific survival in univariate analysis and multivariate analysis [81]. VISTA expression is an independent negative prognostic factor in primary cutaneous melanoma [81]. It could have potential as a marker for adjuvant anti-cancer immunotherapeutic intervention in the future [81]. In contrast to PD-L1, which is primarily expressed by activated and exhausted T-cells, VISTA is more highly expressed on myeloid and granulocytic cells [81]. Its different expression pattern compared to PD-L1 could allow it to have novel implications in cancer immunology [81].

10.15 BRAF

10.15.1 BRAF Function

BRAF is a serine/threonine kinase that is an important component of the mitogen-activated protein kinase pathway [82]. In this pathway, BRAF is a Raf protein located downstream from the oncogene Ras [82]. Activation of this membrane-to-nucleus signaling pathway that controls cell proliferation, differentiation, and apoptosis is associated with melanocyte and melanoma proliferation [82]. BRAF mutations have been discovered in multiple types of carcinomas, most commonly in melanomas [82]. This is likely because alpha-melanocyte-stimulating hormone is a regulator of melanocyte biology that binds to melanocortin receptor I to upregulate the cyclic AMP cascade that activates BRAF and leads to increased proliferation and melanogenesis in response to UV radiation [83]. The most common mutation in melanomas is a 1799T $\rightarrow$ A transversion in exon 15 of BRAF, resulting in a V600E amino acid missense mutation [82]. This mutation increases BRAF kinase activity, allowing for continuous transcription-mediated proliferation and neoplastic growth [82].

10.15.2 BRAF Role as a Pharmacodynamic Biomarker

Determining BRAF mutation status in patients with melanoma has potential to become a pharmacodynamic marker. In a study that compared mutational status of BRAF in 126 melanomas from which the degree of exposure to ultraviolet light differs, melanomas that developed on skin without chronic sun-induced damage had frequent mutations in BRAF, while melanomas that developed on skin with chronic sun-induced damage had infrequent mutations in BRAF [84]. Melanomas that developed on skin with intermittent sun exposure and melanomas that developed from moles had higher incidence of BRAF mutations compared to other types of melanoma [84]. The researchers proposed that patients with melanomas that developed from skin with intermittent sun exposure could have melanocytes with increased susceptibility to UV exposure and a higher probability of acquiring BRAF mutations and proliferating [84]. Thus, these patients would be expected to be more responsive to therapeutic interventions that target the RAS-RAF-ERK pathway involving BRAF such as sorafenib, a Raf kinase inhibitor [84]. Patients with melanomas that developed from skin with chronic sun-induced damage could have melanocytes that are less susceptible and require a high cumulative UV dose to induce melanoma from sun-damaged skin rather than BRAF mutations [84]. Thus, these patients would be less responsive to therapeutic interventions targeting the RAS-RAF-ERK pathway [84].

10.15.3 BRAF Role as a Prognostic Biomarker

Determining BRAF mutation status in patients with melanoma also has potential to become a prognostic marker. In a study that analyzed 140 intermediate thickness melanoma patients, BRAF V600E status is closely associated with sentinel node involvement [85]. Sentinel node involvement was associated with lower recurrence-free survival, melanoma-specific survival, and overall survival [85]. BRAF V600E positivity was associated with worse recurrence-free survival and overall survival [85].

10.16 PRAME

10.16.1 PRAME Function

PReferentially expressed Antigen in Melanoma (PRAME) is a melanoma-associated antigen and repressor of retinoic acid receptor (RAR) signaling. Retinoic acid through RAR signaling induces tumor-suppressive activities including proliferation arrest, differentiation, and apoptosis in many cell types. Impaired RAR signaling has been implicated in carcinogenesis. PRAME interacts with RAR to repress the expression of RAR-target genes [86]. Most normal healthy tissues do not express PRAME except for testis, ovary, placenta, adrenals, and endometrium. PRAME is expressed in cutaneous melanoma, ocular melanoma and various non-melanocytic malignant neoplasms [87].

10.16.2 PRAME Role as a Diagnostic Biomarker

PRAME immunohistochemical expression has the potential to become a diagnostic marker because it is preferentially expressed in melanoma cancer cells. A study examined the immunohistochemical expression of PRAME in 155 primary cutaneous melanomas, 100 metastatic cutaneous melanomas, and 140 cutaneous melanocytic nevi. Diffuse nuclear immunoreactivity for PRAME was present in 87% of metastatic cutaneous melanomas and 83.2% of primary cutaneous melanomas, while 86.4% of cutaneous melanocytic nevi were completely negative for PRAME. Diffuse PRAME expression is rare in melanocytic nevi [87].

Diffuse PRAME immunohistochemical expression can assist in margin assessment of melanoma in situ with adjacent tumor-negative skin [86]. The margins of ten excisions for primary melanomas were evaluated to determine the clearance between melanoma in situ and the nearest side margin using H&E-stained sections and immunostains for PRAME and Sox10 expression. The assessment of margins using immunohistochemistry for PRAME correlated well with margin status and clearance based on routine H&E-stained sections and immunohistochemistry for Sox10. Unlike Sox10 which highlights all melanocytes, PRAME less frequently stains normal melanocytes, so it offers an improved microscopic picture as to where the melanocytic lesion ends. If inflammation, cautery artifacts, or background melanocyte hyperplasia make it difficult to determine the end of a lesion, PRAME could be superior to H&E or immunostains for melanocyte differentiation antigens for assessing margins. A limitation is that rare non-neoplastic melanocytes in solar lentigines and sections from chronically sun-damaged skin can also be PRAME positive. This makes immunohistochemical staining for PRAME less useful in distinguishing a solar lentigo from lentigo maligna [87].

PRAME immunohistochemical staining is useful in the diagnostic interpretation of difficult cutaneous melanocytic tumors with ambiguous microscopic features including melanocytic neoplasms with spitzoid and nevoid features. Definitive diagnosis based on H&E histomorphology is difficult for these ambiguous cutaneous melanocytic tumors. While cytogenetic tests including fluorescence in situ hybridization (FISH), genome-wide array comparative genomic hybridization (CGH), and single nucleotide polymorphism (SNP) array can help assess these tumors, they are expensive and have a prolonged turnaround time. A study examined 110 melanocytic tumors with ambiguous features on H&E examination by at least two dermatopathologists. Each melanocytic tumor was evaluated by FISH for melanoma and/or SNP-array and PRAME immunohistochemistry. A threshold of > 75% of tumor cells positive for PRAME immunohistochemistry was established in support of a melanoma diagnosis. There was an 90% concordance agreement between PRAME immunohistochemistry and cytogenetic (FISH and/or SNP-array) results and a 92.7% concordance agreement between PRAME immunohistochemistry results and final diagnostic interpretation that incorporated all available histomorphologic, clinical, PRAME immunohistochemistry, and cytogenetic data. The sensitivity of diffuse PRAME immunoreactivity for melanoma was 75%, while its specificity was 98.8% in these highly challenging melanocytic tumors [88].

10.17 Commercially Available Biomarker Tests: The DermTech Smart Sticker

10.17.1 The DermTech Smart Sticker Function

A commercially available biomarker test called the DermTech Smart Sticker has been developed as a screening tool to determine if a suspicious lesion should be biopsied for melanoma. The biomarker test was developed to limit the number of biopsies performed. Currently, biopsies are performed as part of the current standard of care for melanoma diagnosis [89]. However, the majority of surgical biopsies are negative for melanoma and can be considered avoidable [89]. In the USA, about 3 million surgical pigmented skin lesions biopsies are performed each year to diagnose fewer than 200,000 new cases of invasive melanoma and melanoma in situ [89]. In addition, patients with early melanoma often have subtle histopathologic changes on initial biopsy [89]. Often earlier lesions with varying degrees of benign cellular atypia and positive margins on initial biopsy are further subject to excisional removal which contributes to additional excisional procedures in up to 30% of patients [89]. The DermTech Smart Sticker was designed to be a highly accurate rule-out assay to aid in the clinician's decision to biopsy atypical melanocytic lesions with one or more ABCDE criteria and suspicion for a melanoma and to aid in early melanoma detection [89].

This biomarker test uses four stickers to collect skin cells from a suspicious lesion [90]. This can be performed at a doctor's office or at home under the supervision of a healthcare professional [90]. This non-invasive adhesive patch-based gene expression rule-out test is called a pigmented lesion assay (PLA) [89]. The stickers are sent to the DermTech gene lab which uses RT-PCR to detect biomarkers' long intergenic non-protein coding RNA 518 (LINC00518) and Preferentially expressed antigen in melanoma (PRAME) [90]. DNA-sequencing technique identifies the presence of Telomerase reverse transcriptase (TERT) mutations [90]. LINC00518 decoys miR-204-5p to upregulate Adaptor-Related Protein Complex 1 Sigma 2 Subunit expression which promotes melanoma cell growth, invasion, migration, and metastasis [91]. PRAME is a melanoma-associated antigen [89]. TERT is a component of telomerase normally repressed in postnatal somatic cells to cause cell senescence [92]. TERT mutations may prevent its repression [92]. TERT encodes a reverse transcriptase that creates a template for telomere addition [92]. Longer telomeres are associated with cancer, including cutaneous melanoma [92]. Positive results for LINC00518, PRAME, or TERT mutations correlate with the presence of melanoma [90].

The results are sent to the patient's physician in less than 5 business days [90]. The physician may then determine next steps based on the test results [90]. If a positive result is found for any of the genomic markers tested, the doctor may recommend surgical biopsy/treatment [90]. It is recommended that positive PLA tests are followed up with a surgical biopsy, whereas negative tests are scheduled for surveillance [89].

10.17.2 The DermTech Smart Sticker Role as a Screening Biomarker

Several studies have been conducted testing the effectiveness of the DermTech Smart Sticker clinically.

One study consisted of 381 patients assessed with the PLA [89]. There were 51 PLA-positive test results that were managed with a surgical biopsy [89]. Of these biopsied lesions, 37% were melanomas which corresponded to a number needed to biopsy of 2.7 [89]. All melanomas were histopathologically classified as melanoma in situ or Stage 1 [89]. There were 330 PLA-negative test results [89]. Of these negative results, 99% were clinically managed with surveillance [89]. Three of the patients with PLA-negative results received follow-up biopsies in the following 3–6 months, and none of them were diagnosed as melanoma histologically [89]. Assuming that PLA-negative results without a follow-up biopsy were true negatives, the estimated sensitivity and specificity of the PLA from these data sets were 95% and 91%, respectively, with a negative predictive value of more than 99% [89]. A limitation to this study is that it was assumed that PLA-negative lesions not biopsied at 3–6 months were true negatives [89]. Of the lesions positive for both LINC00518 and PRAME, 93% were diagnosed histopathologically as melanoma [89]. Of the lesions positive for LINC00518 only, 7% were diagnosed histopathologically as melanoma [89]. Of the lesions positive for PRAME-only, 50% were diagnosed histopathologically as melanoma [89]. PLA results that were positive for both LINC00518 and PRAME were more likely to have a positive histopathologic diagnosis of melanoma [89]. In this study, use of the PLA reduced the number of unnecessary surgical procedures while increasing the detection of melanoma in pigmented lesions in early-stage disease [89].

Another study analyzed use of the DermTech Smart Sticker in 398 validation samples [93]. Each non-invasive adhesive patch biopsy was followed by conventional surgical biopsy of the same pigmented lesion which was assessed by a primary reader and panel of three expert dermatopathologists who provided a consensus diagnosis [93]. LINC00518 and/or PRAME detection differentiated melanoma from non-melanoma samples with a sensitivity of 91% and a specificity of 69% [93].

Another study did a 12-month chart review follow-up of 734 pigmented lesions that had PLA-negative results [94]. Thirteen of the lesions were biopsied in the follow-up period and submitted for histopathologic review [94]. None of the lesions biopsied had a histopathologic diagnosis of melanoma [94]. PLA has a high negative predictive value and can help guide the management of pigmented lesions to avoid unnecessary surgical procedures [94].

The DermTech Smart Sticker's noninvasive nature of tissue collection may be preferable for patients with wound-healing issues, patients with lesions in cosmetically sensitive areas, and patients who are anticoagulated and have a tendency to develop hypertrophic scars [93].

10.18 DecisionDx-Melanoma

10.18.1 DecisionDx-Melanoma Function

DecisionDx-Melanoma is a gene expression profile (GEP) test designed to predict a patient's risk of recurrence and likelihood of sentinel lymph node positivity in Stage I, II, and III melanomas [95]. The purpose of this test is to expand upon the AJCC 8th edition staging to provide improved risk stratification for patients [95].

The greatest number of deaths from melanoma occur in patients who were diagnosed with early-Stage I-III melanoma at the time of initial diagnosis [95]. Despite being initially classified as low risk, two out of three patients who developed metastatic disease and died from their primary melanoma tumor were initially classified as Stage I or II [95]. A substantial percentage of early-stage melanoma patients develop metastases [95]. Currently, practice management decisions are based on assessment of a patient's risk of recurrence, but anatomic/pathologic staging often falls short in identifying patients at risk for metastasis or death [95].

Eligible patients for this test have Stage I-III cutaneous melanoma, were newly diagnosed up to 3 years ago, can have all histological subtypes, and have availability of tissue from their primary biopsy [95]. The DecisionDx-Melanoma test analyzes patient samples for 3 control genes and 28 prognostic genes important for melanoma tumor progression, including migration and metastasis, cellular differentiation, chemokine activity, immune response, and angiogenesis using RT-PCR [95]. The results of the DecisionDx-Melanoma test generate a 31-GEP continuous test score that stratifies patients based on risk of recurrence into three classes [95]. Class 1A has a low risk of recurrence/metastasis within 5 years [95]. Class 1B/2A has increased risk of recurrence/metastasis within 5 years [95]. Class 2B has the highest risk of recurrence/metastasis within 5 years [95]. Using an algorithm, the patient's 31-GEP continuous test score can be combined with clinical and pathologic factors such as Breslow thickness, patient age, ulceration status, and mitotic rate to create two integrated tests result called the i31-sentinel lymph node biopsy (SLNB) and the i31-risk of recurrence (ROR) [95]. The i31-SLNB provides a sentinel lymph node (SLN) positivity risk prediction designed to identify patients at low risk of SLN positivity who can forgo the procedure and patients at high risk of SLN positivity who should be offered a SLNB [95]. The i31-ROR guides intensity of follow-up, surveillance, and referrals based on risk of recurrence and survival outcome prediction [95].

10.18.2 DecisionDx-Melanoma as a Prognostic Biomarker

An increased 31-GEP continuous test score is closely associated with decreased recurrence-free and metastasis-free survival rates. A meta-analysis that examined the 31-GEP looked at data from 1,479 patients [96]. Class 1A patients had a 91.4% five-year recurrence-free rate and 94.1% distant metastasis-free survival rate [96]. Class 2B patients had a 43.6% five-year recurrence-free rate and 55.5% distant metastasis-free survival rate [96]. Class 2 was significantly associated with recurrence ($p < 0.0001$) and distant metastasis recurrence ($p < 0.0001$) [96]. Patients with Class 2B tumors were 2.9 times more likely to experience a recurrence and 2.8 times more likely to experience a distant metastasis [96]. DecisionDx-Melanoma had improved sensitivity and negative predictive value compared to sentinel lymph node biopsy [96]. The 31-GEP continuous test score could identify AJCC Stage I-III patient subsets with high likelihood for recurrence and distant metastasis [96]. When 31-GEP and sentinel lymph node biopsy results were considered together, sensitivity and negative predictive value for distant metastasis-free survival were both improved [96].

Another meta-analysis examined six studies on the 31-GEP [97]. There was a significant association between Class 2 test results and recurrence-free ($p < 0.00001$), distant metastasis ($p < 0.00001$), and overall survival rates ($p < 0.00001$) [97]. DecisionDx-Melanoma test results were associated with sentinel lymph node biopsy status ($p < 0.00001$) [97].

A retrospective study of 901 cutaneous melanoma samples obtained from patients with stages I-III cutaneous melanoma assessed 31-GEP test predictions of 5-year melanoma-specific survival to determine if the 31-GEP could further risk-stratify melanoma-specific mortality within each AJCC 8th edition stage. 31-GEP testing was able to identify a subset of patients with Stage 1 cutaneous melanomas not eligible for adjuvant therapy but with survival rates similar to some patients who were eligible for adjuvant therapy. In the combined Stage I-III cohort, the addition of 31-GEP data significantly stratified melanoma-specific survival ($p < 0.001$) with a higher 5-year melanoma-specific survival in Class 1A patients compared to Class 2B patients [98].

I31-GEP could reduce the number of SLNBs performed and improve the yield of positive SLNBs. Current guidelines recommend offering SLNB to patients with > 10% likelihood of sentinel lymph node (SLN) positivity. Guidelines do not recommend SLNB for patients with T1a tumors without high-risk features who have < 5% likelihood of a positive SLN. The decision to perform SLNB for patients with higher-risk T1 melanomas in which a positive node is expected 5%–10% of the time is less certain. A study found that compared with other covariates in the i31-GEP, the continuous 31-GEP score had the largest likelihood ratio ($p < 0\,0.001$) for predicting SLN positivity. The use of the i31-GEP increased the percentage of patients in the study with T1-T4 tumors predicted to have a 5% SLN-positive likelihood from 8.5% to 27.7% with a negative predictive value of 98% [99].

In patients with T1 tumors originally classified with a likelihood of SLN positivity of 5%-10%, the i31-GEP reclassified 63% of cases as having < 5% or > 10% likelihood of positive SLN. Therefore, the i31-GEP could be applied in the future to better distinguish patients who would benefit from a SLNB from those who can forgo the procedure [99].

A study compared accuracy of the 31-GEP to the web-based AJCC Individualized Melanoma Patient Outcome Prediction using 205 Stage I/II cutaneous melanomas. Of these cases, 21% had discordant GEP and AJCC classification. Of the deaths in these discordant cases, 85% were predicted as high risk by 31-GEP but low risk by AJCC. Therefore, the 31-GEP improves identification of high-risk melanomas when used with the AJCC online prediction tool [100].

10.19 Interpretating Screening and Diagnostic Biomarker Study Findings

In this review, we discussed how measurable levels of antigens, proteins, and antibodies could aid in the screening and diagnosis of melanoma. To know if a biomarker is clinically valuable as a screening or diagnostic tool, it must be tested in situations where the distinction between benign nevi and malignant melanoma is not obvious based on the pre-existing histopathological criteria currently used by pathologists. Many of the studies suggest that specific biomarkers could aid in the screening or diagnosis of melanoma made these claims based on the ability of the biomarkers to distinguish between lesions that were clearly benign nevi or malignant melanoma based on their histopathological findings. Throughout this chapter, we indicated where further studies with less distinct lesions are necessary to determine if these biomarkers can be used clinically as screening or diagnostic tools. Since melanoma is deadly, a screening biomarker must have very high sensitivity, or it is not useful [2].

10.20 Discussion

Biomarkers are used to diagnose and manage multiple diseases including diabetes, prostate cancer, and ovarian cancer. Their use in the evaluation and management of melanoma is still being investigated. Currently, definitive diagnosis of melanoma requires biopsy and evaluation of histopathologic features, but the interpretation of these features can be subjective and unusual melanoma variants can lack these distinctive histopathologic features. Biomarkers could potentially address these limitations in diagnosis and assist in achieving a more precise clinical diagnosis and severity assessment of patients with melanoma.

In this chapter, 14 biomarkers that are closely associated with clinical outcomes in melanoma were analyzed regarding their potential use in melanoma screening, diagnosis, prognosis, monitoring, and pharmacodynamic evaluation. Some biomarkers were grouped into more than one category. Identification of key biomarkers in melanoma involves analysis of their role in the pathogenesis of melanoma.

To screen patients for melanoma, HMB-45 is an immunohistochemical stain that is immunoreactive with both primary and metastatic melanomas to identify patients who qualify for further biopsy and histopathologic examination for melanoma diagnosis.

For diagnosis of melanoma, Ki-67 antibody, cytoplasmic PTEN, and PRAME immunohistochemical staining can facilitate the distinction between benign nevi and malignant melanoma. Loss of P16 expression can distinguish between benign nevi, spitzoid melanoma, desmoplastic melanoma, and malignant cellular blue nevi to aid in correctly diagnosing patients and identifying which patients need further treatment for melanoma. MITF and tyrosinase antibody staining can also be used to differentiate melanomas from other tumor types to correctly diagnose patients. PRAME immunohistochemical staining can help in the diagnostic interpretation of ambiguous melanocytic neoplasms with spitzoid and nevoid features.

Analyzing levels of biomarkers can determine the prognosis of a patient with melanoma to assist in clinical decision-making and further guide treatment. Elevated levels of immunohistochemical staining for Ki-67, MCAM, PHH3, and VISTA indicate increased mitotic activity, increased tumor spread, and decreased ability of the immune system to fight the tumor. Loss of expression of PTEN and p16 identify patients with loss of tumor suppressors and thus worse outcomes. Elevated serum levels of S100B and LDH indicate increased aggressiveness of the tumor. Positivity for tyrosinase mRNA and BRAFB600E provides insight into the mechanism of melanoma progression and predicts worse outcomes. The presence of a dense peri-tumoral and intratumoral inflammatory cell infiltrate predicts better outcomes and provides a way wherein the immune system t defend itself against the tumor.

To monitor patients for progression or regression of melanoma, elevated serum S100B levels and presence of tyrosinase mRNA increase with tumor progression and metastatic spread and decrease with clinical response to therapy.

When determining the best treatment plan for the patient, the presence of inflammatory cells predicts response to PD-L1 therapy and BRAF positivity predicts response to therapies targeting the RAS-RAF-ERK pathway.

There are limitations to the use of biomarkers in melanoma. Some diagnostic biomarkers such as MITF and tyrosinase immunohistochemical staining distinguish melanomas from other tumor types but cannot distinguish melanomas from benign nevi. This is an important distinction to make when determining treatment plan. Levels of certain biomarkers are characteristically altered in some patients with melanoma, but not all patients. This variability limits the use of certain biomarkers, such as MCAM and tyrosinase immunohistochemical staining, for melanoma diagnosis, prognosis, and monitoring. Serum levels of biomarkers that are indicative of pathogenesis in melanoma can also be altered in other cancers including loss of cytoplasmic PTEN expression, elevated serum LDH, and the presence of inflammatory cells, nullifying the precision of these biomarkers over biopsy and histopathologic evaluation for assessing melanoma.

10.21 Conclusion

Melanoma is a malignant tumor originating from melanocytes, cells that sit in the basal layer of the epidermis and synthesize melanin pigment [1]. It is the most deadly form of skin cancer, and the fifth most common cancer in men and women in the USA [2]. Currently, definitive diagnosis requires biopsy and evaluation of histopathologic features, but the interpretation of these features can be subjective and unusual melanoma variants can lack these distinctive histopathologic features. Currently, the only biomarker approved by the AJCC for melanoma staging and classification is serum levels of LDH. While there is potential for biomarkers to have a role in melanoma diagnosis and management, their superiority over biopsy and histopathologic assessment has not been well established and is a high hurdle to overcome.

References

1. Goldsmith HS. Melanoma: an overview. CA Cancer J Clin. 1979;29(4):194–215. https://doi.org/10.3322/canjclin.29.4.194.
2. Siegel RL, Miller KD, Fuchs HE, Jemal A. Cancer statistics. CA Cancer J Clin. 2022;72(1):7–33. https://doi.org/10.3322/caac.21708.
3. Urso C, Rongioletti F, Innocenzi D, Batolo D, Chimenti S, Fanti PL, et al. Histological features used in the diagnosis of melanoma are frequently found in benign melanocytic naevi. J Clin Pathol. 2005;58(4):409–12. https://doi.org/10.1136/jcp.2004.020933.
4. Balch CM, Soong SJ, Gershenwald JE, Thompson JF, Reintgen DS, Cascinelli N, et al. Prognostic factors analysis of 17,600 melanoma patients: validation of the American joint committee on cancer melanoma staging system. J Clin Oncol. 2001;19(16):3622–34. https://doi.org/10.1200/jco.2001.19.16.3622.
5. Cabrera R, Recule F. Unusual clinical presentations of malignant melanoma: a review of clinical and histologic features with special emphasis on dermatoscopic findings. Am J Clin Dermatol. 2018;19(Suppl 1):15–23. https://doi.org/10.1007/s40257-018-0373-6.
6. Eriksson H, Frohm-Nilsson M, Hedblad MA, Hellborg H, Kanter-Lewensohn L, Krawiec K, et al. Interobserver variability of histopathological prognostic parameters in cutaneous malignant melanoma: impact on patient management. Acta Derm Venereol. 2013;93(4):411–6. https://doi.org/10.2340/00015555-1517.
7. Elmore JG, Barnhill RL, Elder DE, Longton GM, Pepe MS, Reisch LM, et al. Pathologists' diagnosis of invasive melanoma and melanocytic proliferations: observer accuracy and reproducibility study. BMJ. 2017;357: j2813. https://doi.org/10.1136/bmj.j2813.
8. Abbas O, Miller DD, Bhawan J. Cutaneous malignant melanoma: update on diagnostic and prognostic biomarkers. Am J Dermatopathol. 2014;36(5):363–79. https://doi.org/10.1097/DAD.0b013e31828a2ec5.
9. Ogata D, Namikawa K, Takahashi A, Yamazaki N. A review of the AJCC melanoma staging system in the TNM classification (eighth edition). Jpn J Clin Oncol. 2021;51(5):671–4. https://doi.org/10.1093/jjco/hyab022
10. Scholzen T, Gerdes J. The Ki-67 protein: from the known and the unknown. J Cell Physiol. 2000;182(3):311–22. https://doi.org/10.1002/(sici)1097-4652(200003)182:3%3c311::aid-jcp1%3e3.0.co;2-9.
11. Booth DG, Takagi M, Sanchez-Pulido L, Petfalski E, Vargiu G, Samejima K, et al. Ki-67 is a PP1-interacting protein that organises the mitotic chromosome periphery. Elife. 2014;3: e01641. https://doi.org/10.7554/eLife.01641.
12. Sobecki M, Mrouj K, Camasses A, Parisis N, Nicolas E, Llères D, et al. The cell proliferation antigen Ki-67 organises heterochromatin. Elife. 2016;5: e13722. https://doi.org/10.7554/eLife.13722.
13. Cuylen S, Blaukopf C, Politi AZ, Müller-Reichert T, Neumann B, Poser I, et al. Ki-67 acts as a biological surfactant to disperse mitotic chromosomes. Nature. 2016;535(7611):308–12. https://doi.org/10.1038/nature18610.
14. Li LX, Crotty KA, McCarthy SW, Palmer AA, Kril JJ. A zonal comparison of MIB1-Ki67 immunoreactivity in benign and malignant melanocytic lesions. Am J Dermatopathol. 2000;22(6):489–95. https://doi.org/10.1097/00000372-200012000-00002.
15. Uguen A, Uguen M, Guibourg B, Talagas M, Marcorelles P, De Braekeleer M. The p16-Ki-67-HMB45 immunohistochemistry scoring system is highly concordant with the fluorescent

in situ hybridization test to differentiate between melanocytic nevi and melanomas. Appl Immunohistochem Mol Morphol. 2018;26(6):361–7. https://doi.org/10.1097/pai.0000000000000428.
16. Gimotty PA, Van Belle P, Elder DE, Murry T, Montone KT, Xu X, et al. Biologic and prognostic significance of dermal Ki67 expression, mitoses, and tumorigenicity in thin invasive cutaneous melanoma. J Clin Oncol. 2005;23(31):8048–56. https://doi.org/10.1200/jco.2005.02.0735.
17. Ladstein RG, Bachmann IM, Straume O, Akslen LA. Ki-67 expression is superior to mitotic count and novel proliferation markers PHH3, MCM4 and mitosin as a prognostic factor in thick cutaneous melanoma. BMC Cancer. 2010;10:140. https://doi.org/10.1186/1471-2407-10-140.
18. Moretti S, Spallanzani A, Chiarugi A, Fabiani M, Pinzi C. Correlation of Ki-67 expression in cutaneous primary melanoma with prognosis in a prospective study: different correlation according to thickness. J Am Acad Dermatol. 2001;44(2):188–92. https://doi.org/10.1067/mjd.2001.110067.
19. Frahm SO, Schubert C, Parwaresch R, Rudolph P. High proliferative activity may predict early metastasis of thin melanomas. Hum Pathol. 2001;32(12):1376–81. https://doi.org/10.1053/hupa.2001.29658.
20. Vogt T, Zipperer KH, Vogt A, Hölzel D, Landthaler M, Stolz W. P53-protein and Ki-67-antigen expression are both reliable biomarkers of prognosis in thick stage I nodular melanomas of the skin. Histopathology. 1997;30(1):57–63. https://doi.org/10.1046/j.1365-2559.1996.d01-558.x.
21. Ma X, Wu Y, Zhang T, Song H, Jv H, Guo W, et al. Ki67 proliferation index as a histopathological predictive and prognostic parameter of oral mucosal melanoma in patients without distant metastases. J Cancer. 2017;8(18):3828–37. https://doi.org/10.7150/jca.20935.
22. Nielsen PS, Riber-Hansen R, Jensen TO, Schmidt H, Steiniche T. Proliferation indices of phosphohistone H3 and Ki67: strong prognostic markers in a consecutive cohort with stage I/II melanoma. Mod Pathol. 2013;26(3):404–13. https://doi.org/10.1038/modpathol.2012.188.
23. Hopkins BD, Hodakoski C, Barrows D, Mense SM, Parsons RE. PTEN function: the long and the short of it. Trends Biochem Sci. 2014;39(4):183–90. https://doi.org/10.1016/j.tibs.2014.02.006.
24. Milella M, Falcone I, Conciatori F, Cesta Incani U, Del Curatolo A, Inzerilli N, et al. PTEN: multiple functions in human malignant tumors. Front Oncol. 2015;5:24. https://doi.org/10.3389/fonc.2015.00024.
25. Cao J, Wan L, Hacker E, Dai X, Lenna S, Jimenez-Cervantes C, et al. MC1R is a potent regulator of PTEN after UV exposure in melanocytes. Mol Cell. 2013;51(4):409–22. https://doi.org/10.1016/j.molcel.2013.08.010.
26. Slipicevic A, Holm R, Nguyen MT, Bøhler PJ, Davidson B, Flørenes VA. Expression of activated Akt and PTEN in malignant melanomas: relationship with clinical outcome. Am J Clin Pathol. 2005;124(4):528–36. https://doi.org/10.1309/yt58wwmta6yr1prv.
27. Němejcová K, Dundr P, Jakša R, Bártů M, Stružinská I, Hojný J, et al. Comprehensive analysis of PTEN in primary cutaneous melanoma. Folia Biol (Praha). 2020;66(1):7–16.
28. Bucheit AD, Chen G, Siroy A, Tetzlaff M, Broaddus R, Milton D, et al. Complete loss of PTEN protein expression correlates with shorter time to brain metastasis and survival in stage IIIB/C melanoma patients with BRAFV600 mutations. Clin Cancer Res. 2014;20(21):5527–36. https://doi.org/10.1158/1078-0432.ccr-14-1027.
29. Peng W, Chen JQ, Liu C, Malu S, Creasy C, Tetzlaff MT, et al. Loss of PTEN promotes resistance to T Cell-mediated immunotherapy. Cancer Discov. 2016;6(2):202–16. https://doi.org/10.1158/2159-8290.cd-15-0283.
30. Oaxaca G, Billings SD, Ko JS. P16 Range of expression in dermal predominant benign epithelioid and spindled nevi and melanoma. J Cutan Pathol. 2020;47(9):815–23. https://doi.org/10.1111/cup.13721.
31. Carlson JA, Ross JS, Slominski A, Linette G, Mysliborski J, Hill J, et al. Molecular diagnostics in melanoma. J Am Acad Dermatol. 2005;52(5):743–75; quiz 75–8. https://doi.org/10.1016/j.jaad.2004.08.034

32. Talve L, Sauroja I, Collan Y, Punnonen K, Ekfors T. Loss of expression of the p16INK4/CDKN2 gene in cutaneous malignant melanoma correlates with tumor cell proliferation and invasive stage. Int J Cancer. 1997;74(3):255–9. https://doi.org/10.1002/(sici)1097-0215(19970620)74:3%3c255::aid-ijc4%3e3.0.co;2-y.
33. Hilliard NJ, Krahl D, Sellheyer K. P16 expression differentiates between desmoplastic Spitz nevus and desmoplastic melanoma. J Cutan Pathol. 2009;36(7):753–9. https://doi.org/10.1111/j.1600-0560.2008.01154.x.
34. Al Dhaybi R, Agoumi M, Gagné I, McCuaig C, Powell J, Kokta V. P16 expression: a marker of differentiation between childhood malignant melanomas and Spitz nevi. J Am Acad Dermatol. 2011;65(2):357–63. https://doi.org/10.1016/j.jaad.2010.07.031.
35. Harms PW, Hocker TL, Zhao L, Chan MP, Andea AA, Wang M, et al. Loss of p16 expression and copy number changes of CDKN2A in a spectrum of spitzoid melanocytic lesions. Hum Pathol. 2016;58:152–60. https://doi.org/10.1016/j.humpath.2016.07.029.
36. Chang LM, Cassarino DS. P16 expression is lost in severely atypical cellular blue nevi and melanoma compared to conventional, mildly, and moderately atypical cellular blue nevi. ISRN Dermatol. 2014;2014: 348417. https://doi.org/10.1155/2014/348417.
37. Mihic-Probst D, Saremaslani P, Komminoth P, Heitz PU. Immunostaining for the tumour suppressor gene p16 product is a useful marker to differentiate melanoma metastasis from lymph-node nevus. Virchows Arch. 2003;443(6):745–51. https://doi.org/10.1007/s00428-003-0897-9.
38. Lade-Keller J, Riber-Hansen R, Guldberg P, Schmidt H, Hamilton-Dutoit SJ, Steiniche T. Immunohistochemical analysis of molecular drivers in melanoma identifies p16 as an independent prognostic biomarker. J Clin Pathol. 2014;67(6):520–8. https://doi.org/10.1136/jclinpath-2013-202127.
39. Bouwhuis MG, Suciu S, Kruit W, Salès F, Stoitchkov K, Patel P, et al. Prognostic value of serial blood S100B determinations in stage IIB-III melanoma patients: a corollary study to EORTC trial 18952. Eur J Cancer. 2011;47(3):361–8. https://doi.org/10.1016/j.ejca.2010.10.005.
40. Skaleinius J. Immunologic phenotyping and S100 as biomarkers for response to anti-PD1 therapy in metastatic melanoma: a retrospective analysis. https://gupea.ub.gu.se/handle/2077/57102 (2018). Accessed.
41. Weide B, Elsässer M, Büttner P, Pflugfelder A, Leiter U, Eigentler TK, et al. Serum markers lactate dehydrogenase and S100B predict independently disease outcome in melanoma patients with distant metastasis. Br J Cancer. 2012;107(3):422–8. https://doi.org/10.1038/bjc.2012.306.
42. Kruijff S, Bastiaannet E, Kobold AC, van Ginkel RJ, Suurmeijer AJ, Hoekstra HJ. S-100B concentrations predict disease-free survival in stage III melanoma patients. Ann Surg Oncol. 2009;16(12):3455–62. https://doi.org/10.1245/s10434-009-0629-8.
43. Kruijff S, Hoekstra HJ. The current status of S-100B as a biomarker in melanoma. Eur J Surg Oncol. 2012;38(4):281–5. https://doi.org/10.1016/j.ejso.2011.12.005.
44. Nikolin B, Djan I, Trifunovic J, Dugandzija T, Novkovic D, Djan V, et al. MIA, S100 and LDH as important predictors of overall survival of patients with stage IIb and IIc melanoma. J buon. 2016;21(3):691–7.
45. Oberholzer PA, Urosevic M, Steinert HC, Dummer R. Baseline staging of melanoma with unknown primary site: the value of serum s100 protein and positron emission tomography. Dermatology. 2008;217(4):351–5. https://doi.org/10.1159/000155878.
46. Schultz ES, Diepgen TL, Von Den Driesch P. Clinical and prognostic relevance of serum S-100 beta protein in malignant melanoma. Br J Dermatol. 1998;138(3):426–30. https://doi.org/10.1046/j.1365-2133.1998.02119.x.
47. Wevers KP, Kruijff S, Speijers MJ, Bastiaannet E, Muller Kobold AC, Hoekstra HJ. S-100B: a stronger prognostic biomarker than LDH in stage IIIB-C melanoma. Ann Surg Oncol. 2013;20(8):2772–9. https://doi.org/10.1245/s10434-013-2949-y.
48. Beyeler M, Waldispuhl S, Strobel K, Joller-Jemelka HI, Burg G, Dummer R. Detection of melanoma relapse: first comparative analysis on imaging techniques versus S100 protein. Dermatology. 2006;213(3):187–91. https://doi.org/10.1159/000095034.

49. Hauschild A, Engel G, Brenner W, Gläser R, Mönig H, Henze E, et al. Predictive value of serum S100B for monitoring patients with metastatic melanoma during chemotherapy and/or immunotherapy. Br J Dermatol. 1999;140(6):1065–71. https://doi.org/10.1046/j.1365-2133.1999.02905.x.
50. Barak V, Leibovici V, Peretz T, Kalichman I, Lotem M, Merims S. Assessing response to new treatments and prognosis in melanoma patients, by the biomarker S-100β. Anticancer Res. 2015;35(12):6755–60.
51. Pearl RA, Pacifico MD, Richman PI, Wilson GD, Grover R. Stratification of patients by melanoma cell adhesion molecule (MCAM) expression on the basis of risk: implications for sentinel lymph node biopsy. J Plast Reconstr Aesthet Surg. 2008;61(3):265–71. https://doi.org/10.1016/j.bjps.2007.04.010.
52. Pacifico MD, Grover R, Richman PI, Daley FM, Buffa F, Wilson GD. Development of a tissue array for primary melanoma with long-term follow-up: discovering melanoma cell adhesion molecule as an important prognostic marker. Plast Reconstr Surg. 2005;115(2):367–75. https://doi.org/10.1097/01.prs.0000148417.86768.c9.
53. Johnson JP, Bar-Eli M, Jansen B, Markhof E. Melanoma progression-associated glycoprotein MUC18/MCAM mediates homotypic cell adhesion through interaction with a heterophilic ligand. Int J Cancer. 1997;73(5):769–74.
54. Mahmood MN, Lee MW, Linden MD, Nathanson SD, Hornyak TJ, Zarbo RJ. Diagnostic value of HMB-45 and anti-melan a staining of sentinel lymph nodes with isolated positive cells. Mod Pathol. 2002;15(12):1288–93. https://doi.org/10.1097/01.mp.0000037313.33138.df.
55. Gown AM, Vogel AM, Hoak D, Gough F, McNutt MA. Monoclonal antibodies specific for melanocytic tumors distinguish subpopulations of melanocytes. Am J Pathol. 1986;123(2):195–203.
56. Busam KJ, Iversen K, Coplan KC, Jungbluth AA. Analysis of microphthalmia transcription factor expression in normal tissues and tumors, and comparison of its expression with S-100 protein, gp100, and tyrosinase in desmoplastic malignant melanoma. Am J Surg Pathol. 2001;25(2):197–204. https://doi.org/10.1097/00000478-200102000-00007.
57. King R, Weilbaecher KN, McGill G, Cooley E, Mihm M, Fisher DE. Microphthalmia transcription factor. A sensitive and specific melanocyte marker for melanoma diagnosis. Am J Pathol 1999;155(3):731–8. https://doi.org/10.1016/s0002-9440(10)65172-3
58. King R, Googe PB, Weilbaecher KN, Mihm MC Jr, Fisher DE. Microphthalmia transcription factor expression in cutaneous benign, malignant melanocytic, and nonmelanocytic tumors. Am J Surg Pathol. 2001;25(1):51–7. https://doi.org/10.1097/00000478-200101000-00005.
59. Feldmeyer L, Tetzlaff M, Fox P, Nagarajan P, Curry J, Ivan D, et al. Prognostic implication of lymphovascular invasion detected by double immunostaining for D2–40 and MITF1 in primary cutaneous melanoma. Am J Dermatopathol. 2016;38(7):484–91. https://doi.org/10.1097/dad.0000000000000453.
60. Zhuang L, Scolyer RA, Murali R, McCarthy SW, Zhang XD, Thompson JF, et al. Lactate dehydrogenase 5 expression in melanoma increases with disease progression and is associated with expression of Bcl-XL and Mcl-1, but not Bcl-2 proteins. Mod Pathol. 2010;23(1):45–53. https://doi.org/10.1038/modpathol.2009.129.
61. Kelderman S, Heemskerk B, van Tinteren H, van den Brom RR, Hospers GA, van den Eertwegh AJ, et al. Lactate dehydrogenase as a selection criterion for ipilimumab treatment in metastatic melanoma. Cancer Immunol Immunother. 2014;63(5):449–58. https://doi.org/10.1007/s00262-014-1528-9.
62. Vereecken P, Cornelis F, Van Baren N, Vandersleyen V, Baurain JF. A synopsis of serum biomarkers in cutaneous melanoma patients. Dermatol Res Pract. 2012;2012: 260643. https://doi.org/10.1155/2012/260643.
63. Balch CM, Gershenwald JE, Soong SJ, Thompson JF, Atkins MB, Byrd DR, et al. Final version of 2009 AJCC melanoma staging and classification. J Clin Oncol. 2009;27(36):6199–206. https://doi.org/10.1200/jco.2009.23.4799.
64. Hofbauer GF, Kamarashev J, Geertsen R, Böni R, Dummer R. Tyrosinase immunoreactivity in formalin-fixed, paraffin-embedded primary and metastatic melanoma: frequency and

distribution. J Cutan Pathol. 1998;25(4):204–9. https://doi.org/10.1111/j.1600-0560.1998.tb01720.x.
65. Orchard GE. Comparison of immunohistochemical labelling of melanocyte differentiation antibodies melan-A, tyrosinase and HMB 45 with NKIC3 and S100 protein in the evaluation of benign naevi and malignant melanoma. Histochem J. 2000;32(8):475–81. https://doi.org/10.1023/a:1004192232357.
66. Visús C, Andres R, Mayordomo JI, Martinez-Lorenzo MJ, Murillo L, Sáez-Gutiérrez B, et al. Prognostic role of circulating melanoma cells detected by reverse transcriptase-polymerase chain reaction for tyrosinase mRNA in patients with melanoma. Melanoma Res. 2007;17(2):83–9. https://doi.org/10.1097/CMR.0b013e3280a60878.
67. Quaglino P, Osella-Abate S, Cappello N, Ortoncelli M, Nardò T, Fierro MT, et al. Prognostic relevance of baseline and sequential peripheral blood tyrosinase expression in 200 consecutive advanced metastatic melanoma patients. Melanoma Res. 2007;17(2):75–82. https://doi.org/10.1097/CMR.0b013e328054c667.
68. Ladstein RG, Bachmann IM, Straume O, Akslen LA. Prognostic importance of the mitotic marker phosphohistone H3 in cutaneous nodular melanoma. J Invest Dermatol. 2012;132(4):1247–52. https://doi.org/10.1038/jid.2011.464.
69. Ikenberg K, Pfaltz M, Rakozy C, Kempf W. Immunohistochemical dual staining as an adjunct in assessment of mitotic activity in melanoma. J Cutan Pathol. 2012;39(3):324–30. https://doi.org/10.1111/j.1600-0560.2011.01858.x.
70. Neagu M, Constantin C, Tanase C. Immune-related biomarkers for diagnosis/prognosis and therapy monitoring of cutaneous melanoma. Expert Rev Mol Diagn. 2010;10(7):897–919. https://doi.org/10.1586/erm.10.81.
71. Hendry S, Salgado R, Gevaert T, Russell PA, John T, Thapa B, et al. Assessing tumor-infiltrating lymphocytes in solid tumors: a practical review for pathologists and proposal for a standardized method from the international immunooncology biomarkers working group: part 1: assessing the host immune response, TILs in invasive breast carcinoma and ductal carcinoma in situ, metastatic tumor deposits and areas for further research. Adv Anat Pathol. 2017;24(5):235–51. https://doi.org/10.1097/pap.0000000000000162.
72. Martinez-Rodriguez M, Thompson AK, Monteagudo C. A significant percentage of CD20-positive TILs correlates with poor prognosis in patients with primary cutaneous malignant melanoma. Histopathology. 2014;65(5):726–8. https://doi.org/10.1111/his.12437.
73. Kakavand H, Vilain RE, Wilmott JS, Burke H, Yearley JH, Thompson JF, et al. Tumor PD-L1 expression, immune cell correlates and PD-1+ lymphocytes in sentinel lymph node melanoma metastases. Mod Pathol. 2015;28(12):1535–44. https://doi.org/10.1038/modpathol.2015.110.
74. Hwang SJE, Park JJW, Wakade D, Chou S, Byth K, Fernandez-Penas P. Cutaneous adverse events of anti-programmed death 1 antibodies combined with anti-cytotoxic T-lymphocyte-associated protein 4 therapy use in patients with metastatic melanoma. Melanoma Res. 2019;29(2):172–7. https://doi.org/10.1097/cmr.0000000000000518.
75. Gellrich FF, Schmitz M, Beissert S, Meier F. Anti-PD-1 and novel combinations in the treatment of melanoma-an update. J Clin Med. 2020;9(1). https://doi.org/10.3390/jcm9010223
76. Bersanelli M, Buti S. From targeting the tumor to targeting the immune system: transversal challenges in oncology with the inhibition of the PD-1/PD-L1 axis. World J Clin Oncol. 2017;8(1):37–53. https://doi.org/10.5306/wjco.v8.i1.37.
77. Tumeh PC, Harview CL, Yearley JH, Shintaku IP, Taylor EJ, Robert L, et al. PD-1 blockade induces responses by inhibiting adaptive immune resistance. Nature. 2014;515(7528):568–71. https://doi.org/10.1038/nature13954.
78. Daud AI, Loo K, Pauli ML, Sanchez-Rodriguez R, Sandoval PM, Taravati K, et al. Tumor immune profiling predicts response to anti-PD-1 therapy in human melanoma. J Clin Invest. 2016;126(9):3447–52. https://doi.org/10.1172/jci87324.
79. Choi JW, Kim YJ, Yun KA, Won CH, Lee MW, Choi JH, et al. The prognostic significance of VISTA and CD33-positive myeloid cells in cutaneous melanoma and their relationship with PD-1 expression. Sci Rep. 2020;10(1):14372. https://doi.org/10.1038/s41598-020-71216-2.

80. Rosenbaum SR, Knecht M, Mollaee M, Zhong Z, Erkes DA, McCue PA, et al. FOXD3 regulates VISTA expression in melanoma. Cell Rep. 2020;30(2):510-24.e6. https://doi.org/10.1016/j.celrep.2019.12.036.
81. Kuklinski LF, Yan S, Li Z, Fisher JL, Cheng C, Noelle RJ, et al. VISTA expression on tumor-infiltrating inflammatory cells in primary cutaneous melanoma correlates with poor disease-specific survival. Cancer Immunol Immunother. 2018;67(7):1113–21. https://doi.org/10.1007/s00262-018-2169-1.
82. Shinozaki M, Fujimoto A, Morton DL, Hoon DS. Incidence of BRAF oncogene mutation and clinical relevance for primary cutaneous melanomas. Clin Cancer Res. 2004;10(5):1753–7. https://doi.org/10.1158/1078-0432.ccr-1169-3.
83. Davies H, Bignell GR, Cox C, Stephens P, Edkins S, Clegg S, et al. Mutations of the BRAF gene in human cancer. Nature. 2002;417(6892):949–54. https://doi.org/10.1038/nature00766.
84. Curtin JA, Fridlyand J, Kageshita T, Patel HN, Busam KJ, Kutzner H, et al. Distinct sets of genetic alterations in melanoma. N Engl J Med. 2005;353(20):2135–47. https://doi.org/10.1056/NEJMoa050092.
85. Manninen AA, Gardberg M, Juteau S, Ilmonen S, Jukonen J, Andersson N, et al. BRAF immunohistochemistry predicts sentinel lymph node involvement in intermediate thickness melanomas. PLoS ONE. 2019;14(4): e0216043. https://doi.org/10.1371/journal.pone.0216043.
86. Lezcano C, Jungbluth AA, Busam KJ. PRAME immunohistochemistry as an Ancillary test for the assessment of melanocytic lesions. Surg Pathol Clin. 2021;14(2):165–75. https://doi.org/10.1016/j.path.2021.01.001.
87. Lezcano C, Jungbluth AA, Nehal KS, Hollmann TJ, Busam KJ. PRAME expression in melanocytic tumors. Am J Surg Pathol. 2018;42(11):1456–65. https://doi.org/10.1097/pas.0000000000001134.
88. Lezcano C, Jungbluth AA, Busam KJ. Comparison of immunohistochemistry for PRAME with cytogenetic test results in the evaluation of challenging melanocytic tumors. Am J Surg Pathol. 2020;44(7):893–900. https://doi.org/10.1097/pas.0000000000001492.
89. Ferris LK, Gerami P, Skelsey MK, Peck G, Hren C, Gorman C, et al. Real-world performance and utility of a noninvasive gene expression assay to evaluate melanoma risk in pigmented lesions. Melanoma Res. 2018;28(5):478–82. https://doi.org/10.1097/cmr.0000000000000478.
90. How It Works: DermTech. DermTech; 2022.
91. Luan W, Ding Y, Ma S, Ruan H, Wang J, Lu F. Long noncoding RNA LINC00518 acts as a competing endogenous RNA to promote the metastasis of malignant melanoma via miR-204-5p/AP1S2 axis. Cell Death Dis. 2019;10(11):855. https://doi.org/10.1038/s41419-019-2090-3.
92. Toussi A, Mans N, Welborn J, Kiuru M. Germline mutations predisposing to melanoma. J Cutan Pathol. 2020;47(7):606–16. https://doi.org/10.1111/cup.13689.
93. Gerami P, Yao Z, Polsky D, Jansen B, Busam K, Ho J, et al. Development and validation of a noninvasive 2-gene molecular assay for cutaneous melanoma. J Am Acad Dermatol. 2017;76(1):114-20.e2. https://doi.org/10.1016/j.jaad.2016.07.038.
94. Ferris LK, Rigel DS, Siegel DM, Skelsey MK, Peck GL, Hren C, et al. Impact on clinical practice of a non-invasive gene expression melanoma rule-out test: 12-month follow-up of negative test results and utility data from a large US registry study. Dermatol Online J. 2019;25(5).
95. DecisionDx-Melanoma Overview. Castle Biosciences; 2022.
96. Greenhaw BN, Covington KR, Kurley SJ, Yeniay Y, Cao NA, Plasseraud KM, et al. Molecular risk prediction in cutaneous melanoma: A meta-analysis of the 31-gene expression profile prognostic test in 1,479 patients. J Am Acad Dermatol. 2020;83(3):745–53. https://doi.org/10.1016/j.jaad.2020.03.053.
97. Litchman GH, Prado G, Teplitz RW, Rigel D. A systematic review and meta-analysis of gene expression profiling for primary cutaneous melanoma prognosis. Skin J Cutan Med 2020.

98. Wisco OJ, Marson JW, Litchman GH, Brownstone N, Covington KR, Martin BJ, et al. Improved cutaneous melanoma survival stratification through integration of 31-gene expression profile testing with the American Joint Committee on Cancer 8th edition staging. Melanoma Res. 2022;32(2):98–102. https://doi.org/10.1097/cmr.0000000000000804
99. Whitman ED, Koshenkov VP, Gastman BR, Lewis D, Hsueh EC, Pak H, et al. Integrating 31-gene expression profiling with clinicopathologic features to optimize cutaneous melanoma sentinel lymph node metastasis prediction. JCO Precis Oncol. 2021;5. https://doi.org/10.1200/po.21.00162
100. Ferris LK, Farberg AS, Middlebrook B, Johnson CE, Lassen N, Oelschlager KM, et al. Identification of high-risk cutaneous melanoma tumors is improved when combining the online American Joint Committee on Cancer individualized melanoma patient outcome prediction tool with a 31-gene expression profile-based classification. J Am Acad Dermatol. 2017;76(5):818-25.e3. https://doi.org/10.1016/j.jaad.2016.11.051.

Chapter 11
Hidradenitis Suppurativa Biomarkers

Raj H. Patel, Jessica N. Pixley, Luna Samman, and Steven R. Feldman

Abstract Hidradenitis suppurativa (HS) is an inflammatory skin condition involving dysregulation of the innate and adaptive immune responses. Although the precise etiology is not yet elucidated, the pathophysiology of HS is multifactorial and associated with genetic and environment factors. There is currently no cure for HS. Biomarkers have been identified in the blood and tissue of patients with the disease, and the levels of which may be informative about diagnosis, prognosis, treatment efficacy, and monitoring comorbidities for this condition. These biomarkers encompass a wide range of molecules and include inflammatory cytokines, chemokine receptors, growth factors, markers of serum inflammation, and imaging features (Napolitano et al. in Clin Cosmet Investig Dermatol 10:105–115, 2017). Together, these biomarkers serve as important indicators of disease progression and response to treatment. The World Health Organization (WHO) categorizes biomarkers into screening, diagnostic, prognostic, monitoring, and pharmacodynamics. The chapter will discuss the role of biomarkers in HS, focusing on diagnosis, prognosis, monitoring, and therapeutic targets.

Keywords IL-1β · CXC chemokine receptors · C5a · G-CSF · Hepcidin · IL-2 · IL-36 · BCL2 · IL-8 · ESR · IL-17 · Doppler · TNF-α · IL-23 · JAK-STAT · S100A · IRAK · Metformin · PDE-4 · Hidradenitis suppurativa · Treatment targets

R. H. Patel · L. Samman
Wake Forest School of Medicine, 4618 Country Club Road, Winston-Salem, NC 27104, USA

J. N. Pixley (✉)
Virginia Commonwealth University, Richmond, VA 23284, USA
e-mail: pixleyjn@vcu.edu

S. R. Feldman
Professor of Dermatology, Pathology and Social Sciences & Health Policy, Wake Forest School of Medicine, 4618 Country Club Road, Winston-Salem, NC 27104, USA
e-mail: sfeldman@wakehealth.edu

R. Norman (ed.), *Biomarkers in Dermatology*,
https://doi.org/10.1007/978-3-031-66513-4_11

11.1 Introduction

Hidradenitis suppurativa (HS) is a chronic, immune-mediated inflammatory skin disease with a worldwide prevalence of approximately 0.4% [2]. The disease is characterized by occlusion of hair follicles in apocrine gland-containing regions of the body and subsequent cycles of inflammation, healing, and scarring [3]. The disease manifests clinically with recurrent nodules and abscesses, formation of sinus tracts, and scarring that affect the intertriginous regions: the axilla and the inframammary, inguinal, pubic, perianal, and gluteal regions. HS has a female predominance and an average age of onset in the second or third decades of life [2]. The disease reduces patients' quality of life, adversely affecting social, occupational, and psychological facets of life [4]. A multifactorial disease, the complete immunopathogenesis of HS, has not yet been completely elucidated. Treatment of HS is difficult, and the course of the disease often unpredictable. Because HS is apparent on physical examination and its severity can most often be determined clinically without the need for laboratory tests, the clinical utility of biomarkers in HS may not be as profound as in conditions with little to no cutaneous manifestations. Because of this, the choice of treatment in HS is usually based upon visual determination of disease severity, frequency of disease flares, and access to care.

However, biomarkers may provide an additional tool to assess disease severity and to monitor the appearance or progression of HS comorbidities that may not have a visually apparent manifestation, such as cardiovascular disease. According to the World Health Organization (WHO), biomarkers are "any substance, structure, or process that can be measured in the body or its products and influence or predict the incidence of outcome or disease [5]." In addition to locating pathogenic processes and monitoring disease progression, they can also be used to evaluate pharmacological response in various diseases. Different classes of biomarkers include screening biomarkers that identify risk of disease development, diagnostic biomarkers for disease identification, prognostic biomarkers for disease progression and response to therapy, as well as biomarkers for comorbidities to identify associated health issues [5]. Although the search for additional biomarkers in HS is ongoing, several diagnostic, prognostic, monitoring, and therapeutic biomarkers for HS allow for a deeper understanding of the pathogenesis of this chronic disease. These biomarkers include various inflammatory cytokines such as interleukin (IL)-1 and tumor necrosis factor (TNF)-α; growth factors such as granulocyte colony-stimulating factor (G-CSF); markers of inflammation such as erythrocyte sedimentation rate (ESR) and hepcidin; and even characteristic imaging features of HS lesions via doppler ultrasound. Several of these also share potential across different classes such as IL-1β and IL-17, which both have the potential for diagnostic and therapeutic utility. The continued investigation of these biomarkers and greater understanding of their various roles ultimately allows for the development of targeted therapeutics for this complex disease.

As an immune-mediated disease, the pathogenesis of HS involves the interaction of inflammatory mediators and immune cells, as well as genes that control their expression. These substances and structures have the potential to serve as important biomarkers to better classify disease severity in some patients, as well as to track disease progression and the development of certain comorbidities which are not easily visualized clinically. In addition, identification of biomarkers for HS has led to the development of new biologics, including adalimumab, ustekinumab, and secukinumab, which have drastically improved the quality of life for HS patients [6]. This chapter will discuss specific biomarkers present in the DNA, blood, and tissue of HS patients as well as their implications on disease susceptibility, diagnosis, prognosis, and identifying risk for comorbidities.

11.2 Methods

11.2.1 Pathogenesis of Hidradenitis Suppurativa

The precise etiology of HS is not fully elucidated but is understood to be influenced by genetic and environmental factors. HS may involve dysregulation of the gamma-secretase/Notch pathway, which has a key role in maintaining the inner and outer root sheath of the hair follicle and skin appendages [7]. Dysregulation of the notch signaling pathway, which plays a key role in maintaining the structure of hair follicles and skin appendages, can lead to the formation of keratin-filled epidermal cysts, impaired apocrine glands, and activation of toll-like receptors (TLR), contributing to the chronic inflammation that characterizes HS. TNF, IL-1, and IL-17 are pro-inflammatory cytokines of which higher levels have been detected in HS lesions [8].

The pathogenesis of HS involves occlusion and inflammation of the hair follicle with both innate and adaptive immune dysregulation [1]; 95% of early HS lesions present with hyperkeratosis, occlusion of the skin follicle, and perifolliculitis [9]. In addition, bacterial colonization behind the blockage is often a common contributor and can worsen the condition [1, 9]. *Staphylococcus lugdunensis* was isolated in 58% of the HS nodules and abscesses, according to a microbiological analysis of 102 HS lesions from 82 patients [10]. Other frequent species predominating in HS lesions were actinomycetes (identified in 24% of abscesses or nodules and in 87% of chronic suppurating lesions), milleri group streptococci, and polymicrobial anaerobic microflora [10].

The formation of an HS lesion begins with follicular occlusion, leading to dilation of the gland followed by rupture, resulting in expulsion of the follicular contents including keratin and bacteria into the nearby dermis, allowing for an intense inflammatory response via neutrophiles and lymphocytes [1]. The pilosebaceous gland is destroyed as a result of the formation of an abscess brought on by the perifollicular inflammatory cellular infiltration.

Both pro-inflammatory (e.g., IL-1β, TNF-α, IL-23, and IL-17) and anti-inflammatory cytokines (e.g., IL-10) are elevated in HS [11]. Increased levels of the pro-inflammatory cytokines are produced by altered TLRs signaling on macrophages and dendritic cells (DCs), the most prevalent cells in HS lesions, which activates DCs and causes them to generate IL-23 to support Th17 cell polarization (IL-17-producing T-helper cells have been identified in the dermis in chronic HS lesions) [1]. The expulsion of the follicular content stimulates the NLRP3 inflammasome and caspase-1, encouraging the production of IL-1 [12, 13]. IL-1β stimulates the synthesis of matrix metalloproteinases (MMPs), which increase the biologic activity of select chemokines that recruit neutrophils within the skin [14]. The recruitment of these cells aids in the generation of inflammatory cytokines and pus in HS skin [15].

TNF-α, a pro-inflammatory cytokine, positively correlates with HS disease severity [16]. TNF-α is produced in HS via macrophages and dendritic cells (DCs) through keratin fiber recognition via toll-like receptors (TLRs) [9, 17]. TNF-α promotes chemokines and boosts endothelial activation, encouraging immune cell infiltration [18]. Hence, HS lesions are characterized by granulocytes, T-cells, B lymphocytes, plasma cells, and monocytes [18, 19]. TNF-α promotes T-cell differentiation into Th1 and Th17 cells, which produce interferon (IFN)-γ and IL-17, respectively [14, 19]. IFN-γ promotes Th1-attracting chemokines (e.g., CXCL-10) that activate dermal endothelial cells, permitting immune cell invasion from the blood vessels [20].

11.3 Diagnostic Biomarkers

11.3.1 Interleukin-1β

Activation of the IL-1β pathway plays a key role in upregulation of the pro-inflammatory signals associated with HS. The hyperactivity of IL-1β generates immune cell infiltration and extracellular matrix degeneration, driving both local and systemic inflammation [21]. IL-1β is released by monocytes and macrophages following proteolytic cleavage which is mediated by the NLRP3 inflammasome, a cytoplasmic innate immune protein complex [22]. CD11c+ CD1a-CD14+ cells represent the primary source of this biomarker in the skin of HS patients [13]. IL-1β is overexpressed in lesional and perilesional skin of HS patients, even when compared with psoriatic lesions. IL-1β and IL-6 both synergistically induce serum amyloid A [21]. Thus, given its crucial role in the pathogenetic cascade of HS, the activity of IL-1β may be beneficially targeted and monitored through blood serum amyloid A (SAA) levels [21]. This allows for the application of IL-1β to be used in both diagnosis and surveillance, while also serving as an indicator of clinical severity. IL-1 targeted biologics have been used in the treatment of various immune-mediated disorders [23]. Anakinra is a recombinant IL-1 receptor antagonist which is efficacious for the treatment of HS [24]. Other IL-1 inhibitors include canakinumab and bermekimab. Canakinumab's effect on HS has been variable (both positive and negative outcomes) and without randomized controlled trials. Bermekimab is a promising first-line option for moderate-severe HS with favorable initial results and is currently undergoing phase 2 studies [25].

11.3.2 CXC Chemokine Receptors

CXC chemokine receptors serve numerous roles in inflammation including as lymphoid chemokines, directing neutrophils to sites of injury, and mediating chronic inflammation [26]. CXCL-10 and CXCL-8 are overexpressed along with other IL-17-associated cytokines in HS patients, emphasizing their role in the modulation of inflammation and immunoregulation [27]. Serum concentrations of receptors including CXCL16 and its receptor, CXCR6, have reduced expression in patients with HS [28]. While the precise pathophysiology of these receptors has not been elucidated, they may serve as diagnostic biomarkers through monitoring of serum concentrations [27]. Clinical applications remain unknown and may be better understood through prospective studies.

11.3.3 Complement 5a (C5a)

Complement 5a (C5a) signaling results in leukocyte activation and skin destruction, driving the development of tunneling and sinus tract formation in patients with HS [29]. C5a is also a traditional activation product of the complement cascade that can allow for neutrophil infiltration and activation in HS lesions [30]. Levels of C5a and C5b-9 circulate at greater levels in the plasma of patients with HS compared with plasma from patients without the disease ($P = 0.0006$, $P = 0.001$, respectively) [30]. These findings confirm systemic complement activation occurs in HS, thus allowing for the theoretical use of C5a as a diagnostic surrogate biomarker.

Levels of C5a in the tissue and serum correlate with disease activity and level of neutrophil infiltration [31], suggesting the potential use of C5a for the monitoring of disease activity in HS patients. Since C5a also stimulates the production of TNF-α, there is also the potential of its utility as a future therapeutic target [30]. C5a pathway dysregulation also occurs in obesity, insulin resistance, and polycystic ovarian syndrome—which could explain a possible epidemiological correlation between these conditions and HS [31]. Prospective studies evaluating the benefit of C5a antagonists are needed to further explore this association and explore further potential for clinical application.

11.3.4 Granulocyte-Colony Stimulating Factor

Granulocyte-Colony Stimulating Factor (G-CSF) is the main regulator of neutrophilic granulocyte survival, development, and function and is highly expressed in lesional skin of HS patients [32], thus serving as a potential diagnostic and therapeutic target [33]. IL-1 and IL-17 induce production of G-CSF through fibroblasts and keratinocytes. G-CSF also upregulates bacterial receptor components and damaged host cells, leading to the production of skin-destructive enzymes [33]. This pathway may also contribute to the persistence of abscesses and purulence. Elevated levels of G-CSF receptor lead to prolonged neutrophil activation and survival, thus playing a role in maintaining the chronic inflammatory state that characterizes HS [33]. It remains unclear whether selectively blocking the action of G-CSF can provide an efficacious treatment approach for HS.

11.3.5 Serum Hepcidin

The chronic inflammation of HS leads to anemia of chronic disease in many patients through upregulation of IL-6 anbd hepcidin. As an important central regulator of iron homeostasis, hepcidin can allow for differentiation between anemia of chronic disease from iron deficiency anemia [34]. Hepcidin levels were lower in anemic patients with reduced iron stores compared to anemia patients with adequate iron stores [34]. Decreased levels of hepcidin were associated with HS [35, 36]. Thus, the hematological state of HS patients may allow for serum hepcidin as a monitoring biomarker of disease activity. Larger clinical studies are needed to further investigate this association and determine reliability as a primary monitoring parameter.

11.3.6 Serum Interleukin-2 Receptor (IL-2-R)

Soluble IL-2 receptor (IL-2-R) serum level is a diagnostic biomarker [37] and provides a sensitive evaluation of clinical staging of HS patients. Levels of IL-2R are elevated in the serum of patients with HS and are frequently associated with various malignant, autoimmune, and infectious processes [38]. The differentiation and proliferation of T-cells is induced through stimulation of IL-2R with IL-2, thus contributing to increased inflammation in HS [39]. Elevation of IL-2R levels is independent from other comorbid and demographic factors such as smoking, body mass index, diabetes mellitus, and family history, thus offering potential utility in measuring disease severity in addition to staging [38]. Further research is needed to clarify its benefits as a biomarker and clinical application.

11.4 Prognostic Biomarkers

11.4.1 Interleukin-36 (IL-36)

IL-36 expression by T-cells, monocytes, and dendritic cells plays an important role in the regulation of the innate and adaptive immune system. This biomarker has been studied in various dermatological and non-dermatological inflammatory conditions such as systemic lupus erythematosus, atopic dermatitis, psoriasis, and rheumatoid arthritis [40]. IL-36 has important prognostic utility as elevated IL-36 levels increase the risk of HS up to 11 times, after controlling for lifestyle factors [40]. The ability of IL-36 to work independently or synergistically to induce G-CSF expression in keratinocytes and fibroblasts allows for the regulation of neutrophils in the pathogenesis of HS [41]. IL-36 also triggers an inflammatory cascade of events inducing T-helper cells and other interleukins resulting in overall increased inflammation and drainage from HS lesions [42]. Future studies investigating its emergence as a prospective therapeutic target for HS are needed to explore its clinical utility.

11.4.2 BCL2 Genetic Variant (rs59532114)

Genetic factors play an important role in the development of HS given the association of family history as a risk factor. BCL2 serves as a regulator of anti-apoptosis, blocking cell death and regulating skin homeostasis in outer root sheath cells of hair follicles [43]. HS patients with a specific genetic variant in the BCL2 gene, rs59532114, are less likely to experience improved disease severity with adalimumab [43]. Thus, this genetic variant serves as an important prognostic factor determining therapeutic efficacy in patients for the only currently approved medication for HS [44]. Larger studies are needed to verify this association and to better understand the therapeutic implications for patients with this variant.

11.5 Monitoring Biomarkers

11.5.1 Interleukin-8 (IL-8)

IL-8 is a potent pro-inflammatory cytokine and chemoattractant of neutrophils and has been used as a biomarker to monitor inflammatory skin diseases including psoriasis and atopic dermatitis [45]. Various cells including neutrophils, T lymphocytes, mast cells, dermal macrophages, endothelial cells, and keratinocytes have binding sites for IL-8, which contribute to its response [46]. In several observational case–control studies, there was a strong linear correlation with disease severity ($P < 0.05$)

[44], which may point to its efficacy as a monitoring biomarker for HS. Therapy with adalimumab has also led to a decrease in Th17 lymphocyte and neutrophil-related inflammatory serum markers such as IL-8 in HS patients [47], further corroborating its effects on the pro-inflammatory cascade. Thus, IL-8 has potential clinical use in the monitoring of therapeutic response and disease progression.

11.5.2 Serum Erythrocyte Sedimentation Rate (ESR)

Inflammatory markers such as erythrocyte sedimentation rate (ESR) and C-reactive protein (CRP) are relatively easy-to-obtain, inexpensive, and non-specific tests for inflammatory conditions. ESR has been studied as a monitoring biomarker for HS due to its reliability as an indicator for disease severity [38]. Given the elevated inflammatory state in HS and release of interleukins and other acute-phase reactants, erythrocyte aggregation is promoted and leads to a correlative increase in ESR [38]. However, comorbid conditions in HS patients may confound use of ESR as a disease monitoring biomarker in HS [38]. In one study comparing CRP levels with ESR in HS patients, ESR elevation was detected at earlier and lower inflammatory states than CRP [48]. This robust sensitivity may allow for ESR to be used as a monitoring biomarker in patients with varying ranges of clinical severity.

11.5.3 Interleukin-17 (IL-17)

Il-17 is a pro-inflammatory cytokine released primarily by macrophages and neutrophils in inflammatory HS lesions. Circulating levels of IL-17 may be used to monitor the response to treatment and to evaluate the degree of inflammation in HS patients [49]. The mRNA expression of IL-17 is significantly increased in cells of both lesional and perilesional skin, and HS patients with higher serum levels of IL-17 generally have more advanced disease [50]. Given this proportional correlation with clinical severity, the use of IL-17 to monitor disease activity and assess response to future therapies is promising [50]. Clinical benefit of anti-IL-17 therapies for the treatment of HS currently remains limited to case reports [50–52]. Clinical trials evaluating secukinumab for the treatment of HS are currently underway with favorable efficacy and safety in a small group of HS patients thus far. Additional larger, controlled studies may allow for greater understanding of the role of IL-17 in the pathogenesis of HS and offer insight into its use in therapeutic intervention.

11.5.4 Doppler Ultrasound-Based Imaging

Ultrasound imaging allows for the visualization of inflammatory skin lesions and assessment of disease severity through well-characterized sonographic findings [53]. Characterization of inflammatory HS lesions through ultrasound-based imaging allows for superior monitoring of disease progression and clinical management [54]. Sonographic epidermal thickness, dermal tunnel diameter, and power doppler intensity are various image-based characteristics that have been identified as biomarkers in HS lesions [53]. Power doppler intensity has strong analytical and clinical validity and is a biomarker of HS disease activity. Vascular distribution of HS lesions is also an effective characteristic of disease classification, which can be evaluated through power doppler signal [55]. This biomarker also correlates with patient pain score ratings and clinical severity assessment, owing to its benefit in disease monitoring. Prospective studies are necessary to further assess the response of these image-based biomarkers to therapeutic intervention.

11.6 Therapeutic Biomarkers

11.6.1 Interleukin-17 (IL-17)

IL-17 is an important regulator in multiple cutaneous inflammatory disorders including HS [52]. Given its involvement in the stimulation of keratinocytes and the pro-inflammatory cascade of HS, IL-17 has been an attractive target for therapeutic intervention [56]. In addition, serum levels of IL-17 correlate with clinical inflammatory activity of HS, pointing to theoretical utility in clinical monitoring [48, 50]. IL-17 gene expression is increased 30-fold in lesional skin of HS patients compared to healthy control skin. Both neutrophils and CD8 T-cells contribute to the production of IL-17 in HS lesional skin [57]. The IL-17 pathway also involves feed-forward signaling of pro-inflammatory mediators including anti-microbial peptides S100A8, S100A9 and human-β-defensin-2 and chemokines chemokine (C-X-C motif) ligand 1 (CXCL1) and IL-8, which have all been upregulated in HS lesional skin [58]. Further, IL-17 has also been implicated in a variety of crucial pro-inflammatory roles in HS lesional skin, including the recruitment of Th17 and myeloid cells, chemotaxis of neutrophils and monocytes, and immune cell infiltration [13, 59]. IL-17 induces and interacts with IL-1β in a positive feedback inflammatory loop, further contributing to the potency of its effects [47, 56]. Various IL-17 inhibitors are efficacious for HS including secukinumab, bimekizumab, brodalumab, sonelokimab, and ixekizumab [52].

11.6.2 Tumor Necrosis Factor-α (TNF-α)

TNF-α represents one of the most important and well-studied therapeutic biomarkers in the pathogenesis of HS. TNF-α may be a primary driver of the chronic inflammatory state of HS and its concentration is higher in both the serum and skin of HS patients compared to healthy volunteers [60]. This biomarker has also been heavily implicated in mediating the immune response. Initial recognition of therapeutic use of this biomarker stemmed from the beneficial use of TNF-α inhibitors for HS patients with inflammatory bowel disease which led to concurrent improvement in their skin lesions [60]. Since then, TNF-α has been an important therapeutic target and the pharmacodynamic focus of various biologics targeting HS including adalimumab, etanercept, infliximab, golimumab, and certolizumab [60]. However, adalimumab remains the only FDA-approved biological treatment for moderate-severe HS. Given the data behind the pro-inflammatory role of TNF-α, prospective studies evaluating this biomarker are focused on the development of biologics targeting this cytokine [61]. These studies have yielded efficacious results, particularly for infliximab and golimumab.

11.6.3 Interleukin-23 (IL-23)

IL-23 plays a critical role in the establishment of chronic tissue inflammation and promotion of a pathogenic CD4+ T-cell population which produces IL-17, IL-17F, IL-6, and TNF [62]. In HS, IL-23 is abundantly expressed by macrophages in the papillary and reticular dermis of affected skin in HS patients [11]. Gene expression of IL-23 in HS patients is increased relative to IL-12 [11]. Given this important role in the inflammatory cascade, biologics to target this pathway have been developed. IL-23 inhibitors include guselkumab, risankizumab, and tildrakizumab. Guselkumab targets the p19 subunit of extracellular IL-23 and provides an efficacious option for patients with moderate-severe HS refractory to other systemic therapeutics [63, 64]. Future studies are needed to better understand the efficacy and optimal dosing of these agents.

11.6.4 Janus Kinases

The Janus-associated kinase/signal transducers and activators of transcription (JAK-STAT) pathway plays a critical role in cytokine signaling that contributes to local and systemic inflammation in HS [65]. HS pathogenesis is driven by multiple JAK/STAT-mediated cytokines, including interleukin (IL)-1β, IL-17, IL-23, IL-10, and TNF-α [66]. Given this versatility, inhibiting JAK-mediated pathways can allow for broader interruption of inflammatory pathways rather than targeting individual cytokines

[66]. Janus kinases have been identified as a therapeutic biomarker and serve as therapeutic targets for JAK inhibitors, which are under investigation as a potential treatment for HS. Hence, evaluating the safety and efficacy of Janus kinase inhibitor INCB054707 has been the subject of a recent clinical trial investigating its pharmacodynamics [66]. In particular, patients who lack response to targeted biologic therapy may benefit from JAK inhibitors [67]. The pathway is activated through binding of an extracellular ligand to various transmembrane receptors, leading to phosphorylation of intracellular molecules and initiation of an intracellular signaling cascade; ultimately regulating transcription [65]. The Janus kinase family is comprised of tyrosine kinases that induce JAK1, JAK2, JAK3, and TYK2 [65]. Of these, JAK1 has been the greatest focus within HS and targeted pharmacotherapy, as it may reduce cytokine signaling specific to HS pathogenesis while limiting JAK2-mediated cytopenia. Several JAK inhibitors including tofacitinib, beprocitinib, INCB054707 (undergoing phase 2 trials), upadicitinib, and ropsacitinib are under investigation use for the treatment of HS [66–69].

11.6.5 S100A Proteins

S100 proteins encompass a group of small, calcium-binding cytosolic proteins that all share structural similarity but have functional discrepancy [70]. This family of proteins are members of the epidermal differentiation complex, a cluster of genes that code for proteins involved in keratinocyte terminal differentiation [71]. Serum levels of various S100 proteins including S100A4, S100A8, S100A9, S100A15, S100S12, and S100A7 are elevated in lesional and perilesional skin of HS patients [72, 73]. These biomarkers are chemoattractants for neutrophils, monocytes, and macrophages and thus contributing to inflammation [72]. Thus, S100 proteins may also be a promising therapeutic target due to their role in the pathogenesis of HS and promotion of inflammation and fibrosis [72]. Further investigation may allow for development of targeted therapeutics and clinical application of this biomarker.

11.6.6 Phosphodiesterase-4 (PDE-4)

Phosphodiesterase-4, present on various epithelial and immune cells, is an intracellular non-receptor enzyme that modulates inflammation and epithelial integrity [74]. Through reducing levels of intracellular cyclic adenosine monophosphate (cAMP), PDE-4 acts as a pro-inflammatory mediator stimulating the production of various cytokines involved in the pathogenetic cascade of HS, including TNF-α, IL-17, IL-23, and IL-10 [75]. PDE-4 is also a therapeutic target of PDE-4 inhibitors. Given this, PDE-4 inhibitors are efficacious in the treatment of various inflammatory dermatological conditions including HS. Apremilast, an oral phosphodiesterase-4 inhibitor which has been conventionally used in the treatment of plaque psoriasis and psoriatic arthritis, has presented an attractive therapeutic option for patients with moderate-severe HS based on preliminary clinical trials [76]. Roflumilast which also works via a similar mechanism also has potential efficacy in the treatment of HS.

11.7 Conclusion

Hidradenitis suppurativa (HS) is a chronic immune-mediated inflammatory skin disease that has a significant impact on patient quality of life. Despite the complex and multifactorial etiology, the search for biomarkers in HS has led to the identification of various molecules that may serve as diagnostic, prognostic, monitoring, and therapeutic targets. These biomarkers allow for an increased understanding of the pathogenesis behind the development of HS, classification of disease severity and staging, and development of targeted therapeutics. However, it is important to note that the utility of biomarkers in HS may not be as profound as in conditions with little to no visually apparent manifestations, and that clinical assessment remains an important tool in the diagnosis and management of this disease. Despite the lack of established biomarkers for routine clinical use in HS [44], continued research efforts toward identifying and validating potential markers hold promise for their eventual incorporation into clinical practice. This emphasizes the need for larger, multi-center studies to validate and reach consensus on suitable markers. Further research is necessary to better understand the role of biomarkers in HS and to identify additional biomarkers that may be useful in diagnosis, prognosis, and treatment.

References

1. Napolitano M, Megna M, Timoshchuk EA, Patruno C, Balato N, Fabbrocini G, et al. Hidradenitis suppurativa: from pathogenesis to diagnosis and treatment. Clin Cosmet Investig Dermatol. 2017;10:105–15. https://doi.org/10.2147/CCID.S111019.
2. Jfri A, Nassim D, O'Brien E, Gulliver W, Nikolakis G, Zouboulis CC. Prevalence of hidradenitis suppurativa: a systematic review and meta-regression analysis. JAMA Dermatol. 2021;157(8):924–31. https://doi.org/10.1001/jamadermatol.2021.1677.
3. Kurzen H, Kurokawa I, Jemec GB, Emtestam L, Sellheyer K, Giamarellos-Bourboulis EJ, et al. What causes hidradenitis suppurativa? Exp Dermatol. 2008;17(5):455–6 (discussion 7–72). https://doi.org/10.1111/j.1600-0625.2008.00712_1.x.
4. Alikhan A, Lynch PJ, Eisen DB. Hidradenitis suppurativa: a comprehensive review. J Am Acad Dermatol. 2009;60(4):539–61 (quiz 62–3). https://doi.org/10.1016/j.jaad.2008.11.911.
5. Califf RM. Biomarker definitions and their applications. Exp Biol Med (Maywood). 2018;243(3):213–21. https://doi.org/10.1177/1535370217750088.
6. Rendon A, Schäkel K. Psoriasis pathogenesis and treatment. Int J Mol Sci. 2019;20(6). https://doi.org/10.3390/ijms20061475.
7. Melnik BC, Plewig G. Impaired Notch-MKP-1 signalling in hidradenitis suppurativa: an approach to pathogenesis by evidence from translational biology. Exp Dermatol. 2013;22(3):172–7. https://doi.org/10.1111/exd.12098.

8. van der Zee HH, Laman JD, de Ruiter L, Dik WA, Prens EP. Adalimumab (antitumour necrosis factor-α) treatment of hidradenitis suppurativa ameliorates skin inflammation: an in situ and ex vivo study. Br J Dermatol. 2012;166(2):298–305. https://doi.org/10.1111/j.1365-2133.2011.10698.x.
9. Pink A, Anzengruber F, Navarini AA. Acne and hidradenitis suppurativa. Br J Dermatol. 2018;178(3):619–31. https://doi.org/10.1111/bjd.16231.
10. Guet-Revillet H, Coignard-Biehler H, Jais JP, Quesne G, Frapy E, Poirée S, et al. Bacterial pathogens associated with hidradenitis suppurativa, France. Emerg Infect Dis. 2014;20(12):1990–8. https://doi.org/10.3201/eid2012.140064.
11. Schlapbach C, Hänni T, Yawalkar N, Hunger RE. Expression of the IL-23/Th17 pathway in lesions of hidradenitis suppurativa. J Am Acad Dermatol. 2011;65(4):790–8. https://doi.org/10.1016/j.jaad.2010.07.010.
12. van der Zee HH, de Ruiter L, van den Broecke DG, Dik WA, Laman JD, Prens EP. Elevated levels of tumour necrosis factor (TNF)-α, interleukin (IL)-1β and IL-10 in hidradenitis suppurativa skin: a rationale for targeting TNF-α and IL-1β. Br J Dermatol. 2011;164(6):1292–8. https://doi.org/10.1111/j.1365-2133.2011.10254.x.
13. Kelly G, Hughes R, McGarry T, van den Born M, Adamzik K, Fitzgerald R, et al. Dysregulated cytokine expression in lesional and nonlesional skin in hidradenitis suppurativa. Br J Dermatol. 2015;173(6):1431–9. https://doi.org/10.1111/bjd.14075.
14. Wolk K, Join-Lambert O, Sabat R. Aetiology and pathogenesis of hidradenitis suppurativa. Br J Dermatol. 2020;183(6):999–1010. https://doi.org/10.1111/bjd.19556.
15. Scala E, Cacciapuoti S, Garzorz-Stark N, Megna M, Marasca C, Seiringer P, et al. Hidradenitis suppurativa: where we are and where we are going. Cells. 2021;10(8). https://doi.org/10.3390/cells10082094.
16. Shah A, Alhusayen R, Amini-Nik S. The critical role of macrophages in the pathogenesis of hidradenitis suppurativa. Inflamm Res. 2017;66(11):931–45. https://doi.org/10.1007/s00011-017-1074-y.
17. Constantinou CA, Fragoulis GE, Nikiphorou E. Hidradenitis suppurativa: infection, autoimmunity, or both? Ther Adv Musculoskelet Dis. 2019;11:1759720X19895488. https://doi.org/10.1177/1759720X19895488.
18. Del Duca E, Morelli P, Bennardo L, Di Raimondo C, Nisticò SP. Cytokine pathways and investigational target therapies in hidradenitis suppurativa. Int J Mol Sci. 2020;21(22). https://doi.org/10.3390/ijms21228436.
19. Sabat R, Jemec GBE, Matusiak Ł, Kimball AB, Prens E, Wolk K. Hidradenitis suppurativa. Nat Rev Dis Primers. 2020;6(1):18. https://doi.org/10.1038/s41572-020-0149-1.
20. Schroder K, Hertzog PJ, Ravasi T, Hume DA. Interferon-gamma: an overview of signals, mechanisms and functions. J Leukoc Biol. 2004;75(2):163–89. https://doi.org/10.1189/jlb.0603252.
21. Witte-Händel E, Wolk K, Tsaousi A, Irmer ML, Mößner R, Shomroni O, et al. The IL-1 pathway is hyperactive in hidradenitis suppurativa and contributes to skin infiltration and destruction. J Invest Dermatol. 2019;139(6):1294–305. https://doi.org/10.1016/j.jid.2018.11.018.
22. Calabrese L, Fiocco Z, Satoh TK, Peris K, French LE. Therapeutic potential of targeting interleukin-1 family cytokines in chronic inflammatory skin diseases. Br J Dermatol. 2022;186(6):925–41. https://doi.org/10.1111/bjd.20975.
23. Arnold DD, Yalamanoglu A, Boyman O. Systematic review of safety and efficacy of IL-1-targeted biologics in treating immune-mediated disorders. Front Immunol. 2022;13:888392. https://doi.org/10.3389/fimmu.2022.888392.
24. Zarchi K, Dufour DN, Jemec GB. Successful treatment of severe hidradenitis suppurativa with anakinra. JAMA Dermatol. 2013;149(10):1192–4. https://doi.org/10.1001/jamadermatol.2013.5377.
25. Amat-Samaranch V, Agut-Busquet E, Vilarrasa E, Puig L. New perspectives on the treatment of hidradenitis suppurativa. Ther Adv Chronic Dis. 2021;12. https://doi.org/10.1177/20406223211055920.

26. Li A, Peng Y, Taiclet LM, Tanzi RE. Analysis of hidradenitis suppurativa-linked mutations in four genes and the effects of PSEN1-P242LfsX11 on cytokine and chemokine expression in macrophages. Hum Mol Genet. 2019;28(7):1173–82. https://doi.org/10.1093/hmg/ddy414.
27. Vossen ARJV, van der Zee HH, Tsoi LC, Xing X, Devalaraja M, Gudjonsson JE, et al. Novel cytokine and chemokine markers of hidradenitis suppurativa reflect chronic inflammation and itch. Allergy. 2019;74(3):631–4. https://doi.org/10.1111/all.13665.
28. Wang Z, Zhao H, Zhai W, Zhang X, Li L, Yuan C, et al. Reduced expression of CXCL16/CXCR6 is involved in the pathogenesis of hidradenitis suppurativa. Exp Dermatol. 2022. https://doi.org/10.1111/exd.14710.
29. Jørgensen AR, Thomsen SF, Karmisholt KE, Ring HC. Clinical, microbiological, immunological and imaging characteristics of tunnels and fistulas in hidradenitis suppurativa and Crohn's disease. Exp Dermatol. 2020;29(2):118–23. https://doi.org/10.1111/exd.14036.
30. Kanni T, Zenker O, Habel M, Riedemann N, Giamarellos-Bourboulis EJ. Complement activation in hidradenitis suppurativa: a new pathway of pathogenesis? Br J Dermatol. 2018;179(2):413–9. https://doi.org/10.1111/bjd.16428.
31. Grand D, Navrazhina K, Frew JW. Integrating complement into the molecular pathogenesis of Hidradenitis Suppurativa. Exp Dermatol. 2020;29(1):86–92. https://doi.org/10.1111/exd.14056.
32. Witte K, Sabat R, Witte-Händel E, Ghoreschi K, Wolk K. Phytotherapeuthics affecting the IL-1/IL-17/G-CSF axis: a complementary treatment option for hidradenitis suppurativa? Int J Mol Sci. 2022;23(16). https://doi.org/10.3390/ijms23169057.
33. Wolk K, Brembach TC, Šimaitė D, Bartnik E, Cucinotta S, Pokrywka A, et al. Activity and components of the granulocyte colony-stimulating factor pathway in hidradenitis suppurativa. Br J Dermatol. 2021;185(1):164–76. https://doi.org/10.1111/bjd.19795.
34. Ghias MH, Johnston AD, Babbush KM, Kutner AJ, Hosgood HD, Lowes MA, et al. Hepcidin levels can distinguish anemia of chronic disease from iron deficiency anemia in a cross-sectional study of patients with hidradenitis suppurativa. J Am Acad Dermatol. 2022;86(4):954–6. https://doi.org/10.1016/j.jaad.2021.03.090.
35. Ponikowska M, Matusiak L, Kasztura M, Jankowska EA, Szepietowski JC. Deranged iron status evidenced by iron deficiency characterizes patients with hidradenitis suppurativa. Dermatology. 2020;236(1):52–8. https://doi.org/10.1159/000505184.
36. Ponikowska M, Matusiak Ł, Kasztura M, Jankowska E, Szepietowski JC. Decreased serum level of interleukin-22 correlates with hepcidin in patients with hidradenitis suppurativa. Acta Derm Venereol. 2021;101(9):adv00558. https://doi.org/10.2340/00015555-3928.
37. Wieland CW, Vogl T, Ordelman A, Vloedgraven HG, Verwoolde LH, Rensen JM, et al. Myeloid marker S100A8/A9 and lymphocyte marker, soluble interleukin 2 receptor: biomarkers of hidradenitis suppurativa disease activity? Br J Dermatol. 2013;168(6):1252–8. https://doi.org/10.1111/bjd.12234.
38. Matusiak Ł, Bieniek A, Szepietowski JC. Soluble interleukin-2 receptor serum level is a useful marker of hidradenitis suppurativa clinical staging. Biomarkers. 2009;14(6):432–7. https://doi.org/10.1080/13547500903075218.
39. Bachmann MF, Oxenius A. Interleukin 2: from immunostimulation to immunoregulation and back again. EMBO Rep. 2007;8(12):1142–8. https://doi.org/10.1038/sj.embor.7401099.
40. Hayran Y, Allı N, Yücel Ç, Akdoğan N, Turhan T. Serum IL-36α, IL-36β, and IL-36γ levels in patients with hidradenitis suppurativa: association with disease characteristics, smoking, obesity, and metabolic syndrome. Arch Dermatol Res. 2020;312(3):187–96. https://doi.org/10.1007/s00403-019-02012-w.
41. Sachen KL, Arnold Greving CN, Towne JE. Role of IL-36 cytokines in psoriasis and other inflammatory skin conditions. Cytokine. 2022;156: 155897. https://doi.org/10.1016/j.cyto.2022.155897.
42. Hessam S, Sand M, Gambichler T, Skrygan M, Rüddel I, Bechara FG. Interleukin-36 in hidradenitis suppurativa: evidence for a distinctive proinflammatory role and a key factor in the development of an inflammatory loop. Br J Dermatol. 2018;178(3):761–7. https://doi.org/10.1111/bjd.16019.

43. Liu M, Degner J, Georgantas RW, Nader A, Mostafa NM, Teixeira HD, et al. A genetic variant in the BCL2 gene associates with adalimumab response in hidradenitis suppurativa clinical trials and regulates expression of BCL2. J Invest Dermatol. 2020;140(3):574–82.e2. https://doi.org/10.1016/j.jid.2019.06.152.
44. Der Sarkissian S, Hessam S, Kirby JS, Lowes MA, Mintoff D, Naik HB, et al. Identification of biomarkers and critical evaluation of biomarker validation in hidradenitis suppurativa: a systematic review. JAMA Dermatol. 2022;158(3):300–13. https://doi.org/10.1001/jamadermatol.2021.4926.
45. Murata S, Kaneko S, Morita E. Interleukin-8 levels in the stratum corneum as a biomarker for monitoring therapeutic effect in atopic dermatitis patients. Int Arch Allergy Immunol. 2021;182(7):592–606. https://doi.org/10.1159/000512965.
46. Kemény L, Ruzicka T, Dobozy A, Michel G. Role of interleukin-8 receptor in skin. Int Arch Allergy Immunol. 1994;104(4):317–22. https://doi.org/10.1159/000236686.
47. Rosi E, Fastame MT, Scandagli I, Di Cesare A, Ricceri F, Pimpinelli N, et al. Insights into the pathogenesis of HS and therapeutical approaches. Biomedicines. 2021;9(9). https://doi.org/10.3390/biomedicines9091168.
48. Jiménez-Gallo D, de la Varga-Martínez R, Ossorio-García L, Albarrán-Planelles C, Rodríguez C, Linares-Barrios M. The clinical significance of increased serum proinflammatory cytokines, C-reactive protein, and erythrocyte sedimentation rate in patients with hidradenitis suppurativa. Mediat Inflamm. 2017;2017:2450401. https://doi.org/10.1155/2017/2450401.
49. Jiménez-Gallo D, de la Varga-Martínez R, Ossorio-García L, Collantes-Rodríguez C, Rodríguez C, Linares-Barrios M. Effects of adalimumab on T-helper-17 lymphocyte- and neutrophil-related inflammatory serum markers in patients with moderate-to-severe hidradenitis suppurativa. Cytokine. 2018;103:20–4. https://doi.org/10.1016/j.cyto.2017.12.020.
50. Matusiak Ł, Szczęch J, Bieniek A, Nowicka-Suszko D, Szepietowski JC. Increased interleukin (IL)-17 serum levels in patients with hidradenitis suppurativa: implications for treatment with anti-IL-17 agents. J Am Acad Dermatol. 2017;76(4):670–5. https://doi.org/10.1016/j.jaad.2016.10.042.
51. Schuch A, Fischer T, Boehner A, Biedermann T, Volz T. Successful treatment of severe recalcitrant hidradenitis suppurativa with the interleukin-17A antibody secukinumab. Acta Derm Venereol. 2018;98(1):151–2. https://doi.org/10.2340/00015555-2794.
52. Kashetsky N, Mufti A, Alabdulrazzaq S, Lytvyn Y, Sachdeva M, Rahat A, et al. Treatment outcomes of IL-17 inhibitors in hidradenitis suppurativa: a systematic review. J Cutan Med Surg. 2022;26(1):79–86. https://doi.org/10.1177/12034754211035667.
53. Grand D, Frew JW, Navrazhina K, Krueger JG. Doppler ultrasound-based noninvasive biomarkers in hidradenitis suppurativa: evaluation of analytical and clinical validity. Br J Dermatol. 2021;184(4):688–96. https://doi.org/10.1111/bjd.19343.
54. Elkin K, Daveluy S, Avanaki KM. Hidradenitis suppurativa: current understanding, diagnostic and surgical challenges, and developments in ultrasound application. Skin Res Technol. 2020;26(1):11–9. https://doi.org/10.1111/srt.12759.
55. Caposiena Caro RD, Solivetti FM, Bianchi L. Power Doppler ultrasound assessment of vascularization in hidradenitis suppurativa lesions. J Eur Acad Dermatol Venereol. 2018;32(8):1360–7. https://doi.org/10.1111/jdv.14745.
56. Fletcher JM, Moran B, Petrasca A, Smith CM. IL-17 in inflammatory skin diseases psoriasis and hidradenitis suppurativa. Clin Exp Immunol. 2020;201(2):121–34. https://doi.org/10.1111/cei.13449.
57. Lima AL, Karl I, Giner T, Poppe H, Schmidt M, Presser D, et al. Keratinocytes and neutrophils are important sources of proinflammatory molecules in hidradenitis suppurativa. Br J Dermatol. 2016;174(3):514–21. https://doi.org/10.1111/bjd.14214.
58. Hotz C, Boniotto M, Guguin A, Surenaud M, Jean-Louis F, Tisserand P, et al. Intrinsic defect in keratinocyte function leads to inflammation in hidradenitis suppurativa. J Invest Dermatol. 2016;136(9):1768–80. https://doi.org/10.1016/j.jid.2016.04.036.

59. Bernardini N, Skroza N, Tolino E, Mambrin A, Anzalone A, Balduzzi V, et al. IL-17 and its role in inflammatory, autoimmune, and oncological skin diseases: state of art. Int J Dermatol. 2020;59(4):406–11. https://doi.org/10.1111/ijd.14695.
60. Savage KT, Flood KS, Porter ML, Kimball AB. TNF-α inhibitors in the treatment of hidradenitis suppurativa. Ther Adv Chronic Dis. 2019;10:2040622319851640. https://doi.org/10.1177/2040622319851640.
61. Markota Čagalj A, Marinović B, Bukvić Mokos Z. New and emerging targeted therapies for hidradenitis suppurativa. Int J Mol Sci. 2022;23(7). https://doi.org/10.3390/ijms23073753.
62. Langrish CL, Chen Y, Blumenschein WM, Mattson J, Basham B, Sedgwick JD, et al. IL-23 drives a pathogenic T cell population that induces autoimmune inflammation. J Exp Med. 2005;201(2):233–40. https://doi.org/10.1084/jem.20041257.
63. Melgosa Ramos FJ, García Ruiz R, Mateu Puchades A, Alfageme RF. Guselkumab effectiveness, and posology in patients with moderate to severe hidradenitis suppurativa: a retrospective bicentric experience. Dermatol Ther. 2022;35(7):e15558. https://doi.org/10.1111/dth.15558.
64. Casseres RG, Kahn JS, Her MJ, Rosmarin D. Guselkumab in the treatment of hidradenitis suppurativa: a retrospective chart review. J Am Acad Dermatol. 2019;81(1):265–7. https://doi.org/10.1016/j.jaad.2018.12.017.
65. Shreberk-Hassidim R, Ramot Y, Zlotogorski A. Janus kinase inhibitors in dermatology: a systematic review. J Am Acad Dermatol. 2017;76(4):745-53.e19. https://doi.org/10.1016/j.jaad.2016.12.004.
66. Alavi A, Hamzavi I, Brown K, Santos LL, Zhu Z, Liu H, et al. Janus kinase 1 inhibitor INCB054707 for patients with moderate-to-severe hidradenitis suppurativa: results from two phase II studies. Br J Dermatol. 2022;186(5):803–13. https://doi.org/10.1111/bjd.20969.
67. Savage KT, Santillan MR, Flood KS, Charrow A, Porter ML, Kimball AB. Tofacitinib shows benefit in conjunction with other therapies in recalcitrant hidradenitis suppurativa patients. JAAD Case Rep. 2020;6(2):99–102. https://doi.org/10.1016/j.jdcr.2019.10.010.
68. Sibbald C, Alhusayen R. Janus kinase inhibitors for hidradenitis suppurativa: expanding the therapeutic toolbox. Br J Dermatol. 2022;186(5):768–9. https://doi.org/10.1111/bjd.21297.
69. Kozera E, Flora A, Frew JW. Real-world safety and clinical response of Janus kinase inhibitor upadacitinib in the treatment of hidradenitis suppurativa: a retrospective cohort study. J Am Acad Dermatol. 2022;87(6):1440–2. https://doi.org/10.1016/j.jaad.2022.07.047.
70. Singh P, Ali SA. Multifunctional role of S100 protein family in the immune system: an update. Cells. 2022;11(15). https://doi.org/10.3390/cells11152274.
71. Coates M, Mariottoni P, Corcoran DL, Kirshner HF, Jaleel T, Brown DA, et al. The skin transcriptome in hidradenitis suppurativa uncovers an antimicrobial and sweat gland gene signature which has distinct overlap with wounded skin. PLoS ONE. 2019;14(5):e0216249. https://doi.org/10.1371/journal.pone.0216249.
72. Kurpet K, Chwatko G. S100 proteins as novel therapeutic targets in psoriasis and other autoimmune diseases. Molecules. 2022;27(19). https://doi.org/10.3390/molecules27196640.
73. Batycka-Baran A, Baran W, Nowicka-Suszko D, Koziol-Gałczyńska M, Bieniek A, Matusiak Ł, et al. Serum concentration and skin expression of S100A7 (psoriasin) in patients suffering from hidradenitis suppurativa. Dermatology. 2021;237(5):733–9. https://doi.org/10.1159/000510689.
74. Li H, Zuo J, Tang W. Phosphodiesterase-4 inhibitors for the treatment of inflammatory diseases. Front Pharmacol. 2018;9:1048. https://doi.org/10.3389/fphar.2018.01048.
75. Wittmann M, Helliwell PS. Phosphodiesterase 4 inhibition in the treatment of psoriasis, psoriatic arthritis and other chronic inflammatory diseases. Dermatol Ther (Heidelb). 2013;3(1):1–15. https://doi.org/10.1007/s13555-013-0023-0.
76. Kerdel FR, Azevedo FA, Kerdel Don C, Don FA, Fabbrocini G, Kerdel FA. Apremilast for the treatment of mild-to-moderate hidradenitis suppurativa in a prospective, open-label, phase 2 study. J Drugs Dermatol. 2019;18(2):170–6.

Chapter 12
Wound Care Biomarkers

Rohan R. Shah, Raquel L. Bruinsma, and Steven R. Feldman

12.1 Introduction

The wound healing process is a physiologic immune response to tissue insult. However, the cellular and molecular mechanisms that contribute to this response are still not completely understood, and there exists many opportunities for this physiologic response to become pathologic resulting in the formation of scars or ulcers [1]. Key processes in the role of wound healing include hemostasis, inflammation, angiogenesis, extracellular matrix (ECM) remodeling, and fibroblast proliferation [1–3]. Issues in any of these processes can prolong wound healing and result in undesirable complications. For instance, angiogenesis, ECM remodeling, and stem cell recruitment are altered in chronic wound healing when compared to normal wound healing [1].

Other abnormalities in the wound healing process can result in scar formation, hypertrophic scars, keloids, ulcerations, or pressure sores [1]. Scar formation is a sequela of prolonged inflammation and has been linked to increased levels of IL-1B and TNF-a in the wound itself leading to elevated metalloproteinases (MMPs) that excessively degrade the ECM, thus impairing stem cell migration [4]. Hypertrophic scars (HTS) on the other hand, are characterized by excess collagen

R. R. Shah
Rutgers, The State University of New Jersey, 57 US Hwy 1, New Brunswick, NJ 08901-8554, USA
e-mail: rs1520@rutgers.edu

R. L. Bruinsma (✉)
Wake Forest School of Medicine, 4618 Country Club Rd, Winston-Salem, NC, USA
e-mail: rbruinsm@wakehealth.edu

S. R. Feldman
Professor of Dermatology, Pathology and Social Sciences & Health Policy, Wake Forest School of Medicine, 4618 Country Club Road, Winston-Salem, NC 27104, USA
e-mail: sfeldman@wakehealth.edu

R. Norman (ed.), *Biomarkers in Dermatology*,
https://doi.org/10.1007/978-3-031-66513-4_12

production by fibroblasts that are contained within the boundaries of the original wound and are commonly associated with burn injuries [5]. Biomarkers seen in HTS formation include increased levels of TGF-B, platelet-derived growth factor (PDGF) and alpha-smooth muscle actin (aSMA) [6]. Keloid formation is characterized by excess collagen production that extends beyond the margins of the original wound and is linked to an increased number of CD301b+ macrophages and CD26+ adipocyte precursor-derived myofibroblasts [7]. Ulceration is associated with various biomarkers including elevated levels of myeloperoxidase (MPO), reduced levels of TGF-B, and significantly increased levels of ADAM12 [8–10]. Pressure sores, often seen in immobile patients, are characterized by prolonged soft tissue compression and necrosis [1]. Biomarkers pertinent to pressure sores include a reduced expression of chemokine ligand 9 (CXCL9) as well as decreased MMP-9/Tissue Inhibitor of Metalloproteases-1 (TIMP-1) ratios in comparison to normal healing wounds [11, 12].

Biomarkers are commonly used in medicine as both diagnostic and prognostic tools to monitor disease progression and evaluate response to treatments. As defined by the World Health Organization, biomarkers are classified as a substance, structure, or process in a patient's body that can affect the outcome of their disease [13]. Biomarkers are not commonly measured in chronic wounds as they are visible lesions that can be diagnosed and monitored via direct inspection. However, since some chronic wounds have certain predilections for specific biomarkers, the use of biomarkers may be able to aid in tailoring treatment options for specific lesions and provide predictions of a wound's likelihood to heal [2].

As an immune process, the pathogenesis of wound healing involves interactions between many inflammatory and immune cells. Alterations at any point of the physiologic process of wound healing can result in the elongation of the process and result in one of several forms of chronic wounds. The transition of acute wounds to chronic wounds can be clinically appreciated via the appearance of unique biomarkers that can help predict the severity, aid in the diagnosis, and potentially guide the treatment of chronic wounds. This chapter will discuss specific biomarkers that are prevalent in normal healing wounds, as well as biomarkers that are uniquely expressed in chronic wounds and their respective subtypes.

12.2 Methods

A literature search was conducted using the PubMed search engine. Keywords used include *wound healing, wound pathogenesis, wound healing biomarkers,* and *skin wound biomarkers.* One article describing the World Health Organization's definition of a biomarker was also reviewed and included in the bibliography. Articles published prior to 2010 not written in English were filtered out. The selected papers were again filtered based on pertinence to the chapter by reviewing their abstracts and conclusions. This resulted in a final total of 25 articles used in this chapter on biomarkers in wound healing. Information regarding each biomarker was categorized into the following classifications: diagnostic, prognostic, and blood biomarkers.

12.3 Markers for Normal Wound Healing

Acute phase proteins: IL-1, IL-6, TNF-a.

One of the earliest processes involved in wound healing is inflammation. Inflammation is characterized by the release of pro-inflammatory cytokines, growth factors, as well as chemokines from platelets and damaged keratinocytes [14]. Three major pro-inflammatory cytokines that we will focus on here are IL-1, IL-6, and TNF-a.

12.3.1 Role of IL-1 in Wound Healing

IL-1 is known to be implicated in the recruitment of neutrophils and macrophages and is an early mediator of acute inflammation. Additionally, of the pro-inflammatory cytokines, IL-1 is the first detectable upregulated cytokine after wound creation [15]. However, although inflammation is an integral step in the pathogenesis of wound formation of healing, prolonged inflammation can result in delayed wound healing [4]. IL-1 in a wound bed is overexpressed in various chronic wound phenotypes ranging from scars, keloids, chronic ulcers, and diabetic ulcers [3, 4, 16].

12.3.2 IL-1 Biomarker Classification

Monitoring IL-1 levels in non-healing wounds has potential to be a prognostic marker for chronic wounds. Although IL-1 levels are not necessarily increased in one specific chronic wound phenotype, their increased levels in such wounds illustrate their role in augmenting a pro-inflammatory state [15]. Recently, the use of IL-1 receptor antagonists (IL-1RA) has been tested to see if its use can speed up the healing process in diabetic wounds. A common IL-1RA drug, Anakinra, has already been approved by the FDA for the treatment of rheumatoid arthritis for its anti-inflammatory properties [16]. IL-1RA treated wounds have significantly reduced wound area compared to placebo treated wounds at 7- and 14-days post-wound creation. Additionally, IL-1RA treated wounds demonstrated significantly less macrophage and neutrophil infiltration 21 days post-wound creation compared to placebo treated wounds, further affirming the anti-inflammatory effects of blocking the effects of IL-1 [16]. These findings not only confirm the role of IL-1 in maintaining a pro-inflammatory phenotype and thus increasing the likelihood of delayed wound healing, but also highlights the importance of IL-1RA in facilitating normal wound healing and thus warrant further investigation for their utility in other chronic wound phenotypes.

12.3.3 Role of IL-6 in Wound Healing

Like IL-1, IL-6 is a pro-inflammatory cytokine involved in the early stages of acute inflammation during wound healing. IL-6 induces the release of pro-inflammatory cytokines from tissue resident macrophages, keratinocytes, endothelial cells, stromal cells and has been found to induce chemotaxis of leukocytes into a wound [17, 18]. Additionally, IL-6 promotes Th17 and Th2 differentiation in CD4+ T-helper cells. This induces differentiation of M1 and M2 macrophages, which subsequently augment the pro-inflammatory and pro-fibrotic responses, respectively [17]. Thus, IL-6 serves a unique role in the wound healing process by indirectly promoting a switch from a pro-inflammatory state to a reparative state by changing the expression of macrophages from an M1 phenotype to a M2 phenotype as the wound healing process ensues. M2 macrophages have been shown to increase pro-fibrotic signaling necessary for scarring by stimulating fibroblast activation and collagen formation [18]. Both levels of IL-6 and alternatively activated M2 macrophages appear to accumulate in keloids [19].

12.3.4 IL-6 Biomarker Classification

Akin to IL-1, IL-6 can serve as another prognostic biomarker for chronic wounds as its presence is not indicative of a single chronic wound phenotype but can be indicative of abnormal wound healing. As previously discussed, IL-6 levels are increased in keloids which leads to increased expression of M2 macrophages resulting in the excess collagen produced in keloids [19]. In addition to keloids, expression of IL-6 has been implicated in the formation of hypertrophic scars (HTS) secondary to the role of IL-6 in promoting both myofibroblast differentiation and persistence [17]. Myofibroblasts have been shown to persist in HTS resulting in contractures [20]. Additionally, persistence of myofibroblasts in HTS has been linked to anti-apoptotic signaling. Interestingly, IL-6 has been shown to induce Bcl2 signaling in fibroblasts in idiopathic primary fibrosis patients, further illustrating the diverse mechanisms in which IL-6 can promote pathologic wound formation [21]. Unsurprisingly, the use of drugs such as corticosteroids and verapamil to reduce expression of IL-6 for the treatment of both hypertrophic scars and keloids have yielded favorable results in improving scar score and warrants further investigation as potential treatment modalities for other chronic wound phenotypes [17].

12.3.5 Role of TNF-A in Wound Healing

TNF-a is a pro-inflammatory cytokine released early in the inflammatory process of wound healing by vascular endothelial cells, keratinocytes, and fibroblasts [22].

TNF-a increases expression of chemokines such as CXCL2 and CCL2 which function to increase infiltration of leukocytes into the wound bed. Moreover, sustained expression of these chemokines secondary to elevated levels of TNF-a has been implicated in impaired wound healing seen in diabetic mice [23]. Additionally, TNF-a regulates the synthesis of extracellular matrix proteins and MMPs which are heavily involved in wound healing [24]. In a study examining the effect of anti-TNF-a mAb on mice wounds, neutralizing the effects of TNF-a was shown to delay wound closure supporting the role of TNF-a in the proliferative phase of wound healing [24]. However, while TNF-a is known to have a supportive role in the process of wound healing, sustained and elevated levels of TNF-a are known to delay the wound healing process and are seen in chronic wound phenotypes such as scars, keloids, and non-healing diabetic wounds [3, 4, 25].

12.3.6 TNF-A Biomarker Classification

TNF-a represents another pro-inflammatory cytokine elevated in a variety of chronic wound phenotypes and thus could serve as a prognostic biomarker for pathologic wounds. TNF-a has been found to be three times higher in diabetic mouse wounds compared to non-diabetic mice, and three times higher in non-healing venous leg ulcers compared to healing ulcers [26, 27]. Potential reasons for impaired wound healing with elevated TNF-a levels may be attributed to increased matrix metalloproteinase (MMP) activity which plays a role in ECM remodeling via collagen removal [5]. Interestingly, a study examining the role of administering TNF-a early in non-diabetic mice found that TNF-a resulted in significant promotion of wound closure 3 days after wound creation compared to mice treated with PBS, but no such difference was seen 7 days after wound creation [24]. These findings highlight the importance of TNF-a in the healing process and warrant further investigation of TNF-a at different time points in the wound healing process to determine potential treatment options for non-healing wounds.

12.3.7 Role of TGF-B in Wound Healing

TGF-B is a growth factor involved in many processes in wound healing ranging from inflammation, stimulating angiogenesis, fibrosis, regulating re-epithelization, and ECM remodeling [9]. TGF-B mediates its signaling by binding to TGF-B receptor II (TGF-b RII) which subsequently heterodimerizes with and phosphorylates TGF-B receptor I (TGF-B RI). This receptor complex then activates the SMAD intracellular signaling pathway to regulate expression of target genes via phosphorylation of SMAD 2 or SMAD3 and subsequent heterodimerization with SMAD 4. Alternatively, TGF-B can induce SMAD6 and SMAD7 which inhibit the phosphorylation and or nuclear translocation of receptor-associated SMADs in a negative feedback loop [9]. The downstream effects of TGF-B signaling are implicated in a variety of chronic wounds such as hypertrophic scars, keloids, and non-healing venous ulcers [6, 7, 9].

12.3.8 TGF-B Biomarker Classification

The varying levels of TGF-B depending on the phenotype of the chronic wound lends itself to best serving as a prognostic biomarker. In keloids, Xin et al. demonstrated that CD26+ fibroblasts possess increased levels of TGF-B alluding to the role of TGF-B in excess collagen deposition [7]. Conversely, non-healing venous ulcers displayed suppression of TGF-B target genes such as TGF-B RI, TGF-B RII and absence of phosphorylated Smad2 in the epidermis of these wounds [9], plasma TGF-b levels may be predictive of whether children develop HTS after a burn injury [28]. Specifically, children whose burns healed well without HTS formation had significantly higher plasma levels of TGF-B for the first two weeks post burn compared to their HTS-forming counterparts [28]. Thus, the different levels of TGF-B can have vastly different implications on chronic wound pathology depending on the type of chronic wound present.

12.3.9 Role of Matrix Metalloproteinases (MMPs) in Wound Healing

Matrix metalloproteinases (MMPs) are involved in both acute and chronic wounds. As proteases, MMPs are involved in ECM remodeling via the removal of excess collagen [5]. However, if the activity of MMPs is not regulated, then the process of wound healing can progress to a chronic wound [29]. MMPs are expressed by multiple cell types within skin such as keratinocytes and fibroblasts. Expression of MMPs can also be induced by multiple cytokines and growth factors such as vascular endothelial growth factor (VEGF), TNF-a, and TGF-B. There are several isoforms of MMPs which are grouped by their substrate preference and domain organization. MMP-1, MMP-3 and MMP-9 are the major chemokine regulators during wound healing, which function to degrade chemokines thus regulating local inflammation. MMP activity is regulated both directly and indirectly, but the major regulators of MMPs are tissue inhibitors of metalloproteinases (TIMPs) [29]. Studies have shown that ratios of MMPs/TIMPs have specific prognostic values for different chronic wound pathologies [12].

12.3.10 Matrix Metalloproteinases (MMPs) Biomarker Classification

Due to the dynamic nature of MMPs and their respective TIMPs, these biomarkers seem to offer the greatest utility as prognostic or predictive biomarkers for chronic wounds. In chronic non-healing wounds, levels of MMP-1 have been found to be elevated suggesting that downregulation of MMP-1 plays an important role in normal tissue remodeling [4]. On the other hand, Ladwig et al. demonstrated that chronic pressure ulcers that healed well over 36 days characterized by > 85% wound reduction in initial wound volume, displayed significantly lower MMP-9/TIMP-1 ratios at the time of data collection compared to wounds that healed poorly with a < 50% volume reduction in initial wound volume [12]. Furthermore, the average ratio of MMP-9/TIMP-1 across 56 ulcers significantly decreased as the chronic pressure ulcers healed [30]. However, a different study showed that MMP-9 knockout mice displayed delayed wound closure, thus raising the question of whether low levels of MMP-9 or high levels of TIMP-1 contributed to the increased wound reduction in chronic pressure ulcers [31].

12.3.11 Role of Platelet Derived Growth Factor (PDGF) in Wound Healing

Platelet-derived growth factor (PDFG) is an early growth factor released initially by platelet degranulation and in later wound stages, by macrophages, fibroblasts and endothelial cells [1]. PDGF is involved in several processes including vascular endothelial proliferation, fibroblast proliferation and migration, intraepithelial collagen deposition, and inflammatory cell recruitment [32, 33]. Due to its pro-fibrotic role in inducing collagen synthesis, the use of PDGF-BB for the treatment of diabetic foot ulcers was cleared by the FDA in 1997 for use as a topical gel, which is known as Regranex [34].

12.3.12 Platelet Derived Growth Factor (PDGF) Biomarker Classification

While PDGF is a known pro-fibrotic growth factor, its utility as a biomarker for pathologic skin wounds has not been vastly investigated. Nevertheless, HTS has been shown to be associated with high levels of PDGF [6]. Additionally, an earlier study conducted in 1997 demonstrated that diabetic mice possessed a significantly lower concentration of PDGF in both wounded and non-wounded skin, thus supporting the use of exogenous PDGF for the treatment of diabetic foot ulcers [35]. Thus,

PDGF appears to have the highest utility as a diagnostic biomarker for both HTS and diabetic foot ulcers.

12.3.13 Role of Vascular Endothelial Growth Factor (VEGF) in Wound Healing

Vascular endothelial growth factor (VEGF) is a growth factor responsible for stimulating angiogenesis in wounds, which is integral for proper wound healing as newly formed wounds are hypoxic and lack nutrients necessary for survival [5]. VEGF is secreted by many cell types such as M2 macrophages, mast cells, fibroblasts, and endothelial cells [5, 35]. Oral wounds possess reduced levels of VEGF compared to cutaneous wounds, which is supported by the decreased angiogenesis seen in oral wounds [36].

12.3.14 Vascular Endothelial Growth Factor (VEGF) Biomarker Classification

The use of VEGF as a biomarker has the highest utility as a diagnostic biomarker for diabetic foot ulcers. It is known that diabetes affects the vasculature of afflicted individuals, and unsurprisingly, diabetic skin is associated with reduced VEGF expression [5]. Furthermore, the use of topical VEGF on diabetic mice wounds accelerated the wound healing process by augmenting angiogenesis in these mice [35]. The use of topical VEGF offers a promising therapeutic option for diabetic patients suffering from non-healing wounds and warrants further investigation for its efficacy in humans.

12.3.15 Role of Fibroblast Growth Factor (FGF) in Wound Healing

Fibroblast growth factor (FGF) is a growth factor essential for wound angiogenesis, granulation tissue formation, and re-epithelization regulation [37]. FGFs are released by a plethora of cells including vascular smooth muscle cells, endothelial cells, and keratinocytes [38]. Of the various FGFs, FGF-2 has been shown to speed up tissue repair when administered to wounds, confirming its importance in wound healing [39].

12.3.16 Fibroblast Growth Factor (FGF) Biomarker Classification

FGF best serves as a predictive biomarker for wound healing. Nissen et al. demonstrated that wounds that possessed high levels of FGF-2 also had increased endothelial cell proliferation [40]. Additionally, studies using gene-knockout mice models demonstrated that reduced FGF-2 expression caused delayed wound healing [37]. Newer studies have looked at other isoforms of FGF and have shown that FGF-7 levels directly correlate with scar formation in mouse embryos and administration of FGF-7 was shown to reduce fibrosis and thus scarring [30].

12.3.17 Role of Epidermal Growth Factor (EGF) in Wound Healing

Epidermal growth factor (EGF) is a growth factor crucial for wound healing via stimulation, proliferation, and migration of keratinocytes, endothelial cells, and fibroblasts [41]. EGF is primarily secreted by platelets, macrophages, and mononuclear cells, and is the most abundant during the earliest stages of wound healing [42, 43]. The receptor for EGF, EGFR, is responsible for mediating re-epithelization and dermal maturation [44].

12.3.18 Epidermal Growth Factor (EGF) Biomarker Classification

The use of EGF as a biomarker would best serve as a prognostic biomarker. Studies have shown decreased levels of both EGF and its receptor in refractory diabetic foot ulcer ("DFU") lesions [45]. Moreover, the topical application of active EGF to DFU lesions has been shown to promote wound healing [46]. Specifically, EGF application to refractory DFU lesions appears to promote wound healing by accelerating granulation tissue production, increasing vascularity and number of fibroblasts, and improving fibroblast morphology [47].

12.3.19 Role of B-catenin and C-MYC in Wound Healing

Nuclear factor, B-catenin, and its downstream target, c-myc, play an important role in the differentiation of epidermal stem cells (ESCs) during the wound healing process (Shi). It has been reported that the B-catenin and c-myc pathway promotes proliferation through regulation of ESC transition from the G1 phase to the S phase of the cell cycle as well as inducing the dedifferentiation of mature epidermal cells to stem cell-like epidermal cells [48, 49]. As such, deficits in B-catenin and c-myc correspond to delayed wound closure [50]. On the other extreme, studies have shown that increased levels of both B-catenin and c-myc are associated with healing impairment [2].

12.3.20 B-catenin and C-MYC Biomarker Classification

Elevated nuclear levels of B-catenin and c-myc are associated with healing impairment and as such would serve best as prognostic biomarkers [2]. Overexpression of these biomarkers has been seen in non-healing edges of chronic wounds and subsequently resulted in a thickened and hyperproliferative epidermis suggesting improper wound healing [2].

12.3.21 Role of CD301b+ Macrophages in Wound Healing

CD301b+ macrophages are a specific subtype of mid-phase macrophages present during the wound healing process. Specifically, they have been shown to facilitate and augment re-epithelialization, dermal proliferation, and fibroblast recruitment during mid-stage repair [51]. While their absence has been shown to impede the normal wound healing process, CD301b+ macrophages are unusually increased in keloids [7, 51].

12.3.22 CD301b+ Macrophage Biomarker Classification

The selective increase of CD301b+ macrophages in keloids also signifies as a diagnostic biomarker [7]. CD301b+ macrophages have been shown to express increased levels of IL-10, TGF-B1, and PDGFB, which are all key mediators in the reparative phase of wound healing and are generally pro-fibrotic [51]. It should be restated that low levels of CD301b+ macrophages have demonstrated poor wound healing and thus future studies should investigate the role of this subtype of macrophages in both keloid formation and other chronic wound subtypes to better elucidate its role in wound healing and its proper classification as a biomarker [51].

12.3.23 Role of CD26+ Fibroblasts in Wound Healing

CD26+ fibroblasts represent a pro-fibrotic lineage of fibroblasts that exhibits a high expression of fibrillin, collagen, and fibronectin suggesting these play a role in the deposition of ECM [52]. The pro-fibrotic role of CD26+ fibroblasts was further reaffirmed from the work of Michalak-Mica et al. who demonstrated that CD26-knockout cells were slower at achieving skin homeostasis in epidermal stratification, slower at producing new ECM, and demonstrated decreased levels of fibronectin compared to their CD26+ counterparts [53].

12.3.24 CD26+ Fibroblast Biomarker Classification

CD26+ expression is increased in keloids and thus the role of CD26+ fibroblasts would be best served as a diagnostic marker for keloids [7]. In keloids, CD26+ fibroblasts exhibit both increased proliferation and invasion in the wound bed [7]. Interestingly, one study has shown that the use of collagen hydrogels containing CD26+ ASCs in the treatment of skin burns in mice resulted in accelerated skin healing as well as improved scar architecture [54]. Thus, more research should be done to investigate the process of elevated CD26+ fibroblast expression resulting in the setting of keloid formation to augment understanding of this chronic wound subtype.

12.3.25 Role of Myeloperoxidase (MPO) in Wound Healing

Myeloperoxidase (MPO) possesses anti-angiogenic properties and is released from neutrophils as part of the first line response to invading pathogens [8, 55]. MPO has been shown to augment activity of neutrophils by increasing reactive oxygen species (ROS) production which exacerbate the pro-inflammatory state during an acute wound [56]. Elevated levels of MPO at a wound site are associated with elevated levels of neutrophils and increased reactive oxygen species (ROS) production contributing to delayed healing [57].

12.3.26 Myeloperoxidase (MPO) Biomarker Classification

The pro-inflammatory role of MPO in the wound healing process lends itself to serving as a prognostic biomarker for chronic wound progression. In DFUs, MPO is expressed at higher levels in chronic wounds compared to acute wounds, which is likely secondary to the pro-inflammatory role MPO plays in wound healing. Another contributor to increased MPO expression in chronic wounds is its anti-angiogenic properties as supported by elevated annexin A5, which is a late apoptotic cell marker exclusively found in diabetic wound exudates and reflects a decreased supply of sustenance needed for cell proliferation and survival [8].

12.3.27 Role of ADAM12 in Wound Healing

ADAM12 is a member of a metalloproteinases (ADAMs) family involved in various physiological functions such as cell adhesions, migration, membrane protein shedding, and proteolysis [58]. In the context of wound healing, ADAM12 interacts with the TGF-B receptor and augments TGF-B signaling by regulating localization of TGF-B receptors to early endosomes [58, 59]. ADAM12 has also been shown to control activation of other growth factors responsible for wound healing such as heparin-binding EGF-like growth factor (HB-EGF) and insulin growth factor (IGF) binding proteins [10].

12.3.28 ADAM12 Biomarker Classification

The increased expression of ADAM12 in various dermatologic conditions lends itself to serving best as a prognostic biomarker. ADAM12 expression is elevated in the non-healing edge of chronic skin ulcers, as well as in basal cell carcinoma (BCC), peripheral tumor margins, and in malignant melanomas [10, 58]. ADAM12-deficient mice exhibited significantly increased keratinocyte migration and proliferation in their wounds compared to their wild-type counterparts, suggesting increased levels of ADAM12 in chronic wounds impairs wound healing by reducing the activity of keratinocytes [58].

12.3.29 Role of Human Cathelicidin Anti-microbial Protein hCAP18 in Wound Healing

Human cathelicidin anti-microbial protein (hCAP18) and its terminal fragment (LL-37) are components of the innate immune system and offer broad-spectrum anti-microbial activity. Levels of hCAP18 and LL-37 peak at 48 h in healing skin wounds and decline to pre-injury levels after wound closure. Specifically, these proteins appear to play an important role in the re-epithelization of wounds as shown by reduced skin re-epithelization in a dose dependent manner once treated with antibodies against LL-37 [60].

12.3.30 Human Cathelicidin Anti-microbial Protein hCAP18 Biomarker Classification

The selective decrease in expression of hCAP18 and LL-37 in chronic ulcers lends itself to serving best as a diagnostic biomarker. Specifically, chronic ulcers have not only shown low levels of hCAP18 in the epithelium, but immunoreactivity for both hCAP18 and LL-37 is also absent in these chronic wounds, hence the utility of these proteins as diagnostic biomarkers for chronic ulcers [60].

12.3.31 Role of Chemokine Ligand 9 (CXCL9) in Wound Healing

Chemokine ligand 9 (CXCL9) is a pro-inflammatory chemokine that is upregulated by TNF-a and secreted by macrophages and dendritic cells at local wound sites [61]. CXCL9 is involved in endothelial cell chemotaxis during the proliferative stage of angiogenesis and reduced activation of CXCL9 can result in delayed wound healing [11].

12.3.32 Chemokine Ligand 9 (CXCL9) Biomarker Classification

The failure of CXCL9 expression to increase in pressure ulcers compared to healthy healing wounds suggests that CXCL9 would serve best as a diagnostic biomarker for pressure ulcers [11]. However, given the broad nature of chemokines and their role in wound healing, it could be the case that levels of CXCL9 have not been identified in other chronic wound pathologies and warrants further research into its expression in other wound healing pathologies.

12.3.33 Role of Hypoxia-Inducible Factors (HIF-1, HIF-2, HIF-3) in Wound Healing

The initial wound healing process is characterized by hypoxic conditions secondary to local disruption of vasculature and subsequent activation of hypoxia-inducible factors (HIFs). HIF-1 is a central mediator in the wound healing response to combat tissue hypoxia by stimulating pro-angiogenic factors such as VEGF. Thus, reduced levels of HIF-1 in wound beds can result in decreased blood flow to the wound and subsequently prolong the wound healing process [62]. In addition to HIF-1, HIF-2 has been shown to share many of the pro-angiogenic roles as HIF-1, while HIF-3 appears to negatively affect vasculogenic function [63].

12.3.34 Hypoxia-Inducible Factors (HIF-1, HIF-2, HIF-3) Biomarker Classification

The nature of HIFs in wound healing and their levels in the wound bed of diabetic foot ulcers being predictive of healing outcomes lends itself to these factors serving best as prognostic biomarkers. As mentioned earlier, the pro-angiogenic properties of HIF-1 and HIF-2 are crucial for the proper healing of wounds, and thus these levels are positively correlated to the likelihood of adequate wound healing in diabetic foot ulcers. Conversely, HIF-3's anti-angiogenic properties serve the opposite role as a prognostic biomarker, and thus lower ratios of (HIF-1 + HIF-2)/HIF-3 are negatively associated with good healing outcomes in diabetic foot ulcers [63].

12.4 Summary

Wound healing represents a complex immunologic process that functions to repair injuries to the body's first line of defense via a nuanced balance of pro-inflammatory and anti-inflammatory processes. Due to the skin being the most superficial organ and injuries being visibly appreciable, the need for biomarkers to monitor injury progression or aid in diagnosis has not been employed. However, advancements in research, biotechnology and the pathophysiology of wound healing have allowed for the detection of many biomarkers that are either unique to different skin pathologies or differentially expressed. These biomarkers range from being diagnostic for certain pathologies to aiding in the prognosis and treatment management for other conditions.

Since cutaneous wound healing represents an expansive process that shares many steps with injuries to other tissues and organs, the presence of many current biomarkers impedes the ability to isolate one pathology from another. For example, elevated levels of pro-inflammatory cytokines such as IL-6 or TNF-a are not diagnostic of any condition due to their role as pro-inflammatory mediators in many pathologic states. However, in the context of specific wound pathologies, such as hypertrophic scars or keloids, levels of IL-6 can be used to gauge the response to treatment as IL-6 not only induces M2 macrophage expression resulting in increased fibrosis, but also promotes myofibroblast differentiation [19].

Unique expression of certain biomarkers such as CD301b+ macrophages, which facilitate and re-augments epithelization following injury, represents the diagnostic utility of biomarkers as these macrophages have been shown to be selectively increased in keloids [7, 51]. Thus, the utility of biomarkers is heavily incumbent upon the understanding of the pathophysiology of a condition to determine where a specific process goes awry so that those components can be measured. With respect to dermatologic conditions, serum biomarkers may be mistakenly overlooked as the manifestation of these conditions and response to treatment are visible changes that can be monitored via direct inspection.

At their core, chronic wounds are due to disruptions in the wound healing process at a cellular level that cannot be objectively measured visually. Ergo the use of biomarkers can not only guide treatment protocols based on measurable differences in biomarkers, but it can also predict the likelihood of certain wounds becoming pathologic allowing clinicians to employ preventative measures from such pathologic wounds developing in the first place. The utility of biomarkers is limited by the presence of unique biomarkers that have been identified for different pathologies. Thus, future research in wound healing should identify new biomarkers that exhibit preferential expression in a certain condition to improve diagnostic measures and our understanding of the pathophysiology behind these conditions. This will inevitably shape the manner in which we effectively treat these pathologies.

Case Example: A 70-year-old male developed a stage II sacral pressure ulcer measuring 1.5 × 4 cm. On the forearms were signs of skin atrophy, skin lacerations, and senile purpura.

Use of biomarkers: Order a blood test to assess for infection and quantify levels of biomarkers such as IL-1 and TNF-alpha. Tissue may be sampled for MMP-9/TMP-1 ratio along with presence of VEGF and FGF. The presence of these wound healing biomarkers can complement the clinical diagnosis of a pressure wound ulcer in this patient. This helps with management as the clinician can have a better sense of the timing for the infection, which is especially helpful for pressure ulcers which are often found days later due to their inconspicuous locations. Additionally, the clinician can delineate whether the pressure ulcer will be able to heal by itself or whether further management is needed. Such wounds all require protective dressings and if infection is suspected, appropriate antibiotics as well.

References

1. Eming SA, Martin P, Tomic-Canic M. Wound repair and regeneration: mechanisms, signaling, and translation. Sci Transl Med. 2014;6:265sr6.
2. Lindley LE, Stojadinovic O, Pastar I, Tomic-Canic M. Biology and biomarkers for wound healing. Plast Reconstr Surg. 2016;138:18S-28S.
3. Karppinen S, Heljasvaara R, Gullberg D, Tasanen K, Pihlajaniemi T. Toward understanding scarless skin wound healing and pathological scarring. F1000Res. 2019;8.
4. Tarnuzzer RW, Schultz GS. Biochemical analysis of acute and chronic wound environments. Wound Repair Regen. 1996;4:321–5.
5. Nguyen AV, Soulika AM. The dynamics of the skin's immune system. Int J Mol Sci. 2019;20.
6. Finnerty CC, Jeschke MG, Branski LK, Barret JP, Dziewulski P, Herndon DN. Hypertrophic scarring: the greatest unmet challenge following burn injury. Lancet. 2016;388:1427–36.
7. Xin Y, Wang X, Zhu M, et al. Expansion of CD26 positive fibroblast population promotes keloid progression. Exp Cell Res. 2017;356:104–13.

8. Krisp C, Jacobsen F, McKay MJ, Molloy MP, Steinstraesser L, Wolters DA. Proteome analysis reveals antiangiogenic environments in chronic wounds of diabetes mellitus type 2 patients. Proteomics. 2013;13:2670–81.
9. Pastar I, Stojadinovic O, Krzyzanowska A, et al. Attenuation of the transforming growth factor β –Signaling pathway in chronic venous ulcers. Mol Med. 2010;16:92–101.
10. Harsha A, Stojadinovic O, Brem H, et al. ADAM12: a potential target for the treatment of chronic wounds. J Mol Med (Berl). 2008;86:961–9.
11. Edsberg LE, Wyffels JT, Brogan MS, Fries KM. Analysis of the proteomic profile of chronic pressure ulcers. Wound Repair Regen. 2012;20:378–401.
12. Ladwig GP, Robson MC, Liu R, Kuhn MA, Muir DF, Schultz GS. Ratios of activated matrix metalloproteinase-9 to tissue inhibitor of matrix metalloproteinase-1 in wound fluids are inversely correlated with healing of pressure ulcers. Wound Repair Regen. 2002;10:26–37.
13. Thijs JL, van Seggelen W, Bruijnzeel-Koomen C, de Bruin-Weller M, Hijnen D. New developments in biomarkers for atopic dermatitis. J Clin Med. 2015;4:479–87.
14. Reinke JM, Sorg H. Wound repair and regeneration. Eur Surg Res. 2012;49:35–43.
15. Dinarello CA. Interleukin-1 and interleukin-1 antagonism. Blood. 1991;77:1627–52.
16. Perrault DP, Bramos A, Xu X, Shi S, Wong AK. Local administration of interleukin-1 receptor antagonist improves diabetic wound healing. Ann Plast Surg. 2018;80:S317–21.
17. Johnson BZ, Stevenson AW, Prêle CM, Fear MW, Wood FM. The role of IL-6 in skin fibrosis and cutaneous wound healing. Biomedicines. 2020;8.
18. Wright HL, Cross AL, Edwards SW, Moots RJ. Effects of IL-6 and IL-6 blockade on neutrophil function in vitro and in vivo. Rheumatology (Oxford). 2014;53:1321–31.
19. Braga TT, Agudelo JSH, Camara NOS. Macrophages during the fibrotic process: M2 as friend and foe. Front Immunol. 2015;6.
20. Moulin V, Larochelle S, Langlois C, Thibault I, Lopez-Vallé CA, Roy M. Normal skin wound and hypertrophic scar myofibroblasts have differential responses to apoptotic inductors. J Cell Physiol. 2004;198:350–8.
21. Moodley YP, Misso NLA, Scaffidi AK, et al. Inverse effects of interleukin-6 on apoptosis of fibroblasts from pulmonary fibrosis and normal lungs. Am J Respir Cell Mol Biol. 2003;29:490–8.
22. Mast BA, Schultz GS. Interactions of cytokines, growth factors, and proteases in acute and chronic wounds. Wound Repair Regen. 1996;4:411–20.
23. Wetzler C, Kämpfer H, Stallmeyer B, Pfeilschifter J, Frank S. Large and sustained induction of chemokines during impaired wound healing in the genetically diabetic mouse: prolonged persistence of neutrophils and macrophages during the late phase of repair. J Investig Dermatol. 2000;115:245–53.
24. Ritsu M, Kawakami K, Kanno E, et al. Critical role of tumor necrosis factor-α in the early process of wound healing in skin. J Dermatol Dermatol Surg. 2017;21:14–9.
25. Xu F, Zhang C, Graves DT. Abnormal cell responses and role of TNF-α in impaired diabetic wound healing. Biomed Res Int. 2013;2013:754802–9.
26. Siqueira MF, Li J, Chehab L, et al. Impaired wound healing in mouse models of diabetes is mediated by TNF-α dysregulation and associated with enhanced activation of forkhead box O1 (FOXO1). Diabetologia. 2010;53:378–88.
27. Wallace HJ, Stacey MC. Levels of tumor necrosis factor-α (TNF-α) and soluble TNF receptors in chronic venous leg ulcers—correlations to healing status. J Investig Dermatol. 1998;110:292–6.
28. Rorison P, Thomlinson A, Hassan Z, Roberts SA, Ferguson MWJ, Shah M. Longitudinal changes in plasma transforming growth factor beta-1 and post-burn scarring in children. Burns. 2010;36:89–96.
29. Caley MP, Martins VLC, O'Toole EA. Metalloproteinases and wound healing. Advances in wound care (New Rochelle, N.Y.). 2015;4:225–34.
30. Takaya K, Aramaki-Hattori N, Sakai S, Okabe K, Asou T, Kishi K. Fibroblast growth factor 7 suppresses fibrosis and promotes epithelialization during wound healing in mouse fetuses. Int J Mol Sci. 2022;23.

31. Monaghan M, Browne S, Schenke-Layland K, Pandit A. A collagen-based scaffold delivering exogenous MicroRNA-29B to modulate extracellular matrix remodeling. Mol Ther. 2014;22:786–96.
32. Jian K, Yang C, Li T, et al. PDGF-BB-derived supramolecular hydrogel for promoting skin wound healing. J Nanobiotechnol. 2022;20.
33. Zubair M, Ahmad J. Role of growth factors and cytokines in diabetic foot ulcer healing: a detailed review. Rev Endocr Metab Disord. 2019;20:207–17.
34. Beer H, Longaker MT, Werner S. Reduced expression of PDGF and PDGF receptors during impaired wound healing. J Investig Dermatol. 1997;109:132–8.
35. Galiano RD, Tepper OM, Pelo CR, et al. Topical vascular endothelial growth factor accelerates diabetic wound healing through increased angiogenesis and by mobilizing and recruiting bone marrow-derived cells. Am J Pathol. 2004;164:1935–47.
36. Glim JE, van Egmond M, Niessen FB, Everts V, Beelen RHJ. Detrimental dermal wound healing: what can we learn from the oral mucosa? Wound Repair Regen. 2013;21:648–60.
37. Ortega S, Ittmann M, Tsang SH, Ehrlich M, Basilico C. Neuronal defects and delayed wound healing in mice lacking fibroblast growth factor 2. Proc Natl Acad Sci PNAS. 1998;95:5672–7.
38. Lawrence WT, Diegelmann RF. Growth factors in wound healing. Clin Dermatol. 1994;12:157–69.
39. Chuma H, Mizuta H, Kudo S, Takagi K, Hiraki Y. One day exposure to FGF-2 was sufficient for the regenerative repair of full-thickness defects of articular cartilage in rabbits. Osteoarthritis Cartilage. 2004;12:834–42.
40. Nissen LJ, Cao R, Hedlund E, et al. Angiogenic factors FGF2 and PDGF-BB synergistically promote murine tumor neovascularization and metastasis. J Clin Investig. 2007;117:2766–77.
41. Wenczak BA, Lynch JB, Nanney LB. Epidermal growth factor receptor distribution in burn wounds. Implications for growth factor-mediated repair. J Clin Inv. 1992;90:2392–401.
42. Singla S, Singla S, Kumar A, Singla M. Role of epidermal growth factor in healing of diabetic foot ulcers. Indian J Surg. 2012;74:451–5.
43. Steed DL. Modifying the wound healing response with exogenous growth factors. Clin Plast Surg. 1998;25:397–405.
44. Tokumaru S, Higashiyama S, Endo T, et al. Ectodomain shedding of epidermal growth factor receptor ligands is required for keratinocyte migration in cutaneous wound healing. J Cell Biol. 2000;151:209–19.
45. McDonnell J, Redekop K, Verboom P, Lovas K, Kalo Z. Pdg15: the cost of treating diabetic foot ulcers (dfu) with apligraf in the netherlands. Value Health. 2001;4:508.
46. Robson MC. Invited discussion: recombinant human epidermal growth factor (EGF) to enhance healing for diabetic foot ulcers. Ann Plast Surg. 2006;56:399–400.
47. Zhang J, Hu W, Diao Q, et al. Therapeutic effect of the epidermal growth factor on diabetic foot ulcer and the underlying mechanisms. Exp Ther Med. 2019;17:1643–8.
48. Katoh M, Katoh M. Notch ligand, JAG1, is evolutionarily conserved target of canonical WNT signaling pathway in progenitor cells. Int J Mol Med. 2006;17:681–5.
49. Zhang C, Chen P, Fei Y, et al. Wnt/β-catenin signaling is critical for dedifferentiation of aged epidermal cells in vivo and in vitro. Aging Cell. 2012;11:14–23.
50. Shi Y, Shu B, Yang R, et al. Erratum to: Wnt and notch signaling pathway involved in wound healing by targeting c-myc and Hes1 separately. Stem Cell Res Ther. 2015;6:254.
51. Shook B, Xiao E, Kumamoto Y, Iwasaki A, Horsley V. CD301b+ macrophages are essential for effective skin wound healing. J Investig Dermatol. 2016;136:1885–91.
52. Tabib T, Morse C, Wang T, Chen W, Lafyatis R. SFRP2/DPP4 and FMO1/LSP1 define major fibroblast populations in human skin. J Investig Dermatol. 2018;138:802–10.
53. Michalak-Micka K, Klar AS, Dasargyri A, Biedermann T, Reichmann E, Moehrlen U. The influence of CD26+ and CD26− fibroblasts on the regeneration of human dermo-epidermal skin substitutes. Sci Rep. 2022;12:1944.
54. Barrera J, Trotsyuk A, Maan ZN, et al. Adipose-derived stromal cells seeded in pullulan-collagen hydrogels improve healing in murine burns. Tissue Eng Part A. 2021;27:844–56.

55. Hasmann A, Wehrschuetz-Sigl E, Marold A, et al. Analysis of myeloperoxidase activity in wound fluids as a marker of infection. Ann Clin Biochem. 2013;50:245–54.
56. Lau D, Brümmer J, Daiber A, et al. Myeloperoxidase mediates neutrophil activation by association with CD11b/CD18 integrins. Proc Natl Acad Sci PNAS. 2005;102:431–6.
57. Murthy S, Gautam MK, Goel S, Purohit V, Sharma H, Goel RK. Evaluation of in vivo wound healing activity of bacopa monniera on different wound model in rats. Biomed Res Int. 2013;2013:972028–9.
58. Kawaguchi M, Hearing VJ. The roles of ADAMs family proteinases in skin diseases. Enzym Res. 2011;2011: 482498.
59. Atfi A, Dumont E, Colland F, et al. Disintegrin and metalloproteinase ADAM12 contributes to TGF-β signaling through interaction with the type II receptor. J Cell Biol. 2007;178:201–8.
60. Heilborn JD, Nilsson MF, Kratz G, et al. The cathelicidin anti-microbial peptide LL-37 is involved in re-epithelialization of human skin wounds and is lacking in chronic ulcer epithelium. J Invest Dermatol. 2003;120:379–89.
61. Bünemann E, Hoff N, Buhren BA, et al. Chemokine ligand-receptor interactions critically regulate cutaneous wound healing. Eur J Med Res. 2018;23:4.
62. Hong WX, Hu MS, Esquivel M, et al. The role of hypoxia-inducible factor in wound healing. Adv Wound Care. 2014;3:39–399.
63. Thom SR, Hampton M, Troiano MA, et al. Measurements of CD34+/CD45-dim stem cells predict healing of diabetic neuropathic wounds. Diabetes. 2016;65:486–97.

Chapter 13
Biomarkers in Acne and Rosacea

Julian Melchor, Raquel L. Bruinsma, and Steven R. Feldman

Abstract Acne vulgaris and rosacea are common, chronic inflammatory conditions. While both can present with papules and pustules on the face, they have their own distinctive pathophysiology, clinical presentation, and treatment plans. While AV is clinically diagnosed, treatments options may vary depending on the clinical severity and what the patient can tolerate. Some current medications can be financially burdensome, have unwanted side effects, or have a treatment schedule that can be difficult for some patients to maintain. Targeting certain biomarkers in acne vulgaris and rosacea can potentially provide more feasible treatment options for patients with acne and rosacea. This chapter will focus on the specific biomarkers involved in acne vulgaris and rosacea which could potentially expand our current understanding and methodology in diagnosis, prognosis, and managing treatment for patients with these skin disorders. A literature review was conducted of ten biomarkers using the classification standards from the World Health Organization. These ten biomarkers were selected based on their involvement in the pathogenesis of AV or rosacea, as well as their current usage as treatment targets for other dermatological conditions.

Keywords Biomarkers · Acne · Rosacea · Acne vulgaris · Biomarkers for acne · Biomarkers for rosacea · IL-17 · IL-33 · Diagnosis · Treatment · Pathophysiology · Dermcidin · microRNA · IGF-1

J. Melchor
College of Medicine, Florida State University, 1115 W Call St, Tallahassee, FL 32306, USA
e-mail: jm15v@med.fsu.edu

R. L. Bruinsma (✉)
Wake Forest School of Medicine, 4618 Country Club Rd, Winston-Salem, NC, USA
e-mail: rbruinsm@wakehealth.edu

S. R. Feldman
Professor of Dermatology, Pathology and Social Sciences & Health Policy, Wake Forest School of Medicine, 4618 Country Club Road, Winston-Salem, NC 27104, USA
e-mail: sfeldman@wakehealth.edu

R. Norman (ed.), *Biomarkers in Dermatology*,
https://doi.org/10.1007/978-3-031-66513-4_13

13.1 Introduction

13.1.1 Acne Vulgaris

Acne vulgaris (AV) is a chronic inflammatory disease mainly involving the pilosebaceous unit [1]. AV is one of the most common dermatologic conditions worldwide, affecting almost 650 million people around the globe [2]. Some key features of its pathophysiology involve abnormal follicular keratinization, hyperseborrhoea, *Propionibacterium acnes* (P.acnes) proliferation in the pilosebaceous unit, alterations of sebum fatty acid composition, dysregulation of the hormone microenvironment, and many other causes [1, 2]. Acne can result in substantial scarring, post-inflammatory hyperpigmentation, local discomfort, financial burden for treatment costs, and negative psychosocial effects on the quality of life of affected individuals [2, 3].

Acne can appear in a multitude of different severities. Typically, it presents as comedones, papules, and pustules, which can progress to nodules and cysts [3]. Other symptoms include scars, erythema, and hyperpigmentation and even can be associated with other psychological disorders such as depression and anxiety [2, 3]. Acne scars have the potential of being seen in about 43%-95% of AV patients [4]. Early and effective treatment is essential for patients as it has the potential of markedly impacting an individual's quality of life [2]. Treatment options range from multiple different agents based on the severity of disease [2, 5].

There are an array of different medication options available for patients with acne [5]. Treatment options range from topical retinoids, topical and systemic antibiotics, benzoyl peroxide, isotretinoin, and several other agents such as antiandrogens and corticosteroids [5]. Research on acne biomarkers may lead to earlier detection of worsening prognosis and more effective treatment options [5].

13.2 Rosacea

Rosacea is a chronic inflammatory skin disorder primarily affecting the nose, cheeks, chin, forehead, and eyes [6]. There are more than 16 million individuals affected by this disorder in the United States alone, with an 18% peak incidence and 5% prevalence worldwide [7]. Rosacea classically presents with persistent erythema, papules and pustules, episodes of flushing, telangiectasias, and rhinophyma [6, 7]. While rosacea tends to effect males and females equally, some symptoms seem to have a gender- and age-specific preference [7]. While rhinophyma typically presents in males, flushing and erythema tend to appear first in patients of younger ages [7]. Rosacea typically affects the face, and thus, it can have a negative impact on the patient's self-esteem and quality of life [6].

The pathophysiology of rosacea is thought to include a dysregulated and over functioning immune system or a potential neurocutaneous origin [6]. Activation of the

Table 13.1 Biomarkers in acne vulgaris and rosacea

Acne vulgaris biomarkers	Rosacea biomarkers
Interleukin-17	Interleukin-17
Insulin-like growth Factor-1	Interleukin-33
Noncoding RNA	Noncoding RNA
Dermcidin	Chemokines
Irisin	Thiol disulfide homeostasis

innate and adaptive immune systems can trigger rosacea. Environmental factors can also trigger rosacea [7]. Rosacea is a clinical diagnosis, with clinical subtypes such as erythematotelangiectatic, papulopustular, phymatous, ocular, and granulomatous rosacea [6, 7]. Primary features of diagnosis include persistent central erythematous distribution on the face and phymatous changes [6, 7]. Determining the subtype is an important step in treatment, as treatments are based on rosacea subtype to optimize the patient's outcomes. Treatments can either be topical or systemic, such as topical metronidazole, oral doxycycline, topical ivermectin, minocycline, encapsulated benzoyl peroxide cream, and some biologic agents [6]. Even with the multitude of medication options, new advances in therapies are crucial for expanding treatment options and improving outcomes for patients [6, 7].

13.3 Biomarkers

Biomarkers are defined by the World Health Organization (WHO) as "any substance, structure, or process that can be measured in the body or its products and influence or predict the incidence of outcome or disease" [8]. Biomarkers not only have the potential to be an additional tool in the creation of new treatment options, but also assessing different disease severities. The U.S Food and Drug Administration (FDA) have approved for biomarkers use in the treatment development process [8], meaning further research utilizing these biomarkers can potentially lead to new developments in treatment, aiding clinical diagnosis, and monitoring disease severity for an array of pathologies. This chapter will focus on the specific biomarkers involved in acne vulgaris and rosacea that could potentially expand our current understanding and methodology in diagnosis, prognosis, and managing treatment for patients with these skin disorders (Table 13.1).

13.4 Methods

A literature review was conducted through PubMed. The keywords used were *biomarkers, acne, rosacea, acne vulgaris, biomarkers for acne, and biomarkers for rosacea.* One hundred and seventy-eight search results were found for acne, and

53 search results were found for rosacea. Articles obtained for this chapter were then limited to those published after 2015 in English, yielding 88 search results for acne and 30 search results for rosacea. Prescreening these search results then included reviewing the titles of the articles, abstracts, and relevance to the objective of the chapter. After screening and eliminating those who did not fit the inclusion criteria, 24 articles total were included in the final screened results. Biomarkers in this chapter were classified using the WHO definitions for biomarker classifications such as screening, prognostic, monitoring, pharmacodynamic, and diagnostic biomarkers.

13.5 Acne Vulgaris

13.5.1 Biomarkers

13.5.1.1 Interleukin-17

Interleukin-17 (IL-17) is a pro-inflammatory cytokine who promotes antimicrobial responses, barrier maintenance, and pathologic inflammation throughout the human body [9]. The T-helper (Th) 17 pathways, which involve activated T-cells that mainly secrete IL-17, are important players in the inflammatory response [4]. Mast cells also contribute in the role of IL-17 secretion in acne [10]. IL-17 has the ability to induce the expression of other pro-inflammatory cytokines and chemokines, as well as activate neutrophils [4]. While the role IL-17 plays in the pathogenesis of AV is not entirely understood, current literature suggests it has a vital role in a multitude of other dermatologic diseases. Specifically, mast cells, APCs, and T-cells are the observed cellular players in the acne immune response [9].

Though acne vulgaris has a multifactorial etiology, *Propionibacterium acnes* is one of the main contributors in its pathogenesis [10]. Repeated exposure to *P. acnes* has the ability to activate immune cells due to its pro-inflammatory potential, specifically promoting the release of IL-17 and other major cytokines [4, 9]. Th17 cells were also seen in increased numbers amongst acne patients, with predictions in which these cells are involved in the formation of closed comedones [9]. Thus, the presence of IL-17 within AV lesions has the potential to indicate the role of this major cytokine's involvement in acne's pathogenesis.

There has been evidence vitamin D3 has a potential role in IL-17 levels amongst patients with acne. Vitamin D3 decreases the expression of retinoic acid receptor (RAR) alpha, which decreases the generation of Th17 cells and thus IL-17 [10]. Elsadek et al. (2018) discovered a negative correlation between the serum and tissue IL-17 levels when compared to serum and tissue vitamin D3 levels. It is believed vitamin D3 inhibits the generation of Th17 cells by decreasing the retinoic acid receptor alpha, as well as direct IL-17 suppression within these IL-17 secreting cells [10]. The results explained how milder cases of AV patients had higher Vitamin D3 levels and lower IL-17 levels. This inhibition by Vitamin D3 has also been recorded to play a role in the *P. acnes*-induced Th17 expression in AV [10]. This correlation could be a potential target for future acne pharmaceuticals. Not only is there a potential usage for vitamin D3 as a topical or systemic agent for AV patients, but so are IL-17 inhibitors in combination with vitamin D3 [10].

IL-17 has the potential to serve as a prognostic biomarker and treatment target for patients with AV. IL-17 levels were higher in patients with acne compared to those without [4]. Those patients with increased disease severity were observed to have higher levels of IL-17, especially those with acne scarring lesions [4, 10]. IL-17 expression within the acne lesions were also increased [10]. This is potentially due to a more robust inflammatory response. Ebrahim et al. (2018) stated using a cutoff for IL-17 levels at $\geq$ 9.51 pg/mL and $\geq$ 12.59 pg/mL allowed their researchers to predict and detect the severity of AV amongst their study subjects. Those with acne scars were observed to have higher levels of IL-17 in their serum compared to their nonscarring counterparts [4]. Even though the functional role of this cytokines involvement in AV remains understudied, there is a potential for this biomarker to allow clinicians to predict the severity of their patient's disease [4, 9]. With the assistance of the Th cell response, it has been observed mast cells play an early role in acne with IL-17 secretion [9]. Neutrophils then take over as the main IL-17 producer in the later stages of diseases [9]. These early mast cells are a potential target for acne therapeutics in future studies. While the presentation of AV can be widely variable amongst different patient populations, biomarkers such as these can assist in forming a treatment plan that can be more patient centered and specific to their disease progression.

13.5.1.2 Insulin-Like Growth Factor-1

Insulin-like growth factor-1 (IGF-1) is a polypeptide hormone who binds to its tyrosine kinase receptor and mediates a multitude of different intracellular signaling pathways [11]. Some of the pathways involved contribute to the regulation of protein synthesis, glucose transport, cell proliferation, and cell survival [11]. IGF-1 has also been seen to play a role in sebaceous gland growth, proliferation, and function, a major player in the pathogenesis of AV [12]. Diet is an additional factor which induces and aggravates acne [13]. It is hypothesized that the increased glucose in the blood causes this rise in IGF-1 levels, which then directly affects androgen and lipid metabolism involved in AV [13].

There is a highly polymorphic microsatellite region within the IGF-1 gene that influences the expression of IGF-1 [12]. Increased plasma levels of IGF-1 were observed in AV patients compared to healthy patients [11]. Rahaman et al. (2016) discussed how 192/192 homozygote patients were observed to have higher levels of IGF-1 and more severe acne compared to the non-192/non-192 patients. The studies genotype data exhibited a 4.29 times odds risk of forming acne lesions within the 192/192 homozygote group compared to the non-192/non-192 group [12]. This suggests the possible role IGF-1 can play in acne's pathogenesis, which may even have a genetic basis.

IGF-1 has the potential to become a prognostic biomarker and treatment target for patients with AV. Increased levels of IGF-1 have been traced from either the systemic circulation or local synthesis on acne-prone skin [11]. While numerous factors, such as diet, age, and lifestyle, can affect IGF-1 levels, the majority of this variability has a genetic basis [12]. Diet, in particular, could be a target for future acne therapies. Diets containing high glycemic loads have an increased level of IGF-1, potentially promoting acne development and severity [13]. The increased IGF-1 has the potential to increase sebaceous gland production and inflammatory markers, leading to this hypothesis [13]. It has also been discovered IGF-1 was higher in acne scar patients compared to active acne patients, suggesting its role in the pathogenesis of acne scar tissue formation [11]. With the multitude of ways IGF-1 can play a role in AV, this biomarker may shine a light on future medical treatments for AV and play a role as a prognostic biomarker for patients at risk for acne scars.

13.5.1.3 Noncoding RNAs

Micro-(mi) RNAs are noncoding endogenous RNA molecules which aid in gene expression by posttranscriptional modification [14]. These molecules have been identified in numerous skin conditions, suggesting a role in their pathogenesis. Literature shows patients with AV who tend to scar produce a more prolonged and robust inflammatory response than those patients who do not scar. Ghumra et al. (2021) studied this phenomenon, and discovered miR-223, miR-21, and miR-150 were miRNAs that were upregulated in patients with AV who had acne scars. Additionally, miR-223 and miR-21 were increased in the early stages of mild scarring. Therefore, miRNAs have the potential to be used as a prognostic biomarker for acne patients who are prone to scarring. These miRNAs could allow clinicians to identify those patients at greatest risk of scarring prior to the event, in order to initiate preventative therapy regardless of their acne severity [14]. Therefore, miRNAs have the potential to become a future prognostic biomarker for patients at risk for acne scars.

Circular (circ) RNA are noncoding biological molecules who have recently been of focus as a potential biomarker for a variety of human diseases [15]. These molecules have the ability to regulate transcription, alternative splicing and gene expression, and were first discovered in viruses, plants, and animals [16]. Liang et al. (2018) discovered these circRNAs were highly expressed in the lesional skin of patients with severe acne. These subtypes of circRNAs detected in acne skin were also identified to be those that function in inflammation, metabolism, and immune responses. These findings suggest a potential biomarker for future pharmaceuticals to target and pharmacodynamic biomarker for acne therapies. Further studies with a large patient population and detailed mechanism of action of circRNAs can assist in discovering the role circRNAs play in the pathogenesis of AV.

13.5.1.4 Dermcidin

Dermcidin (DCD) is an antimicrobial peptide found in the dermis of the skin [17]. Antimicrobial peptides inhibit the growth of pathogenic microorganisms on the skin, play a role in wound healing, and boost the cutaneous immunological response [18]. DCD is mainly secreted from eccrine sweat glands and sebaceous glands in the absence of inflammatory markers in the skin [17, 18]. It is hypothesized that these peptides become enzymatically broken down and form a layer on the skins surface, potentially preventing the colonization of microorganisms [17]. *Propionibacterium granulosum*, *Staphylococcus epidermidis*, and *Malassezia furfur* are some of the microorganisms who play a role in the pathogenesis of AV [18]. *P. acnes*, a well-known player of AV pathogenesis, is involved in inflammatory acne by skin colonization and release of inflammatory markers during comedogensis [17].

DCD has the potential to become a pharmacodynamic biomarker and treatment target for future AV patients. DCD was decreased in those patients with AV compared to healthy subjects without acne [17, 18]. Upon treatment with isotretinoin, a vitamin A derivative used in the treatment of AV, concentrations of DCD began to improve [18]. This suggests that DCD may play an anti-inflammatory role in AV, and isotretinoin may increase DCD levels during the treatment course. DCD has also demonstrated promising microcidal activity against various microorganisms, some including *E. coli*, *E. faecalis*, *S. aureus*, and *P. acnes* [17]. Nakano et al. (2015) suggested that DCD has a concentration-dependent antibacterial activity against *P. acnes*, and inflammatory AV patients do not have adequate immunologic control to suppress the growth of the *P. acnes* microenvironment. Increasing concentrations of DCD may assist in the anti-inflammatory response against these microorganisms and inflammatory AV. Future studies with a larger sample size and analysis of DCD concentrations will help researchers get a better understanding of the relationship between DCD and AV. DCD demonstrates the potential to become a promising pharmacodynamic biomarker for future treatments of AV.

13.5.1.5 Irisin

Irisin is an adipomyokine released from adipocytes and myocytes due to stimuli such as physical activity [19, 20]. This adipomyokine acts as a link between muscles and adipose tissue to other organs and tissues of the body [20]. Recent studies have shown the multitude of potential roles irisin may participate in. It is anti-inflammatory, antioxidant, and anti-diabetic effects, and maintaining balance between resorption and formation of bone and functioning of the nervous system are just some of the functional roles irisin can partake in throughout the human body [19, 20]. Serum irisin levels also were noticeably decreased in patients with severe AV, especially those with insulin resistance [19]. Additionally, this adipomyokine has been discovered in chronic inflammatory conditions and patients with chronic conditions involving insulin resistance.

Acne is an inflammatory condition with multifactorial etiology most commonly seen in patients undergoing puberty. During puberty, there is a rise in androgens and insulin levels which increase a patient's risk for AV. These rising androgens levels increase sebaceous gland size, sebum production, and proliferation of keratinocytes, while the rising insulin levels can ultimately increase androgen synthesis [19]. Mustafa et al. (2018) found AV patients had more insulin resistance compared to healthy controls, and these AV patients also had decreased serum irisin levels. This negative correlation between insulin resistance and serum irisin levels in AV patients suggests a possible prognostic role in the pathogenesis of AV and comorbid disease. The anti-inflammatory and anti-diabetic effects of irisin could be a potential target in future research for AV studies. With the minimal studies in the current literature establishing this potential role as a prognostic biomarker in AV, continued research on the functional role of irisin in AV with population-based studies would help further investigate this phenomenon.

13.6 Rosacea

13.6.1 Biomarkers

13.6.1.1 Interleukin-17

Interleukin-17 (IL-17) is a pro-inflammatory cytokine who is mainly released by Th17 T-helper cells (CD4+) in response to stimuli. IL-17 is an important mediator of the pathogenic response amongst many inflammatory skin disorders [21]. While there are around six members within this cytokine family, they mainly promote secretion of other chemokines, cytokines, angiogenic factors, and antimicrobial proteins [21, 22]. Some of these inflammatory markers include CXCL8, CCL20, GM-CSF, C-CSF, IL-6, and many others [21]. This response is what potentiates the chronic inflammation seen in these particular inflammatory conditions.

Though the etiology of rosacea is multifactorial, abnormalities in inflammation and vascularity are current theories behind its pathogenesis. IL-17 levels were increased within the serum of patients with rosacea compared to healthy subjects, with a correlation between the IL-17 levels and edema severity [21]. Hayran et al. (2022) suggested that future studies involving the role IL-17 may play in the pathogenesis of rosacea can provide an expansion in current treatment options. Skin disorders, such as psoriasis and hidradenitis suppurativa, are chronic inflammatory skin conditions that have IL-17-associated pathogenesis and treatment options effectively targeting the IL-17 pathway. Treatment involves a multitargeted approach to prevent symptoms and disease burden amongst patients [21, 22]. There are a number of treatment options available, but the need for newly updated treatment remedies is suggested by clinicians and there are no current medications targeting the IL-17 pathway [22]. With the involvement of the IL-17 pathway in a multitude of chronic inflammatory conditions, including skin disorders and current treatments targeting this cytokine, a trial for rosacea patients with IL-17 as a therapeutic target and pharmacodynamic biomarker is promising. Future studies comparing the response of current or new IL-17 inhibitors on patients with rosacea is warranted to observe if this potential biomarker can be a successful therapeutic target for patients suffering from rosacea.

13.6.1.2 Interleukin-33

Interleukin-33 (IL-33) is a pro-inflammatory cytokine inducer of the T-helper 2 cell-mediated response [23]. This cytokine is normally expressed in endothelial and epithelial cells and has been reported to enhance keratinocyte VEGF expression [23, 24]. IL-33 has been reported in various diseases, including a multitude of skin disorders such as psoriasis, vitiligo, and atopic dermatitis [23]. It is suggested IL-33 is released from keratinocytes once ultraviolet (UV) light activates the inflammasome complexes within these cells [23]. With rosacea being a common chronic inflammatory skin disorder with multiple etiologies, UV light can act as one of the many triggers [24]. These rosacea triggers can cause patients to have a flare of symptoms such as flushing, telangiectasias, erythema, papules, and pustules [23, 24].

Patients with rosacea were found to have increased expression of IL-33 in their skin, especially those with the erythematotelangiectatic and papulopustular subtypes [24]. Suhng et al. (2018) suggested IL-33 may have a potential role in the angiogenesis and vasodilation of skin in patients with rosacea. In this study, there was an increased release of IL-33 within cells exposed to UV radiation who had an abundance of LL-37, another marker involved in rosacea pathophysiology. This UV radiation was found to stimulate the release of IL-1 family of cytokines from keratinocytes, which IL-33 is a part of this cytokine family. There is a potential in which LL-37, in the presence of pro-inflammatory cytokines, may be the cause of UV sensitivity in patients with rosacea. IL-33 may also partake in activation of mast cell degranulation and worsening rosacea symptoms [24]. With telangiectasias and erythema being such prominent vascular symptoms of rosacea and some of its subtypes, IL-33 could be a potential diagnostic and prognostic biomarker. IL-33 expression in patients can assist clinicians in diagnosis of rosacea, especially those subtypes with vascular symptoms. Additionally, clinicians can use IL-33 as a prognostic biomarker for those patients with symptom progression who are either not responding to treatment or having clinically worsening symptoms. Future research with a large population sample and analysis of IL-33's role in the pathophysiology of rosacea is necessary for a more detailed understanding.

13.6.1.3 Noncoding RNAs

As stated previously in this chapter, microRNAs (miRNAs) are small noncoding RNA molecules who aid in gene expression. Specifically, miRNAs play a role in RNA silencing, targeting messenger RNA, and posttranscriptional processing [25]. They have emerged in the recent literature as potential pathobiologic, diagnostic, and therapeutic candidates as biomarkers of inflammatory and autoimmune diseases [26]. This is mainly due to the discovery of miRNA expression being altered in inflammatory skin disorders, metabolic diseases, and some cancers [26]. Long noncoding RNAs (lncRNAs) are another subset of nucleotides who have a multitude of biologic functions, who also play a role in some pathological conditions such as cancer, autoimmune, and inflammatory diseases [25]. These lncRNAs are involved in the immune response, epidermal development, and leukocyte-mediated cytotoxic regulation [25].

Evidence supports microRNAs and lncRNAs aid in the progression of inflammatory skin disorders both individually and as a unit by modulating specific pathological pathways [25]. Seo et al. (2021) demonstrated that nine miRNAs were upregulated, and seven miRNAs were downregulated in the skin of patients with papulopustular rosacea compared to those healthy subjects. Two of the miRNAs in this study, miRNA-21-3p and miRNA-31-5p, who are involved in angiogenesis and inflammation, were upregulated amongst these rosacea patients. The miRNA-21 was one of the microRNAs suggested previously in this book chapter to be a potential prognostic AV biomarker found upregulated in AV patients prone to acne scarring. Wang et al. (2020) suggested that miRNAs and lncRNAs play an essential role in the pathogenesis of rosacea. Specifically, lncRNAs contribute to the signaling pathways involved in rosacea such as ferroptosis, PPAR, NOD-like, NF-Kb, and JAK-STAT pathways, while miRNAs are involved in JAK-STAT signaling and enhancing T-cell activation. Not only are these pathways potential therapeutic targets for the development of future therapies, but lncRNAs and microRNAs may act as diagnostic and pharmacodynamic biomarkers for rosacea. Even though the diagnosis of rosacea is clinical, the array of subtypes can make it challenging. These noncoding RNAs may aid in the diagnosis of the specific subtypes of rosacea and become targets for pharmaceuticals to alleviate symptoms or prevent disease. More studies on the role these noncoding RNAs play in rosacea's pathogenesis and potential clinical trials are needed to further validate this relationship.

13.6.1.4 Chemokines

Chemokines are a family of cytokine-like proteins who play a vital role in inflammation and regulating leukocyte trafficking [27, 28]. These proteins are divided into four subfamilies, such as the CC subfamily and CXC subfamily and regulate the recruitment process of organ-specific leukocyte subsets [28]. They perform a multitude of biological functions in inflammatory diseases and have suggested to impact patients with rosacea [27]. Additionally, specific effector memory T-cells have been seen to preferentially express particular cytokines [28]. Chemokines have also been seen involved in embryogenesis, tumor progression, tumor metastasis, and promotion of angiogenesis [28].

Chemokines have been suggested to play a role in the pathophysiology of rosacea, specifically CCL3, CXCL8, CXCL9, and CXCL10 (Fig. 13.1) [27]. Liu et al. (2022)

found that these particular proteins were increased in patients with rosacea compared to healthy controls. This study found that CCL3, CXCL8, and CXCL9 were positively increased using the Investigators Global Assessment to assess papules and pustules, while CXCL9 and CXCL10 were positively increased using the Clinicians Erythema Assessment to assess persistent erythema. Specifically, CXC2 and CXCR3 were expressed in the skin of patients with rosacea. The authors suggested these chemokines are not only positively correlated with disease severity, but could be a potential clinical aid as a diagnostic or prognostic biomarker for rosacea patients. With the clinical manifestations and disease severity of rosacea having a large variability within the population, using clinical diagnosis alone can be challenging. The aid of serum biomarkers can allow clinicians to have a more specific diagnostic or prognostic tool for their patients. These chemokines have also been implicated in other comorbid conditions that can be related to rosacea, such as neurological disorders and gastrointestinal disorders [27]. This makes using these chemokines as biomarkers more of a challenge, and thus, specific subfamilies of chemokines need to be found for specific subtypes of rosacea. Future studies and clinical trials are needed in order to better understand the role chemokines play in the pathogenesis of rosacea, as well as the potential use of these proteins to become diagnostic and prognostic biomarkers.

13.6.1.5 Thiol Disulfide Homeostasis

Thiols are antioxidants who play a vital role in the elimination of reactive oxygen species (ROS) [30]. These thiols can be oxidized into disulfides under oxidative stress and can be reversibly reduced back into thiols to maintain a thiol disulfide homeostatis [30, 31]. Thiols are the main compound associated with antioxidant defense, protein metabolism, regulation of redox metabolism and protect keratinocytes from oxidative stress [30, 32]. A variety of diseases have been associated with oxidative stress, which is an imbalance of antioxidants and oxidants [31, 32]. Some inflammatory and generative diseases have seen a shift of homeostasis favoring disulfides, while some proliferative diseases have shifted homeostasis toward thiols [30]. This homeostatic dysregulation of ROS and oxidative stress can cause molecular and cellular abnormalities to occur, causing irreversible damage to DNA, proteins, and lipids [31]. Damage from oxidative stress has been implicated in the pathophysiology of rosacea, including inflammation, vascular changes, and tissue damage [30]. It is believed that maintaining this thiol disulfide homeostasis plays a homeostatic role in protecting cells from harmful redox reactions, leading to potential damage and disease.

Current literature has investigated the role of the thiol disulfide homeostasis in dermatological disease [30]. The inflammatory process and vascular changes commonly seen in rosacea patients are thought to occur due to ROS deactivating the body's natural defenses [30, 31]. These ROS have been observed to cause harmful damage to keratinocytes, fibroblasts, and endothelial cells [32]. This oxidative stress

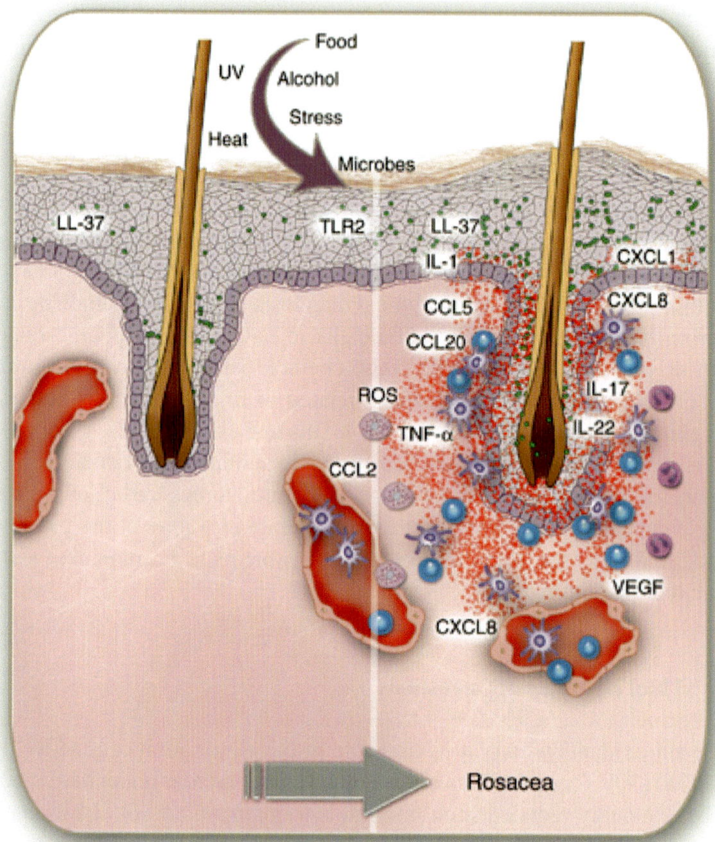

Fig. 13.1 Inflammatory process, including chemokines, of rosacea within the skin [29]

can affect the onset and progression of rosacea [31]. The skin has several antioxidant methods in order to protect itself from oxidative stress and damage, with the thiol disulfide homeostasis being one of these pathways [30]. Sener et al. (2019) determined that the disulfide level was increased in rosacea patients. Not only did this study suggest the role this homeostasis plays in the inflammatory pathway in rosacea, but also has the potential to become a therapeutic biomarker and biomarker of oxidative damage in patients with rosacea (Fig. 13.2). Pektas et al. (2022) also discovered the increased disulfide levels and decreased thiol levels in patients with rosacea compared to healthy controls. This study found an increased ROS and oxidative stress in the skin samples of rosacea patients, as well as decreased number of antioxidants. Additionally, the subtype of rosacea did not affect the parameters of oxidative stress within the study, which is a very important finding. The thiol disulfide homeostasis has a promising potential to become either a prognostic biomarker or pharmacodynamic biomarker for oxidative stress and damage. While rosacea can

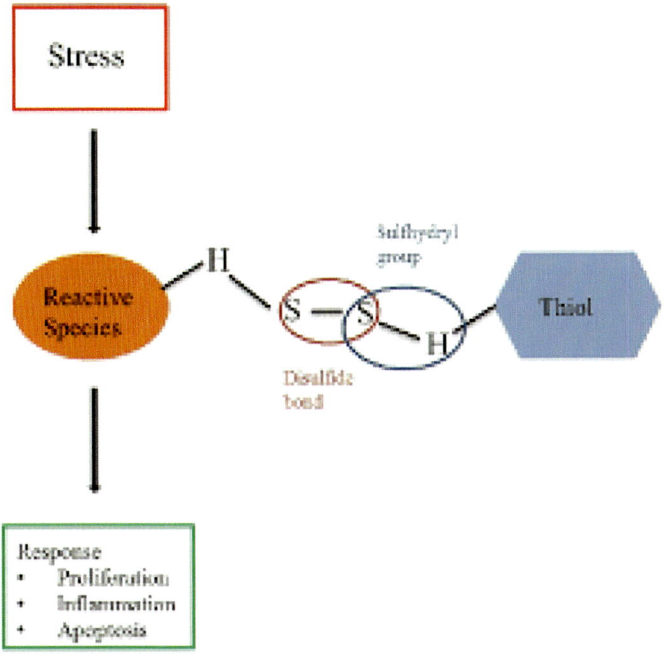

Fig. 13.2 Thiol disulfide homeostasis mechanism [33]. Reproduced with permission from ©2019 [33] distributed under the terms of the Creative Commons Attribution License

be diagnosed clinically, biomarkers such as these can aid clinicians in adjusting and regulating treatment plans depending on the severity of oxidative damage in each patient. Future studies with a large population size, including all the different subtypes of rosacea, are needed to better understand the role this homeostasis plays in the pathophysiology of rosacea.

13.7 Discussion

Acne vulgaris and rosacea are chronic inflammatory skin diseases which are vastly prevalent around the globe. AV is a multifactorial condition mainly involving the pilosebaceous unit and is clinically classified as mild, moderate, or severe manifestation. Clinical presentations of AV can vary from closed or open comedomes, inflammatory papules, nodules, pustules, and cysts [5]. There are a multitude of treatment options available for AV patients, mainly depending on their disease severity, tolerability, and preference for patients and clinicians to select from. Each of these pharmacological agents target-specific areas involved in the pathogenesis of AV, some of these include topical antibiotics, systemic antibiotics, isotretinoin, topical retinols, antiandrogens, and many others [5]. Intolerable adverse effects or ineffective clinical improvement can occur using these treatment options, which can lead to a necessary trial of other pharmaceuticals and patient frustration. Rosacea is another inflammatory skin condition mainly affecting the cheeks, nose, chin, and forehead. Severity and subtypes of rosacea vary amongst patients, such as papulopustular, ocular, or granulomatous rosacea. Clinical manifestations of rosacea generally involve flushing, erythema, phymatous changes, papules, pustules, and telangiectasias with some other subtype specific symptoms [6]. Diagnosis is mainly clinical, with treatment options varying depending on patients' symptoms. These pharmacological agents also pose the same issue as AV medications do with treatment efficacy and adverse effects.

It is important for clinicians to be able to understand, diagnose, and effectively treat these common conditions for the benefit of their patients. In order to do so, extensive research on the pathophysiology and future improvement of treatment options is crucial. Biomarkers have been extensively studied in recent years and play a large role in the diagnosis and management of a variety of chronic diseases. While their use in dermatologic diseases is less known, there is a potential for use as a diagnostic, prognostic, or even a pharmacodynamic marker for AV and rosacea.

In this chapter, ten biomarkers were associated with the pathophysiology and clinical outcomes of patients with AV and rosacea. These biomarkers were analyzed based on their potential for use as diagnostic, prognostic, and pharmacodynamic biomarkers, as well as their clinical use for screening and monitoring symptoms. Some of these biomarkers were analyzed in more than one of these categories based on their characteristics and pathophysiological involvement. Mainly, these biomarkers in AV and rosacea were targeted due to their involvement in the inflammatory signaling pathways and immunological response. For the purposes of our study and this chapter, the biomarkers selected showed promising evidence which emphasized possible usage for future diagnosis, management, prognosis, and treatment involvement for AV and rosacea patients.

The biomarkers individually analyzed for their involvement in AV were insulin-like growth factor-1, dermcidin, and irisin, while those analyzed for their involvement in rosacea were interleukin-33, chemokines, and thiol disulfide homeostasis. Interleukin-17 and several types of noncoding RNAs were analyzed for their involvement in both AV and rosacea. Interleukin-17 is a well-known pro-inflammatory cytokine involved in both inflammatory skin conditions. In AV, IL-17 has the potential to become a prognostic biomarker and therapeutic target for future pharmaceuticals. This cytokine was increased in the skin lesions of those patients with acne scars compared to those without acne scars. The use of IL-17 can assist clinicians in creating a preventative treatment strategy specifically for those at a higher risk of acne scars. The use of this biomarker as a therapeutic target and a pharmacodynamic biomarker can be used for those with rosacea. IL-17 was increased in the serum of rosacea patients and demonstrates promising therapeutic results for other chronic inflammatory diseases. Noncoding RNAs, such as microRNAs, circRNAs and lnRNAs, are endogenous molecules who aid in gene expression. MicroRNAs can be a prognostic biomarker for AV patients, as well as a diagnostic biomarker and pharmacodynamic biomarker for those patients with rosacea. With the variety of studies investigating their involvement in other autoimmune and inflammatory disorders, future studies on these noncoding RNA's roles in AV and rosacea are promising. IGF-1, dermcidin, and irisin also show promising results as potential prognostic and pharmacodynamic biomarkers, as well as therapeutic targets for future AV patients. IL-33, chemokines, and thiol disulfide homeostasis also display hopeful usage as prognostic, diagnostic, and pharmacodynamic biomarkers for rosacea patients.

While biomarkers have promising evidence to be used for patients with AV and rosacea, there are some limitations to their use as well. Most of the biomarkers elevated in AV and rosacea were also increased in other inflammatory or skin conditions. This could lead to false positive readings and confusing laboratory results for clinicians to analyze, potentially causing more harm and confusion rather than benefiting patients. Additionally, while some of these biomarkers were specific to a particular subtype of AV or rosacea, others were not. Specific biomarkers for subtypes of these conditions can be more of use for providers since they can provide more targeted use for a specific patient population, without getting confused for another inflammatory skin disorder or disease state. Lastly, levels of these biomarkers and a patient's clinical presentation can vary, posing a challenge for diagnostic criteria. All these factors can threaten the future use of these biomarkers for clinical aid. Currently, diagnosis of AV and rosacea remain clinical, with prognosis and treatment depending on clinical presentation and severity.

Biomarkers have the ability to be very beneficial for the future of medicine and clinical management of particular diseases. Specifically, with dermatologic disorders, there are potential diagnostic usages to limit clinical variability, assessment of severity, and significant insight on the treatment response with particular or new pharmaceutical targets. With the lack of biomarkers for diagnosis and prognosis to date for AV and rosacea patients, the diagnosis is largely based on clinical manifestations. Clinically, there can be some variability in the diagnosis of acne and rosacea depending on the perception of the provider. Additionally, current therapeutic remedies can have intolerable adverse effects and unfeasible prices to sustain a treatment plan. With the profound negative effects these inflammatory conditions can have on patient's self-esteem, quality of life, and psychosocial impact, it is important to find a treatment option that works best for these individuals. More extensive studies and large clinical trials further analyzing the pathophysiological role of biomarkers in acne and rosacea are needed.

13.8 Conclusion

Acne vulgaris and rosacea are both chronic inflammatory conditions affecting a significant portion of the population worldwide. While the diagnosis of acne and rosacea is mainly clinical, the use of biomarkers has the potential to confirm diagnosis, explore the patient's prognosis, and provide new therapeutic targets for pharmaceuticals. Advancements of use with these biomarkers can provide clinicians and researchers the opportunity to help patients with these chronic skin diseases, but they do pose some limitations as well. Even with this, there are still potential uses for biomarkers in the diagnosis, prognosis, and response to treatment of acne and rosacea. The spectrum of disease and clinical presentation for acne and rosacea is vast, and thus, use of biomarkers can aid in clinical assessment of these conditions. As multifactorial diseases, there are multiple causes for symptom onset and possible treatment for these conditions, and thus, a wide variety of tools are ideally needed for management. With promising advances in research and a better understanding of their roles in these skin diseases, there could be a future where these biomarkers can provide a significant change and impact for this patient population.

References

1. B D. What is new in the pathophysiology of acne, an overview. J Eur Acad Dermatol Venereology JEADV. (2017, September 31). https://pubmed.ncbi.nlm.nih.gov/28805938/. Retrieved 14 Aug 2022.
2. Moradi Tuchayi S, Makrantonaki E, Ganceviciene R, Dessinioti C, Feldman SR, Zouboulis CC. Acne vulgaris. Nat Rev Dis Primers (2015, September 17). https://pubmed.ncbi.nlm.nih.gov/27189872/. Retrieved 14 Aug 2022.
3. Sing Heng AH, Chew FT. Systematic review of the epidemiology of Acne Vulgaris. Sci Rep. (2020, April 1). https://pubmed.ncbi.nlm.nih.gov/32238884/. Retrieved 14 Aug 2022.
4. Ebrahim AA, Mustafa AI, El-Abd AM. Serum interleukin-17 as a novel biomarker in patients with acne vulgaris. J Cosmet Dermatol. (2019, December 18). https://pubmed.ncbi.nlm.nih.gov/30964235/. Retrieved 09 Sep 2022.
5. Oge LK, Broussard A, Marshall MD. Acne vulgaris: diagnosis and treatment. Am Fam Phys. (2019, October 15). https://pubmed.ncbi.nlm.nih.gov/31613567/. Retrieved 15 Aug 2022.
6. Van Zuuren EJ, Arents BWM, Van Der Linden MMD, Vermeulen S, Fedorowicz Z, Tan J. Rosacea: new concepts in classification and treatment. Am J Clin Dermatol. (2021, July 22). https://pubmed.ncbi.nlm.nih.gov/33759078/. Retrieved 16 Aug 2022.
7. Buddenkotte J, Steinhoff M. Recent advances in understanding and managing rosacea. F1000Research. (2018, December 3). https://pubmed.ncbi.nlm.nih.gov/30631431/. Retrieved 16 Aug 2022.
8. Strimbu K, Tavel JA. What are biomarkers? Curr Opin HIV AIDS. (2010, November). https://www.ncbi.nlm.nih.gov/pmc/articles/PMC3078627/. Retrieved 15 Aug 2022.
9. Eliasse Y, Leveque E, Garidou L, Battut L, McKenzie B, Nocera T, Redoules D, Espinosa E. Il-17 + mast cell/T helper cell axis in the early stages of Acne. Front Immunol. (2021, September 28). https://pubmed.ncbi.nlm.nih.gov/34650562/. Retrieved 13 Sep 2022.
10. Abd-Elmaged WM, Nada EA, Hassan MH, Elsadek BEM, Abdelrahim EA, Ahmed NS, Toghan R, Ahmed HTI. Lesional and circulating levels of interleukin-17 and 25-hydroxycholecalciferol in active acne vulgaris: correlation to disease severity. J Cosmet Dermatol. (2019, April). https://pubmed.ncbi.nlm.nih.gov/30070012/. Retrieved 13 Sep 2022.
11. Assaf HA, Abdel-Maged WM, Elsadek BEM, Hassan MH, Adly MA, Ali SA. Survivin as a novel biomarker in the pathogenesis of acne vulgaris and its correlation to insulin-like growth factor-I. Dis Markers. (2016, October 10). https://pubmed.ncbi.nlm.nih.gov/27803511/. Retrieved 14 Sep 2022.
12. Rahaman SMA, De D, Handa S, Pal A, Sachdeva N, Ghosh T, Kamboj P. Association of insulin-like growth factor (IGF)-1 gene polymorphisms with plasma levels of IGF-1 and acne severity. J Am Acad Dermatol. (2016, October). https://pubmed.ncbi.nlm.nih.gov/27476104/. Retrieved 14 Sep 2022.

13. Kim H, Moon SY, Sohn MY, Lee WJ. Insulin-like growth factor-1 increases the expression of inflammatory biomarkers and sebum production in cultured sebocytes. Ann Dermatol. (2017, November 1). https://pubmed.ncbi.nlm.nih.gov/28223742/. Retrieved 14 Sep 2022.
14. Ghumra W, Lee N, Whitehouse H, Bhutani R, Lagos D, Layton AM. MicroRNAs as biomarkers of atrophic scarring in acne: a cross-sectional analysis of 41 patients. Clin Exp Dermatol. (2021, December). https://pubmed.ncbi.nlm.nih.gov/34101224/. Retrieved 14 Sep 2022.
15. Chen L, Wang C, Sun H, Wang J, Liang Y, Wang Y, Wong G. The bioinformatics toolbox for circrna discovery and analysis. Briefings Bioinf. (2021, March 22). https://pubmed.ncbi.nlm.nih.gov/32103237/. Retrieved 15 Sep 2022.
16. Liang J, Wu X, Sun S, Chen P, Liang X, Wang J, Ruan J, Zhang S, Zhang X. Circular RNA expression profile analysis of severe acne by RNA-Seq and Bioinformatics. J Eur Acad Dermatol Venereology JEADV. (2018, April 6). https://pubmed.ncbi.nlm.nih.gov/29573483/. Retrieved 14 Sep 2022.
17. Nakano T, Yoshino T, Fujimura T, Arai S, Mukuno A, Sato N, Katsuoka K. Reduced expression of dermcidin, a peptide active against propionibacterium acnes, in sweat of patients with acne vulgaris. Acta Dermato-Venereologica. (2015, September). https://pubmed.ncbi.nlm.nih.gov/25673161/. Retrieved 15 Sep 2022.
18. Alatas ET, Polat AK, Kalayci M, Dogan G, Belli AA. Plasma dermcidin levels in acne patients, and the effect of isotretinoin treatment on dermcidin levels. Dermatol Ther. (2019, September). https://pubmed.ncbi.nlm.nih.gov/31364786/. Retrieved 15 Sep 2022.
19. Mustafa AI, El-Shimi OS. Serum irisin: a prognostic marker for severe acne vulgaris. J Cosmet Dermatol. (2018, September 20). https://pubmed.ncbi.nlm.nih.gov/30238599/. Retrieved 20 Sep 2022.
20. Korta P, Pochec E, Mazur-Bialy A. Irisin as a multifunctional protein: implications for health and certain diseases. Medicina (Kaunas, Lithuania). (2019, August 15). https://pubmed.ncbi.nlm.nih.gov/31443222/. Retrieved 20 Sep 2022.
21. Hayran Y, Sen O, Oguz EF, Yucei C, Eren F, Cakmak SK, Yalcin B. Serum IL-17 levels in patients with rosacea. J Cosmet Dermatol. (2022, March). https://pubmed.ncbi.nlm.nih.gov/33877738/. Retrieved 20 Sep 2022.
22. Ali AA, Vender R, Vender R. The role of IL-17 in papulopustular rosacea and future directions. J Cutan Med Surg. (2019, November). https://pubmed.ncbi.nlm.nih.gov/31402691/. Retrieved 20 Sep 2022.
23. Jeon HW, Na EY, Yun SJ, Lee S-C, Lee J-B. Citron essential oils alleviate the mediators related to rosacea pathophysiology in epidermal keratinocytes. Ann Dermatol. (2018, December). https://pubmed.ncbi.nlm.nih.gov/33911504/. Retrieved 20 Sep 2022.
24. Suhng E, Kim BH, Choi YW, Choi HY, Cho H, Byun JY. Increased expression of IL-33 in rosacea skin and UVB-irradiated and LL-37-treated HaCaT cells. Exp Dermatol. (2018, September). https://pubmed.ncbi.nlm.nih.gov/29873850/. Retrieved 20 Sep 2022.
25. Wang L, Lu R, Wang Y, Wang X, Hao D, Wen X, Li Y, Zeng M, Jiang X. Identification of long noncoding RNA associated Cerna networks in rosacea. BioMed Res Int. (2020, February 24). https://pubmed.ncbi.nlm.nih.gov/32185228/. Retrieved 20 Sep 2022.
26. Seo SM, Hong JY, Lee HJ, Yang NG, Chung EH, Lee SY, Park YL, Lee SH, Lee SH, Lee DW, Shin MJ, Ryu S, Kim JE. Differential expression of micrornas in the skin tissue of patients with severe papulopustular rosacea. J Dermatol Sci. (2021, March). https://pubmed.ncbi.nlm.nih.gov/33386184/. Retrieved 20 Sep 2022.
27. Liu T, Li J, Deng Z, Chen M, Sha K, Xiao W, Xie H, Zhao Z. Increased serum levels of CCL3, CXCL8, CXCL9, and CXCL10 in rosacea patients and their correlation with disease severity. J Dermatol. (2022, May). https://pubmed.ncbi.nlm.nih.gov/35233832/. Retrieved 22 Sep 2022.
28. Gerber PA, Buhren BA, Steinhoff M, Homey B. Rosacea: the cytokine and chemokine network. J Invest Dermatol Symp Proc. (2011, December). https://pubmed.ncbi.nlm.nih.gov/22076326/. Retrieved 22 Sep 2022.
29. Gerber PA, et al. Rosacea: the cytokine and chemokine network. J Invest Dermatol Symp Proc 2011;15(1):40–7. https://doi.org/10.1038/jidsymp.2011.9.

30. Sener S, Akbas A, Kilinc F, Baran P, Erel O, Aktas A. Thiol/disulfide homeostasis as a marker of oxidative stress in rosacea: a controlled spectrophotometric study. Cutan Ocul Toxicol. (2019, March). https://pubmed.ncbi.nlm.nih.gov/30173569/. Retrieved 24 Sep 2022.
31. Pektas SD, Cinar N, Pektas G, Akbaba G, Kara A, Hancer HS, Duman DD, Neselioglu S, Erel O, Aksoy DY. Thiol/disulfide homeostasis and its relationship with insulin resistance in patients with rosacea. J Cosmet Dermatol. (2022, June). https://pubmed.ncbi.nlm.nih.gov/34564928/. Retrieved 24 Sep 2022.
32. Georgescu SR, Mitran CL, Mitran MI, Matei C, Popa GL, Erel O, Tampa M. Thiol-disulfide homeostasis in skin diseases. J Clin Med. (2022, March 9). https://pubmed.ncbi.nlm.nih.gov/35329832/. Retrieved 24 Sep 2022.
33. Leimkuhler M, et al. Systemic oxidative stress and antioxidant capacity in cancer patients. J Transl Sci. 2020;6(5). https://doi.org/10.15761/jts.1000372.

Chapter 14
Digital and Minimally Invasive Biomarkers in Dermatology

Jalal Ibrahim, Jesse Wesenberg, and Robert Norman

Abstract In the field of medicine, quality of patient care and preservation of patient health are paramount. As such, new technologies and techniques are constantly being developed and improved upon to better optimize patient responses to therapies and interventions. One of the major emergent domains of modern medical research deals with digital biomarkers and their application in clinical and nonclinical settings. From established techniques involving routine laboratory testing to the introduction of wearable smart devices and microtechnologies, digital biomarker collection and analysis aims to revolutionize medical practice and research studies. In the field of dermatology, such biomarkers may allow physicians and researchers to better manage acute and chronic inflammatory conditions, cut down time-to-recognition of cancers and other time-sensitive conditions, increase compliance to medication use, optimize research design, and improve overall patient health.

Keywords Digital biomarkers · Minimally invasive · Biosensors · Prescription digital therapeutics · Liquid biopsy · Proinflammatory · Cytokines · Chemokines · Genomic · Proteomic · Atopic dermatitis · Psoriasis · Melanoma · Acne vulgaris · Point-of-care testing · Microelectromechanical systems · Digital spatial profile · Smart watches

---

J. Ibrahim · J. Wesenberg
Lake Erie College of Osteopathic Medicine, Bradenton, FL, USA
e-mail: jibrahim80070@med.lecom.edu

J. Wesenberg
e-mail: jwesenberg28482@med.lecom.edu

R. Norman (Deceased) (✉)
Professor of Dermatology, Nova Southeastern University, Tampa, USA
e-mail: skindrrob@aol.com

R. Norman (ed.), *Biomarkers in Dermatology*,
https://doi.org/10.1007/978-3-031-66513-4_14

14.1 Introduction

Historically, the monitoring of patient welfare, progression of disease processes, and drug discovery and development have all depended on temporally limited assessments performed at select physical facilities [1]. Patients often relied on retroactive treatment of pathological processes only recognized after the appearance of substantial and specific symptoms. In many pathologies, as in the instance of several insidious forms of cancer, patient welfare has already been compromised by the time such symptoms have presented. Even more benign cases sometimes progress and cause more substantial and prolonged harm to the patient before being recognized in the clinical setting. Regarding drug testing and development, data from human test subjects has also only been collected during set times at clinical settings. This potentially puts patients at risk for adverse effects occurring in the interim and drastically limits data collection.

Over the past several decades, these drawbacks have led to research into various biomarkers as a means to provide more continuous patient data both for drug development and for patient welfare [1]. Biomarkers are simply defined as "A defined characteristic that is measured as an indicator of normal biological processes, pathological processes or responses to an exposure or intervention [2]." These special biomarkers give more opportunities for both physicians and patients themselves to monitor and assess both active and prospective conditions that may afflict them. Such biomarkers can be used as diagnostic tools and to determine the severity of ailments within the human body, permitting dramatically quicker medical responses and interventions. Essentially, with the use of novel technologies, biomarkers can be measured digitally to assess disease presence and progression continuously and objectively. Definitions of the various biomarkers will be discussed in the next section.

14.2 Digital Biomarkers

14.2.1 Definitions

As a complex, rapidly-emerging medical field, the Food and Drug Administration (FDA) has put in a great deal of effort into formulating and consolidating common definitions to be used in the "Biomarkers, EndpointS, and other Tools," or BEST, resource [3]. Under this system of classification, there are six different subtypes to biomarkers according to their application process: diagnostic, monitoring, pharmacodynamic/response, predictive, prognostic, and safety biomarkers. It is integral to remember that these subtypes have varying degrees of overlap depending on the specific biomarker in question. Utilized together, these different subtypes of biomarkers can paint a comprehensive picture of the patient's current health status, risk of disease development, remission, or progression, and response to various treatments.

14.2.1.1 Diagnostic Biomarkers

Diagnostic biomarkers are those which can be measured in order to determine the presence or absence of a pathological process or to diagnostically differentiate between different subtypes of a particular ailment [3]. For instance, elevated levels of the S100 family of proteins are 90% sensitive for melanoma, a well-known aggressive and highly malignant form of skin cancer [4]. As such, IHC staining for S100 proteins can be an invaluable diagnostic tool for melanoma even before clinical signs and symptoms develop. Diagnostic biomarkers have also proved useful in redefining diagnostic criteria and classification of diseases [3].

As a relatively new area of diagnostic medicine, these biomarkers have continuously evolving interpretation criteria as we discover more about them. For instance, troponin I and troponin H have both been incorporated into modern medicine as diagnostic biomarkers for acute myocardial infarction. Though they have revolutionized our treatment methodology and diagnostic capabilities for MI, patient-to-patient variations and other confounding variables can eclipse the lower limits of diagnostic criteria, resulting in misclassification and misdiagnosis. As such, physicians must be aware of this potential drawback and use a combination of both diagnostic biomarker detection and traditional methods of detection (e.g., CK-MB, associated symptoms, etc., for diagnosing MI) in order to make a definitive diagnosis.

14.2.1.2 Monitoring Biomarkers

Monitoring biomarkers are quite special as they can be used serially to monitor the status of a disease or medical condition for evidence of patient exposure to a specific medicinal or environmental product or to measure the degree of patient response to medical intervention [3]. These biomarkers are helpful to establish the relationships between environmental exposure and disease development, disease progression and severity, and response to pharmacologic, surgical, or non-medicinal intervention. Given it is a broad topic, there is a great degree of overlap between monitoring biomarkers and other subtypes of biomarkers.

An example of one such monitoring biomarker exists in patients being treated with a statin (e.g., atorvostatin), an HMG-CoA reductase inhibitor which is used primarily to combat elevated levels of low-density lipoprotein (LDL). Following treatment, we can continuously measure the patient's LDL cholesterol levels to determine the efficacy of the pharmacologic intervention [3]. The information provided through such continuous biomarker monitoring provides us with a large volume of data that may be used to assess the treatment efficacy in real time and make adjustments to the intervention plan as necessary.

Although monitoring biomarkers are very broad and emergent topic, they also give physicians better opportunities to more easily determine any safety thresholds for any medications a patient can withstand, also known as a therapeutic index [3]. By analyzing such biomarkers, we can easily adapt dosages, frequency of administration, or even the specific drug being utilized in order to minimize the potential risk of any developing any negative outcomes during pharmacologic treatment. There are many more examples of monitoring biomarkers, ranging from assessing HbA1C levels for diabetic patients or INR levels for patients taking warfarin [3]. As you move forward and read about the other types of biomarkers, you will notice that they all overlap in some way, but each have very different indicators as to how well a patient's health can be accessed via digital biomarkers.

14.2.1.3 Pharmacodynamic/Response Biomarkers

With regard to monitoring biomarkers, pharmacodynamic/response biomarkers are quite similar in terms of how they are applied. Pharmacodynamic/response biomarkers assess the actual quantifiable changes induced within the patient in response to a medical product or environmental agent [3]. This is an extremely useful tool for clinical practice and therapeutic development and improvement as it gives physicians early indications as to how quickly or drastically a patient is affected by pharmacologic therapy. An example of this type of biomarker may be observable in a patient taking medication for diabetes, such as metformin. If measurements were taken for the biomarkers associated with diabetes, including serum insulin and glucose levels, HbA1c, glycation end products, etc., both before and after treatment with metformin, a physician could ascertain the efficacy of the current dosing regimen. If desirable change is achieved, the dosage could be maintained. If the patient was either overmedicated or undermedicated, adjustments could be made to dosages in real time rather than relying on data collected during sporadic follow-up visits.

Prescription digital therapeutics are an application of pharmacodynamic/response biomarkers that give patients and physician more power over their health needs. "Digital therapeutics (DTx) is one such category of digital health solutions that provides evidence-based software-driven therapeutic interventions for the prevention and management of a medical disorder or disease." [5] Dtx utilize pharmacodynamic/response biomarker analysis in real time to give feedback on the patient's response to a specific medical intervention and compare this data to a global dataset comprised of many other patients. This gives physicians the ability to apply evidence-based software-driven therapeutic interventions and adapt the patient's therapy to optimize their therapeutic response. Between pharmacodynamic biomarkers and digital therapeutics, physicians are able to expand their dataset regarding a patient's health and better optimize therapeutic interventions. In a dermatologic viewpoint, PDTx can help close gaps between any shortages dermatologist may have and the ever-rising skin disease burdens [6]. They can be used in many dermatologic cases that include skin cancer and inflammatory disease management, and they can be coupled with other devices such as microelectricalmechanical systems (MEMS) to produce the best possible treatment and outcome for patients.

14.2.1.4 Predictive Biomarkers

Predictive/risk biomarkers are those which, when measured, may indicate the likelihood of experiencing a favorable outcome versus an unfavorable outcome after exposure to a medication or to an environmental effect [3]. The primary difference identifying such a cause-effect relationship requires rigorous studies with a high degree of scrutiny for potential bias. As such, appropriately randomized studies with control groups, treatment groups, and alternative treatment groups must be compared to truly grasp the degree of correlation between exposure and outcome. Needless to say, such studies prove both difficult to design and financially demanding.

Once identified, however, such predictive/risk biomarkers are highly useful both for designing more focused studies and for active clinical practices. In studies, predictive/risk biomarker levels can be used to narrow down the patient pool to only those who are predisposed to respond to the treatment in question. Thus, the data yielded from such studies may establish a much more clear relationship between treatment and prognosis. In clinical practice, many predictive/risk biomarkers are already commonplace especially in the emergency department setting. Blood pressure levels denote which antihypertensive regimens may be effective, hemoglobin levels can indicate a need for a blood transfusion, and STEMI presentation can indicate a need for acute reperfusion. Using such predictive/risk biomarkers allows a more tailored treatment approach to each individual patient presentation especially when many predictive/risk biomarkers are measured and collectively treated as a whole (e.g., combining LDL/HDL/TAG levels with Troponin I/T for use in identifying atherosclerotic myocardial infarction).

14.2.1.5 Prognostic Biomarkers

Prognostic biomarkers are exclusively used to assess the chances of a specific clinical event occurring or the risk of disease recurrence and/or disease progression in patients with an underlying disease or condition [3]. While similar to predictive/risk biomarkers, prognostic biomarkers are more useful for assessing the evolution of a pathologic process over time rather than the risk for disease development or likelihood of successful treatment.

This subtype of digital biomarker is essential when it comes to identifying high-risk patients for both statistical analysis and for targeted medical intervention. Researchers may use prognostic biomarkers to formulate inclusion and exclusion criteria for a given clinical trial, allowing a more narrowed focus on high-risk individuals. This increases the rates of events recorded during the trial, eliminating the lower-yield subjects from the study from the very start. Additionally, practicing physicians can utilize these biomarkers to devise a picture of a patient's condition in a diseased state.

Potential risks and adverse outcomes can be identified early on, allowing physicians to make proactive decisions regarding the different avenues of treatment that may be taken. This can be very important in hospital settings to determine the optimal length of admission and appropriate time for patient discharge, and it can also help identify patients that may benefit from costly, intense evaluation and those who are less likely to respond.

14.2.1.6 Safety Biomarkers

Safety biomarkers are measured before, during, and after an exposure to a medication or a medical intervention in order to ensure the safety of the patient [3]. This is useful for determining any adverse events during or after a medical procedure or after beginning a new medication or a different dosage of a previous medication. Some examples of this would be to monitor the levels via biomarkers for the liver, kidney, or heart via a liver function test, urinalysis, metabolic panel, ECG, and/or specific enzyme monitoring to ensure that organ function is preserved during and after treatment. This use of safety biomarkers gives physicians a good understanding of systemic and organ-specific responses to therapy, allowing them to identify toxicities or other complications in a timely manner to ensure the safety of the patient.

A great example of an appropriate use of safety biomarkers is after giving a patient an antiarrhythmic drug for heart issues; a physician would request electrocardiogram (ECG) monitoring, analyzing for the presence of QT interval prolongation [3]. Early detection of such a change in heart conduction could allow the physician to intervene quickly to minimize the patient's risk of developing a lethal arrhythmia such as torsades de pointes. All of the other subtypes of digital biomarkers utilize different approaches to ensure patient safety, and thus they may all also fit under the category of safety biomarkers.

Digital therapeutics also play a role in safety biomarkers. By giving real-time feedback on ongoing medical interventions, DTx help assess the therapeutic benefit and risk of medications through both pharmacodynamic/response biomarkers and safety biomarkers [5].

14.2.1.7 Susceptibility/Risk Biomarkers

Susceptibility/risk biomarkers assess an apparently healthy patient's potential for developing a specific medical condition [3]. The primary difference between this classification of biomarkers and prognostic biomarkers is that susceptibility/risk biomarkers deal with the onset of a disease or disorder while prognostic biomarkers assess prognosis once a patient is diagnosed.

14.2.2 Applications of Digital Biomarkers

As discussed previously, traditional methods of patient evaluation rely on scheduled office, hospital, or clinic visits [1]. The most direct and obvious drawbacks to such a practice arise from the fact that the patient must first recognize their symptoms, then they must schedule an appointment, and, finally, they must wait until the appointment to finally be seen by an examiner.

To begin with, this places great reliance on the patient's ability to recognize their own symptoms and decide to be seen despite the fact that the average patient has very limited medical education. Not only does a varying degree of time pass between onset of illness and recognition of symptoms, but there is also a substantial lag between recognition of symptoms and eventual examination under this system. In addition, there is a substantial lack in the total quantity of data that could be collected, having been almost entirely restricted to these evaluations. While other forms of data collection, including questionnaire-based self-reports, are sometimes used, they vary drastically in their reliability [7].

The use of biomarkers, particularly those that can be measured reliably in the home setting, can provide a complementary form of data collection when used in conjunction with traditional data sources, and they can also enhance the specificity of the data obtained from traditional data sources [1, 8]. Biomarkers collected via minimally or noninvasive methods, including sweat, tears, urine, breath, and the skin surface itself, can provide abundant, continuous forms of data collection with very minimal impact on the patient's routine [7]. While such novel technologies are still very much under development, they are still able to provide exponentially increased quantities of patient data over a much broader spectrum of time.

Additional biomarkers collected in the setting of office, hospital, or clinic visits can also enhance data collection performed in such settings. Current research tying specific biomarker levels with specific pathologies allows for increased diagnostic accuracy in the clinical setting. Thus, the direct effects of emerging biomarker are twofold, both increasing the total quantity of patient data recorded and increasing the reliability of the data collected.

So, what are the tangible benefits to utilizing digital biomarker measurements? As alluded to previously, one of the primary advantages for biomarkers use is a drastic reduction in time-to-recognition of pathological processes. Physicians would be granted substantially higher volume and breadth of data over a longer spectrum of time, including the times between clinical evaluations. Combined with traditional methods of evaluation, data from biomarker analysis could reduce lag time between contraction of an ailment and treatment and allow real-time analysis of both positive and adverse effects of therapies [8]. Quicker diagnosis and quicker treatment both grant the patient increased longevity and improved health [9]. For example, studies have shown that as little as a 6 month delay in recognition of rheumatoid arthritis can result in substantial variations in patient outcomes decades down the road [10]. Additionally, such biomarkers help to establish inclusion and exclusion criteria for research in order to narrow down the focus of research and more accurately determine the efficacy of various treatments and interventions. Finally, analysis of biomarkers can help reduce medical costs in the long run by allowing specific therapies to be targeted to those patients who would benefit the most from them [3].

14.2.3 Potential Benefits and Risks of Digital Biomarkers

Digital biomarkers are a rising tool granting both physicians and patients the ability to assess patient health status and complications regarding medical interventions or disease development and progression [10]. Modern technology has made measuring levels of glucose, cytokines, or other markers much easier, to the point that a patient can measure their own levels outside of the clinical setting. Of course, this is a relatively new innovation in medicine that can pair well with the traditional methods involved in medical testing and data collection. However, we must keep in mind that such digital biomarkers have inherent risks to consider as well as their benefits.

As stated before, digital biomarkers are new and upcoming, so a lot of research is being done to compare the benefits to the risks. There are a great many benefits to utilizing digital biomarkers for patient health assessment. The first and most important benefit to digital biomarkers is that patients can use a variety of portable and/or wearable devices, ranging from watches to phones to skin-patch monitors that allow them to measure their biomarker levels from the comfort of their home [9]. Even sweat, saliva, and tears can be collected and processed to measure their relevant biomarker data. This saves time for both patients and physicians when it comes to determining the health status of a patient or whether there are any complications with a particular treatment regimen that a patient is receiving. For instance, diabetic patients are easily able to monitor their glucose levels at home to both assess the minute-to-minute variations in their levels as well as to assess the efficacy of their insulin regimens and adjust accordingly.

Another advantage of utilizing digital biomarkers over traditional methods of data collection is that biomarkers are objective measurements that cannot be skewed by observer bias [10]. This ensures more accurate data collection in situations where bias can introduce complications. Most importantly, a combination of traditional medicine and digital biomarkers can give the physician a more complete picture on the patient's health status, which, as a result, gives them more knowledge on how to proceed. They can help identify candidates for medical and/or surgical intervention who are more likely to respond well to treatment, serve as diagnostic tools for even the rarest pathological processes, and ensure continuous monitoring of a patient's health status.

Now that we have reviewed some of the benefits of utilizing digital biomarkers, let us discuss the risks. Since the utilization of digital biomarkers are new and unfamiliar to most people, this will cause some potential risks, some that may be known now and some that may only be discovered in the future through research. The risks associated with biomarkers are mostly associated with how little is known about them. We do not know how accurate these biomarkers are nor whether or not they are reliable to determine the exact health status of the patient, and they present complicated issues regarding assuring patient privacy and cybersecurity [9]. These are all questions that need to be answered to ensure that no harm befalls patients who are treated on the basis of biomarker analysis.

14.3 Methods of Biomarker Collection

Given the foundation of these diverse groups of digital biomarkers, it is important to address their methods of collection. As technology advances, physicians discover more avenues by which they can measure biomarkers digitally via various different biosensors [11]. Such biosensors can fit into any number of different classifications based on their respective methods of measurement. These categories include those that utilize bioreceptors, others that use transducers, optical and mechanical biosensors, and miniaturized biosensors based on point-of-care testing, or POCT. Some of these biosensors have even been implemented in portable and wearable devices capable of monitoring key biomarker levels in real time. It is likely that these different classifications will grow in number as research and development produces novel technologies capable of measuring biomarkers.

Utilizing these emerging biosensor technologies, physicians have opened the door to a great number of potential methods to collect patient data via digital biomarkers [12]. Liquid biopsies, including blood and urine samples, cerebrospinal fluid (CSF) samples, and even extracellular fluid collected from paracentesis and similar procedures, have long been in use in the medical field [13]. Through decades of research and refinement, the biomarker analysis of such samples has expanded to encompass such a broad spectrum of diagnostic, monitoring, and prognostic criteria that they have become the defacto laboratory tests for the majority of medical evaluations. In the modern day, there are numerous other minimally invasive samples that can be collected both within and outside of traditional clinically settings for similar biomarker analysis [12]. These include sweat, hair, saliva, tears, and even the patient's breath! Various other biosensors, including electrocardiography, electroencephalography, electromyography, and microelectricalmechanical systems (MEMS), measure electrical fields and electric potentials in order to assess the underlying tissues. In the context of dermatology, such technologies will help limit time-to-recognition of disease processes, augment our ability to monitor dermatologic conditions in afflicted patients, and evaluate the efficacy of various medical, surgical, and lifestyle interventions.

14.3.1 Liquid Biopsy

The gold standard of methods of digital biomarker collection is liquid biopsy. Liquid biopsy is a very important biomarker used today to monitor and/or diagnose a variety of different ailments and illnesses from anemia to meningitis and even cancer. The most common liquid biopsy used is blood, but other fluids such as urine, ascites fluid, or CSF can all be valid components to measure levels within a patient [13].

From a dermatologic stance, numerous diagnostic and monitoring biomarkers can be yielded from blood serum samples. Individuals with psoriasis tend to experience Th17-dominated chronic immune responses, resulting in increased presence of proinflammatory cytokines interleukin-17 (IL-17), IL-22, and IL-23 alongside elevated thymus activation-regulated chemokine (TARC) and other proinflammatory chemokines [14]. Genomic biomarkers that can be prognostic indicators of psoriasis include HLA-C*06:02, LCE3D, IL-23R, IL-23A, NFKBIL1, and proteomic biomarkers, such as IL-17A, IgG aHDL, and GlycA, can also be useful in this regard [15]. Regarding atopic dermatitis (AD), there is quite a significant overlap in biomarkers with psoriasis. While Th2 immune responses are most commonly associated with AD, it has been demonstrated that Th22, Th17, and Th1 responses all also play roles in AD pathogenesis [16]. The clinical severity of AD correlates strongly with serum levels of TARC, S-100 proteins, CCL22, IgE, Eosinophil count, IL-22, IL-4, IL-5, IL-13, and more [16, 17]. With respect to acne vulgaris, serum soluble intercellular adhesion molecule-1 (sICAM-1) levels can indicate both presence and severity of the disease in patients with active outbreaks [18].

In relation to cancer patients, liquid biopsy analysis gives physicians a deeper look at how a patient is truly doing via quantitative measurements obtained from the blood. By analyzing such data, a physician is able to determine whether or not the patient has had any sort of malignant growth [13]. This technique is minimally invasive and gives quite accurate measurements on the biomarkers associated with the cancer cells, and it can give a glimpse into the spread of the cancer before the patient develops additional symptoms. These biomarkers give physicians a clearer image of the progression of the patient's cancer, showing if it has metastasized or not. This is extremely applicable in the setting of dermatology as melanoma is an insidious skin cancer that, without knowing specific measurements beforehand, can lead to severely poor prognosis.

By analyzing liquid biopsy samples for circulating tumor DNA (ctDNA), circulating tumor cells (CTCs), and circulating extracellular nucleic acids (cell-free DNA), a dermatologist may be able to identify melanoma before it can metastasize and cause serious damage [13]. Additional biomarkers for melanoma detection, diagnosis, and progression include the melanocytic markers Melan-A, MART-1, HMB-45, and S-100 protein, as well as the proliferative markers Ki-67 and phosphohistone H3 (PHH3) [4, 19].

Another liquid biopsy technique that is actively utilized is urine. Urine as a source for biomarker analysis is much broader than the blood biopsy for cancer markers, but it still gives physicians an idea if somehow has any diseases or infections [20]. Levels of epithelial cells, kidney-derived cells, white blood cells (WBCs), red blood cells (RBC), urothelial cells, genetic material (in the form of cell-free DNA or cfDNA), proteins, peptides, and inorganic compounds can be taken from sampled urine to help diagnose diseases and provide prognostic data on the disease [21].

cfDNA, released by healthy or diseased cells throughout the body into systemic circulation, is filtered through the kidneys and excreted into the urine [21]. cfDNA is excreted in particularly high amounts in the presence of diseased states because in such states, DNA digestion via phagocytes is incomplete. Thus, urine biopsies may be performed to assess and detect a plethora of diseases, from systemic immune diseases to various cancers, as long as appropriate genomic biomarkers are known

[20, 21]. As with the blood, the genomic biomarkers associated with diseases such as psoriasis and atopic dermatitis can also be pulled from the urine [15, 17, 21].

Presence of elevation of RBCs, WBCs, proteins, glucose, ketones, and nitrites can also be indicative of pathological conditions [21]. Urine is an excellent test for such biomarkers since it is easily accessible, noninvasive, and can be used to diagnose or monitor a wide range of physiological diseases [20]. Changes in urine protein or elevations in urine RBCs can indicate dysfunction of the urinary tract cells [20, 21]. The process to determine the levels of the protein in urine is with liquid chromatography coupled with mass spectrometry. Urine glucose could be indicative of diabetes mellitus, and ketonuria can be indicative of diabetic ketoacidosis or other causes of elevated ketogenesis in the body [21]. Elevated nitrites in the urine is one of the primary diagnostic criteria for urinary tract infection (UTI).

14.3.2 Biological/Chemical Sensing

There are several other sources of reliable biomarker data aside from traditional liquid biopsies. Such sources can vary from breath, hair, saliva, tears, and sweat, all of which pose noninvasive or minimally invasive methods of collection. These forms of biological and chemical sensing experience some overlap with liquid biopsy for biomarker collection, and in some instances, certain biomarkers that cannot be obtained via serum or urine samples can be obtained through one of the aforementioned avenues.

First up, we will explore biomarkers that can be taken from the breath. While some illnesses can produce actual smells in the patient's breath (e.g., sweet smelling breath in ketosis), there are actual devices that, when expired into, can quantitatively measure certain biomarkers found within the breath. Breath samples give physicians the opportunity to discover any volatile biomarkers that could indicate either infectious or non-infectious diseases, such as malaria, lung disease, or tuberculosis [22]. They can determine this by using the breath sample from a patient, reproducing the sample, and utilizing gas chromatography-mass spectrometry (GC–MS) to determine the chemical makeup of the breath. This method has been demonstrated to be quite successful in determining if children from the ages 4–15 have malaria or not, and it has the potential to be much more encompassing [22]. Another method of breath biomarker collection studied by Nowak, et al. involves the use of secondary electrospray ionization high-resolution mass spectrometry (SESI-HRMS) [23]. They determined that SESI-HRMS analysis could prove useful in screening for obstructive sleep apnea (OSA). These methods are also undergoing further research and analysis to expand its success with other diseases that can relate to breath biomarkers. This is quite applicable to the geriatric population, as OSA is extremely prevalent among older patients. Breath biomarkers may prove exceedingly useful as it is very simple and it does not require much experience or cooperation on the patient's front.

The next method of collection comes from hair samples of patients. This source of biomarkers is still in the process of becoming common practice, but for now most of the research has been conducted on pediatric populations. Such hair biomarkers can give physicians a clear measurement of environmental exposures, whether it be from secondhand smoke or chronic stress via cortisol concentrations [24]. Thus, hair sampling can be used to gauge the degree of external toxin exposure and for measuring specific levels of cortisol in patients suspected of (or at risk for developing) Addison disease or Cushing disease. Additionally, the quantity and protein composition of hair can give insight into the patient's nutrition status, including diagnosis of kwashiorkor malnutrition. Since protein malnutrition affects all tissues of the body including the integument, this could be applicable in the field of dermatology. Collecting hair as an indicator of someone's health is gaining popularity in the medical field, so it is important to develop methods to gear hair sampling to encompass the entire population and not just children.

Physicians and other health providers have also used saliva as another way of measuring the health status in patients. Collecting saliva is a much less invasive alternative to blood serum to measure certain biomarkers such as stress and inflammation, such as assessing the levels of cortisol and proinflammatory cytokines [24]. Additionally, much of the same diagnostic data that can be obtained via blood samples can also be obtained from saliva. As such, the same genomic and proteomic biomarkers associated with psoriasis, AD, acne vulgaris, and melanoma can also be collected from saliva samples.

Interestingly, while diagnosis of acne rosacea still very much depends on a full medical history and physical examination, a study conducted by Fernández et al. revealed a potential diagnostic biomarker for its diagnosis [25]. Their studies showed that analysis of gingival crevicular fluid for extracellular metalloproteinase-9 (MMP-9) levels demonstrated a sensitivity of 72.22% and specificity of 81.58% for the diagnosis of rosacea.

Tears are another emerging diagnostic tool in health care. Though an unusual method of diagnosis, recent technologic advancements have enabled biomarker detection from tear samples. Tears come from the lacrimal sac, which is adjacent to the lacrimal film [26]. As an important glandular excretion, tear analysis has been attracting a lot of attention from a vast spectrum of physicians as a potential biomarker for assessing ocular and systemic diseases. The methods of collection with tears utilize the high-performance liquid chromatography-mass spectrometry (LC–MS) [26]. This LC–MS gives effective ways to measure tear proteomics which can help physicians understand the status of a patient's health, in relation to their eyes or other systemic issues. There is still more research to be done with the use of tears as a biomarker, but tear collection proves to have potential in diagnostic medicine.

Last but definitely not least is the use of sweat as a useful biomarker in health care, specifically dermatology. Sweat has been used as biomarkers since long before the term "biomarker" was coined. While the main function of sweat is to help maintain temperature homeostasis, it can also be collected and analyzed to provide detailed information about a person's metabolic state, skin protein composition, and information about skin cells including keratinocytes and melanocytes [27]. As alluded to before, kwashiorkor malnutrition could result in skin barrier disruption due to deficiency of integral skin proteins. In the clinical setting, diaphoresis, or excessive sweat production, is a common symptom of pyretic illness, MI, endocrine disorders such as hyperthyroidism, diabetes, and more. Sweat has also been used to indicate certain fatal conditions such as cystic fibrosis or to assess levels of lipids, protein, and electrolytes, all of which are components of sweat. Additionally, transepidermal water loss (TEWL), measured empirically by placing an enclosed chamber probe into the skin, is a novel method of diagnosing and assessing the severity of AD [28]. It is not uncommon to see TEWL equivalent to 2 or 3 magnitudes higher than normal in patients with AD, and it is this TEWL that accounts for skin dryness in AD patients.

While sweat has the potential to be another useful and noninvasive form of biomarker collection, there has historically been a lack of proper laboratory infrastructure that has prevented proper clinical implementation [27]. However, with the development of smartphone-based biosensors, physicians can obtain a patient-driven sweat analysis both inside and outside the clinical setting. Not only could this provide an alternative to standard blood sampling in patients with poor peripheral vascularity or in patients with poor cooperation, but it could also enable more continuous monitoring of specific biomarkers in the home setting. One such device, a sweat sensor developed by Goa Lab, is shown below (Fig. 14.1) [29]. A wearable "smart wristband" that employs flexible nanorobots capable of both stimulating sweat production and analyzing small samples for biomarkers, this technology has the benefit of being about to track a person's metabolic state, stress levels, and potential other health conditions and transmit the data wirelessly to a physician with very little impact on the patient.

14.3.3 Electrocardiography (ECG)

The electrocardiogram, or ECG, has proved invaluable in cardiovascular diagnosis and monitoring over the past century since it saw its first implementation. Myocardial depolarization and repolarization produce electric fields that can be measured via externally attached electrodes in order to assess cardiac function [30]. As such, the ECG effectively qualifies and quantifies cardiac electrical biomarkers in order to be used as a diagnostic and assessment tool. While its primary use involves cardiac disease and injury, some aspects of ECG monitoring can be applied to evaluate the status and progression systemic diseases including rheumatic fever and scleroderma.

In the hospital and emergency setting, ECGs are commonly used to assess cardiac rate, rhythm, and wave form in an effort to understand the patient's cardiovascular status [30]. In addition to evaluation for heart disease and heart stress, cardiac pulse rate can be measured to help determine the effects of anxiety, cardiovascular stimulation or depression, acute infection, or other systemic pathologies.

Heart rhythm can be analyzed to determine the presence or absence of critical cardiac tachyarrhythmias and bradyarrhythmias, including escape rhythms, atrial fibrillation, ventricular tachycardia, and more. Such arrhythmias can be either primary, standalone conditions or may be secondary to other significant conditions such as myocardial infarction, congestive heart failure, and even psoriasis vulgaris, which carries an increased risk of developing atrial fibrillation [31]. Recently, smart

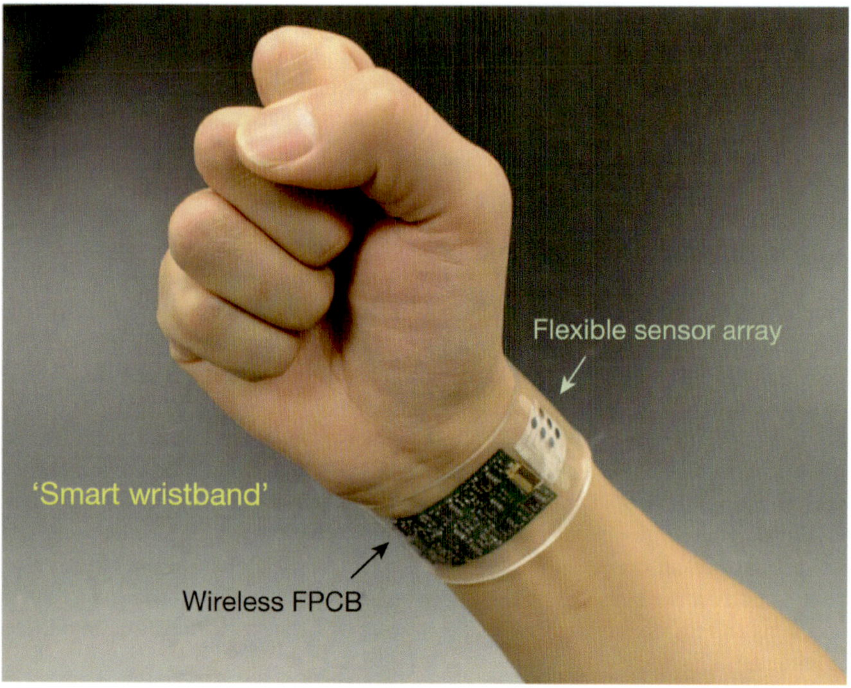

Fig. 14.1 Flexible "Smart Wristband" fixed with flexible nanorobots and circuit board. *FPCB* flexible printed circuit board. Photo by Wei Gao—UC Berkley

watches with ECG monitoring technology have been made available to the public (Fig. 14.2) [8]. Though their accuracy and reliability are questionable, studies have shown that they are fairly sensitive in detecting atrial fibrillation, the most common arrhythmia. As the technology advances and improves, such smart watches may be instrumental in self-monitoring of patients with various cardiovascular conditions.

Wave form can help determine presence of underlying heart disease and injury including ventricular hypertrophy, pericarditis, myocardial infarction, cardiac arrest, and others [30]. Additionally, wave forms, such as the T wave morphological changes seen in hyperkalemia or as an adverse reaction to antiarrhythmics such as digoxin, can be key indicators of electrolyte abnormalities or adverse pharmaceutical reactions.

Overall, the ECG provides valuable diagnostic, monitoring, safety, and prognostic biomarker data both about the cardiovascular system and various other bodily systems to help ensure proper patient care and health management.

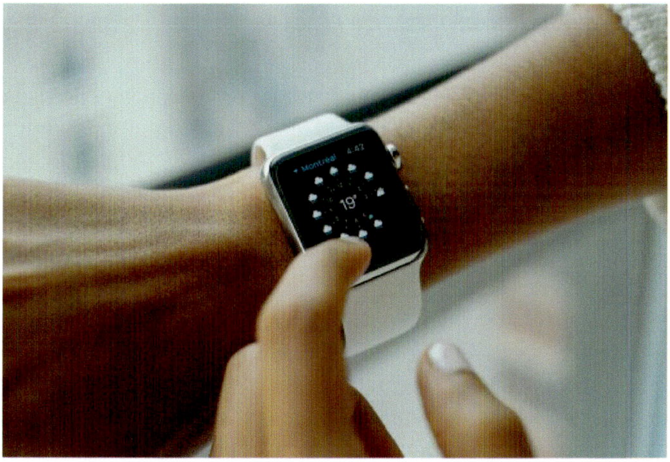

Fig. 14.2 Smart watches such as this one have been integrated with ECG technology capable of sensing and alerting the user when they experience certain arrhythmias

14.3.4 Electromyography (EMG)

Electromyography, or EMG, is a valuable tool that utilizes electrodes to measure neuromuscular activity to assess the health of muscles throughout the body and diagnose muscular disorders [32]. This process generally involves a three-step process: measuring baseline activity at rest, individual motor unit electric potential analysis with slight muscle contraction, and interference pattern analysis. Traditional methods of EMG analysis involve the insertion of needle electrodes that can measure both spontaneous myocyte action potentials and those induced by movement of the electrodes themselves. This data is used to determine the type, severity, and chronicity of any potential underlying muscle disease. The amplitude, frequency, and wave form seen in an EMG can all give insight into the characteristics of potential neurological or neuromuscular impairment.

While utilizing needle electrode EMG measurements can be extremely useful in isolating specific nerves and muscles, sometimes it is of use to take non-specific global measurements of neuromuscular activity [32]. One method of global EMG measurement can be conducted via the skin in a process called surface EMG. As such, surface EMG is much less invasive and capable of long-term measurements that prove useful in assessing conduction velocity and neuromuscular junction fatigue.

14.3.5 Electroencephalography (EEG)

Electroencephalography (EEG) is a diagnostic and prognostic tool used to recognize and evaluate neurological conditions related to vascular compromise, trauma, infectious processes, metabolic abnormalities, and delirium [33]. While EEG remains the gold standard for monitoring critical brain injuries and abnormalities, its application in the hospital setting depends on access and training, both of which are quite financially taxing. Additionally, EEG use is very limited in the emergency setting, where the time it takes to order an EEG, transport the patient, conduct the EEG, and wait for its interpretation could delay intervention and compromise patient health.

As stated previously, EEG is useful in monitoring and diagnosing a variety of neurological deficits or injuries. One of the primary indications of EEG is to evaluate a patient for nonconvulsive status epilepticus (NCSE) [33]. Due to the need to detect NCSE early to properly treat patients and prevent them from developing seizures, researchers have developed new reduced montage rapid response EEG (RRLM-EEG) technologies. In practice, RRLM-EEG used to augment bedside examination resulted in dramatically increased sensitivity (from 77.8% to 100%) and specificity (63.9% to 89%) [33]. The same technology can be applied to emergency neurological conditions including strokes. Though computed tomography (CT) scans still remain the primary diagnostic tools for strokes, RRLM-EEG can be utilized to assessment of post-stroke seizures. In addition, a recent study conducted by Wilkinson, et al. utilized EEG as a method for prehospital stroke diagnosis [34]. They found that analyzing the EEG for the delta/alpha ratio (DAR), the (delta + theta)/(alpha + beta) ratio (DBATR), and the pairwise-derived brain symmetry index (pdBSI) were all effective in both predicting the likelihood of stroke occurrence and the severity of the ischemic stroke once it occurred.

Dementia is another crucial neurological condition with a prognosis that heavily depends on early diagnosis and intervention [35]. When a disease or condition results in cognitive impairment, as occurs during dementia, diagnosis depends on a combination of medical history, physical examination, laboratory studies, and, of course, neuroimaging. EEG can help physicians recognize and differentiate between Alzheimer's disease and vascular dementia, and it does so at a lower cost to the hospital than other neuroimaging techniques. When rapid recognition and therapy are paramount in preserving patient health and preventing functional and mental impairment down the road, such EEG studies, especially with the introduction of RRLM-EEG, play a pivotal role in combating neurological disorders [33, 35].

14.3.6 Microelectromechanical Systems (MEMS)

Advancements in electronics miniaturization have led to the development of microelectromechanical systems (MEMS) capable of analyzing electric potential and electrical and magnetic fields [36]. Of note, these technologies are referred to as Microsystems Technology in Europe and Micro Machines in Japan. Not only do these devices allow for easy incorporation of state-of-the-art digital technologies in portable and wearable devices, they also have applications in drug synthesis and delivery, microsurgery, genomic sequencing and alteration, and more. While most MEMS are transducers, they can be manufactured to specialize in measurement of pressure, distance, temperature, humidity, sound, and just about any other measurement you could think of.

Just as the possible specializations of various MEMS are expansive, the applications of such technologies are equally vast [36]. Miniaturized biosensors allow for direct extraction of biomarkers from desired sources, including measurements taken directly from living cells! Thus, they have advantages over traditional macroscopic sensing in disease diagnosis in that they can save time, reduce costs, and reduce contamination resulting in higher sensitivity and specificity during testing. In other words, they are capable of sampling the same inflammatory cytokines and chemokines, proteins, and genomic markers associated with psoriasis, AD, and melanoma that can be taken from blood samples. Additionally, skin microsensors can be designed to measuring electrical field disturbances within the stratum corneum that have been shown to correlate with AD [28].

14.3.7 Portable and Wearable Devices

One of the more interesting applications of MEMS is use in portable and wearable devices. These devices are able to measure levels of certain markers for patients outside a clinic with minimal impact on the patient. This gives the patient more flexibility in their schedule, and it give physicians and researchers a continuous stream of patient health data. These devices give real-time physiological measurements of the patient's status via their sweat, tears, or glucose levels, essentially looking at the levels of the hormones or metabolites [37]. All the patient has to do is to wear a flexible, comfortable and noninvasive device which will be able to measure the specific biomarker the physician would like to see.

Certain wearable devices can be attached directly onto the patient's skin and can monitor levels of heart rate, vitals, or glucose [38]. An example would be the Dexcom device that is used to measure glucose in diabetic patients. This device has changed the lifestyle of such individual, allowing them to alter their insulin dosing in response to spikes and troughs in blood sugar. Such wearable devices can also be coupled with smartphone applications, allowing patients and physicians alike to view biomarker data collected over time. Still other devices, such as the smartwatches discussed

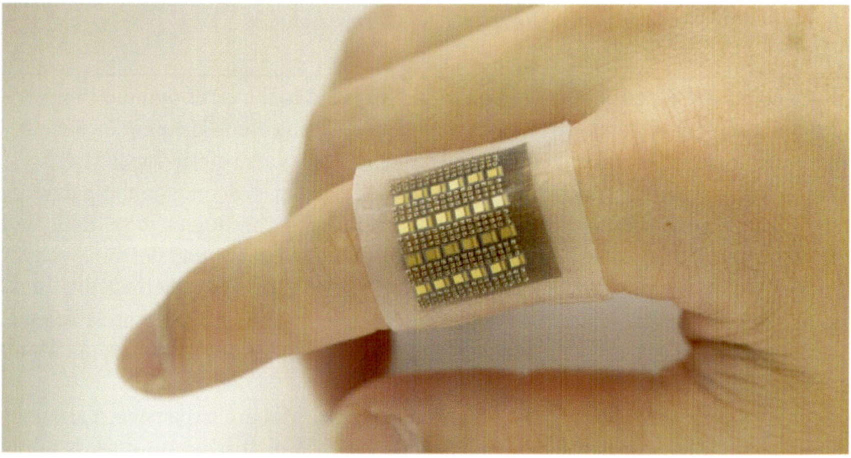

Fig. 14.3 Photoacoustic skin sensors such as that depicted above could be useful in diagnosing tumors, monitoring peripheral perfusion, and diagnosing angiopathies. Photo by Xiaxiang Gao for the Jacobs School of Engineering at UC San Diego

previously, are able to identify key arrhythmias and keep track of heart rate [8]. By measuring your own heart rate when you exercise, such smartwatches are able to provide detailed information on the effects of the exercise itself, and identifying atrial fibrillation at onset can help prevent serious complications.

Another example of a wearable device, skin-adhesive electronic patches can help evaluate conditions relating to the skin superficially and deep by measuring hemoglobin concentration, temperature, and even the biomarkers present in such areas [39]. Hemoglobin measurements, in addition to diagnosing anemia, could be used to monitor perfusion throughout the body. By utilizing photoacoustic patches, in-vivo 3D imaging of blood vessels can be created to identify occlusions and other angiopathies (Fig. 14.3).

Other devices are able to bloody cysts that may be at risk of developing into malignant tumors, and they can compound this finding by uncovering biomarkers related to malignant and premalignant tumors [39]. From a dermatology stance, this could help identify melanoma before it becomes malignant and causes substantial damage systemically. As addressed previously, this time-to-recognition of melanoma could make an astronomical difference on maintaining patient health. As time progresses, more and more devices will be accessible to patients to assess their dermatologic conditions and determine whether they need to be checked by a doctor due to abnormal levels. These devices and digital biomarkers are not only changing the game for dermatology, but for all of health care.

14.3.8 Digital Spatial Profiler

The last method of collection that will be discussed is digital spatial profilers. Digital spatial profiling (DSP) is a platform that allows high-plex profiling at the protein and RNA level [40]. Whereas traditional cancer treatments tend to focus primarily on tumoral cells, this type of platform focuses on the tumor microenvironment to give a more comprehensive understanding of tumor biological behavior and allow for precision oncology intervention. The tumor microenvironment, composed of malignant cells as well as the surrounding non-malignant cells and tissues ranging from immune cells to stromal cells to extracellular matrix, is altered by cancer cells to avoid anti-tumoral homeostasis mechanisms and optimize the environment for tumoral cell growth and proliferation.

An extremely practical application of DSP is the identification, staging, and treatment of melanoma [40]. As shown by studies, such as that conducted by Toki et al., DSP utilization has led to the discovery of numerous biomarkers associated with melanoma [40, 41]. In addition to its viability in discovering such biomarkers, DSP can be used to analyze tumor microenvironment samples to enhance the specificity and sensitivity of testing for melanomas and other cancer types, and they can be used during and after cancer treatment to gauge the efficacy of the treatments.

Key Points

- The field of medicine, from dermatology to emergency medicine to surgery, is constantly evolving to better ensure patient safety, maintenance of health, and optimize therapeutic response.
- Use of digital biomarkers can help detect, prevent, and effectively treat dermatologic conditions and thus provide longevity to patient lives and ensure improved patient health.
- Medical practice historically has relied on office, clinic, or hospital visits with physical examination and laboratory/radiological tests to obtain patient data.
- Digital biomarkers in dermatology and all other medical fields, used in conjunction with traditional patient data collection, can provide a more expansive and continuous stream of data in order to diagnose illness more rapidly, track the progression of a disease process, and monitor patient response to therapies.
- Different subsets of digital biomarkers include diagnostic, monitoring, pharmacodynamic/response, predictive, prognostic, safety, and susceptibility/risk.
- Methods of dermatologic biomarker collection range from traditional blood and urine biopsy to new microelectromechanical systems that can be incorporated into microsensors.
- Wearable smart devices and portable POCT biosensors can be utilized to analyze sweat, saliva, breath, tears, electric fields, and more as a form of noninvasive biomarker sampling in both clinical and nonclinical settings.
- Digital spatial profiling samples the microenvironment of tumor cells, allowing a more comprehensive analysis of biomarkers for cancer diagnosis and staging. This can be incorporated into melanoma recognition and intervention.

References

1. Baran SW, Bratcher N, Dennis J, Gaburro S, Karlsson EM, Maguire S, Makidon P, Noldus LPJJ, Potier Y, Rosati G, Ruiter M, Schaevitz L, Sweeney P, LaFollette MR. Emerging role of translational digital biomarkers within home cage monitoring technologies in preclinical drug discovery and development. Front Behav Neurosci. 2022;14(15): 758274. https://doi.org/10.3389/fnbeh.2021.758274.PMID:35242017;PMCID:PMC8885444.
2. Spring S. Best (biomarkers, endpoints, and other tools). Food and Drug Administration (US) 2016.
3. Califf RM. Biomarker definitions and their applications. Exp Biol Med (Maywood). 2018;243(3):213–21. https://doi.org/10.1177/1535370217750088.PMID:29405771;PMCID:PMC5813875.
4. Hessler M, Jalilian E, Xu Q, Reddy S, Horton L, Elkin K, Manwar R, Tsoukas M, Mehregan D, Avanaki K. Melanoma biomarkers and their potential application for in vivo diagnostic imaging modalities. Int J Mol Sci. 2020;21(24):9583. https://doi.org/10.3390/ijms21249583.PMID:33339193;PMCID:PMC7765677.
5. Dang A, Arora D, Rane P. Role of digital therapeutics and the changing future of healthcare. J Family Med Prim Care. 2020;9(5):2207–13. https://doi.org/10.4103/jfmpc.jfmpc_105_20.PMID:32754475;PMCID:PMC7380804.
6. Tahseen D, Nambudiri VE. Prescription digital therapeutics in dermatology. J Am Acad Dermatol. 2022;86(1):193–4. https://doi.org/10.1016/j.jaad.2021.01.057.
7. Sim D, Brothers MC, Slocik JM, Islam AE, Maruyama B, Grigsby CC, Naik RR, Kim SS. Biomarkers and detection platforms for human health and performance monitoring: a review. Adv Sci (Weinh). 2022;9(7):e2104426. https://doi.org/10.1002/advs.202104426. Epub 2022 Jan 12. PMID: 35023321; PMCID: PMC8895156.
8. Garcia-Gancedo L, Bate A. Digital biomarkers for post-licensure safety monitoring. Drug Discov Today. 2022;27(11):103354. https://doi.org/10.1016/j.drudis.2022.103354. Epub ahead of print. PMID: 36108916.
9. Coravos A, Khozin S, Mandl KD. Developing and adopting safe and effective digital biomarkers to improve patient outcomes. NPJ Digit Med. 2019;2(1):14. https://doi.org/10.1038/s41746-019-0090-4. Epub 2019 Mar 11. Erratum in: NPJ Digit Med. 2019 May 10;2:40. PMID: 30868107; PMCID: PMC6411051.
10. Plant D, Barton A. Adding value to real-world data: the role of biomarkers. Rheumatology (Oxford). 2020;59(1):31–8. https://doi.org/10.1093/rheumatology/kez113.PMID:31329972;PMCID:PMC6909909.
11. Kulkarni MB, Ayachit NH, Aminabhavi TM. Biosensors and microfluidic biosensors: from fabrication to application. Biosensors (Basel). 2022;12(7):543. https://doi.org/10.3390/bios12070543.PMID:35884346;PMCID:PMC9313327.
12. Senf B, Yeo WH, Kim JH. Recent advances in portable biosensors for biomarker detection in body fluids. Biosensors (Basel). 2020;10(9):127. https://doi.org/10.3390/bios10090127.PMID:32961853;PMCID:PMC7559030.
13. Nikanjam M, Kato S, Kurzrock R. Liquid biopsy: current technology and clinical applications. J Hematol Oncol. 2022;15(1):131. https://doi.org/10.1186/s13045-022-01351-y.PMID:36096847;PMCID:PMC9465933.
14. Honma M, Nozaki H. Molecular pathogenesis of psoriasis and biomarkers reflecting disease activity. J Clin Med. 2021;10(15):3199. https://doi.org/10.3390/jcm10153199.PMID:34361983;PMCID:PMC8346978.
15. Ramessur R, Corbett M, Marshall D, Acencio ML, Barbosa IA, Dand N, Di Meglio P, Haddad S, Jensen AHM, Koopmann W, Mahil SK, Ostaszewski M, Rahmatulla S, Rastrick J, Saklatvala J, Weidinger S, Wright K, Eyerich K, Ndlovu M, Barker JN, Skov L, Conrad C, Smith CH; BIOMAP consortium. Biomarkers of disease progression in people with psoriasis: a scoping review. Br J Dermatol. 2022;187(4):481–93. https://doi.org/10.1111/bjd.21627. Epub 2022 Jul 11. PMID: 35482474; PMCID: PMC9796834.

16. Brunner PM, Guttman-Yassky E, Leung DYM. The immunology of atopic dermatitis and its reversibility with broad-spectrum and targeted therapies. J Allergy Clin Immunol. 2017;139(4):S65–76. https://doi.org/10.1016/j.jaci.2017.01.011.
17. Renert-Yuval Y, Thyssen JP, Bissonnette R, Bieber T, Kabashima K, Hijnen D, Guttman-Yassky E. Biomarkers in atopic dermatitis-a review on behalf of the international eczema council. J Allergy Clin Immunol. 2021;147(4):1174-1190.e1. https://doi.org/10.1016/j.jaci.2021.01.013. Epub 2021 Jan 28 PMID: 33516871.
18. Mustafa AI, Ebrahim AA, Abel Halim WAL, Fawzy E, Abdou AF. Serum Soluble Intercellular Adhesion Molecule-1 (sICAM-1): a novel potential biomarker in severe acne vulgaris. Indian J Dermatol. 2022;67(5):512–17. https://doi.org/10.4103/ijd.ijd_387_21. PMID: 36865840; PMCID: PMC9971765.
19. Davis LE, Shalin SC, Tackett AJ. Current state of melanoma diagnosis and treatment. Cancer Biol Ther. 2019;20(11):1366–79. https://doi.org/10.1080/15384047.2019.1640032. Epub 2019 Aug 1. PMID: 31366280; PMCID: PMC6804807.
20. Thomas CE, Sexton W, Benson K, Sutphen R, Koomen J. Urine collection and processing for protein biomarker discovery and quantification. Cancer Epidemiol Biomarkers Prev. 2010 Apr;19(4):953–9. https://doi.org/10.1158/1055-9965.EPI-10-0069. Epub 2010 Mar 23. PMID: 20332277; PMCID: PMC2852495.
21. Chen CK, Liao J, Li MS, Khoo BL. Urine biopsy technologies: cancer and beyond. Theranostics. 2020;10(17):7872–88. https://doi.org/10.7150/thno.44634.PMID:32685026;PMCID: PMC7359094.
22. Berna AZ, DeBosch B, Stoll J, Odom John AR. Breath collection from children for disease biomarker discovery. J Vis Exp. 2019;(144). https://doi.org/10.3791/59217. https://doi.org/10.3791/59217. PMID: 30829338; PMCID: PMC6596991.
23. Nowak N, Engler A, Thiel S, Stöberl AS, Sinues P, Zenobi R, Kohler M. Validation of breath biomarkers for obstructive sleep apnea. Sleep Med. 2021;85:75–86. https://doi.org/10.1016/j.sleep.2021.06.040. Epub 2021 Jul 3 PMID: 34280868.
24. Condon EM, Londono Tobon A, Mayes LC, Sadler LS. Acceptability and feasibility of hair and salivary biomarker collection among multiethnic school-age children. Matern Child Health J. 2020;24(7):865–74. https://doi.org/10.1007/s10995-020-02926-2.PMID:32356128; PMCID:PMC7378972.
25. Fernández J, Jiménez C, Benadof D, Morales P, Astorga J, Cáceres F, Hernández M, Fernández A, Valenzuela F. MMP-9 levels in the gingival crevicular fluid of Chilean rosacea patients. Int J Mol Sci. 2022;23(17):9858. https://doi.org/10.3390/ijms23179858.PMID:36077255;PMCID: PMC9455966.
26. Ponzini E, Santambrogio C, De Palma A, Mauri P, Tavazzi S, Grandori R. Mass spectrometry-based tear proteomics for noninvasive biomarker discovery. Mass Spectrom Rev. 2022;41(5):842–60. https://doi.org/10.1002/mas.21691. Epub 2021 Mar 24. PMID: 33759206; PMCID: PMC9543345.
27. Brasier N, Eckstein J. Sweat as a source of next-generation digital biomarkers. Digit Biomark. 2019;3(3):155–65. https://doi.org/10.1159/000504387.PMID:32095774;PMCID: PMC7011725.
28. Todorov A, Torah R, Ardern-Jones MR, Beeby SP. Electromagnetic sensing techniques for monitoring atopic dermatitis—current practices and possible advancements: a review. Sensors (Basel). 2023;23(8):3935. https://doi.org/10.3390/s23083935.PMID:37112275;PMCID:PMC10144024.
29. American Cancer Society. Like on-the-skin labs, sweat sensors assess biomarkers; 2023. https://www.cancer.org/research/acs-research-news/on-the-skin-labs-sweat-sensors.html
30. Dubin, D. Rapid interpretation of EKG's. 6th ed. Cover Publishing Company; 2000
31. Bacaksiz A, Erdogan E, Tasal A, Vatankulu MA, Kul S, Sevgili E, Ertas G, Dizman D, Onsun N, Uysal O. Electrocardiographic P-wave characteristics in patients with psoriasis vulgaris. Ups J Med Sci. 2013;118(1):35–41. https://doi.org/10.3109/03009734.2012.744372. Epub 2012 Nov 15. PMID: 23153368; PMCID: PMC3572669.

32. Stålberg E, van Dijk H, Falck B, Kimura J, Neuwirth C, Pitt M, Podnar S, Rubin DI, Rutkove S, Sanders DB, Sonoo M, Tankisi H, Zwarts M. Standards for quantification of EMG and neurography. Clin Neurophysiol. 2019;130(9):1688–729. https://doi.org/10.1016/j.clinph.2019.05.008. Epub 2019 Jun 10 PMID: 31213353.
33. Davey Z, Gupta PB, Li DR, Nayak RU, Govindarajan P. Rapid response EEG: current state and future directions. Curr Neurol Neurosci Rep. 2022;22(12):839–46. https://doi.org/10.1007/s11910-022-01243-1. Epub 2022 Nov 25. PMID: 36434488; PMCID: PMC9702853.
34. Wilkinson CM, Burrell JI, Kuziek JWP, Thirunavukkarasu S, Buck BH, Mathewson KE. Predicting stroke severity with a 3-min recording from the Muse portable EEG system for rapid diagnosis of stroke. Sci Rep. 2020;10(1):18465. https://doi.org/10.1038/s41598-020-75379-w. PMID:33116187;PMCID:PMC7595199.
35. Al-Qazzaz NK, Ali SH, Ahmad SA, Chellappan K, Islam MS, Escudero J. Role of EEG as biomarker in the early detection and classification of dementia. *ScientificWorldJournal.* 2014;906038. https://doi.org/10.1155/2014/906038. Epub 2014 Jun 30. PMID: 25093211; PMCID: PMC4100295.
36. Chircov C, Grumezescu AM. Microelectromechanical Systems (MEMS) for biomedical applications. Micromachines (Basel). 2022;13(2):164. https://doi.org/10.3390/mi13020164.PMID: 35208289;PMCID:PMC8875460.
37. Kim J, Campbell AS, de Ávila BE, Wang J. Wearable biosensors for healthcare monitoring. Nat Biotechnol. 2019;37(4):389–406. https://doi.org/10.1038/s41587-019-0045-y. Epub 2019 Feb 25. PMID: 30804534; PMCID: PMC8183422.
38. Beduk T, Beduk D, Hasan MR, Guler Celik E, Kosel J, Narang J, Salama KN, Timur S. Smartphone-based multiplexed biosensing tools for health monitoring. Biosensors (Basel). 2022;12(8):583. https://doi.org/10.3390/bios12080583.PMID:36004979; PMCID:PMC9406027.
39. Gao X, Chen X, Hu H, Wang X, Yue W, Mu J, Lou Z, Zhang R, Shi K, Chen X, Lin M, Qi B, Zhou S, Lu C, Gu Y, Yang X, Ding H, Zhu Y, Huang H, Ma Y, Li M, Mishra A, Wang J, Xu S. A photoacoustic patch for three-dimensional imaging of hemoglobin and core temperature. Nat Commun. 2022;13(1):7757. https://doi.org/10.1038/s41467-022-35455-3.PMID:36522334;PMCID:PMC9755152.
40. Hernandez S, Lazcano R, Serrano A, Powell S, Kostousov L, Mehta J, Khan K, Lu W, Solis LM. Challenges and opportunities for immunoprofiling using a spatial high-plex technology: the NanoString GeoMx® digital spatial profiler. Front Oncol. 2022;29(12): 890410. https://doi.org/10.3389/fonc.2022.890410.PMID:35847846;PMCID:PMC9277770.
41. Toki MI, Merritt CR, Wong PF, Smithy JW, Kluger HM, Syrigos KN, Ong GT, Warren SE, Beechem JM, Rimm DL. High-plex predictive marker discovery for melanoma immunotherapy-treated patients using digital spatial profiling. Clin Cancer Res. 2019;25(18):5503–12. https://doi.org/10.1158/1078-0432.CCR-19-0104. Epub 2019 Jun 12. PMID: 31189645; PMCID: PMC6744974.

Index

R. Norman (ed.), *Biomarkers in Dermatology*, https://doi.org/10.1007/978-3-031-66513-4

V

GPSR Compliance

The European Union's (EU) General Product Safety Regulation (GPSR) is a set of rules that requires consumer products to be safe and our obligations to ensure this.

If you have any concerns about our products, you can contact us on ProductSafety@springernature.com

In case Publisher is established outside the EU, the EU authorized representative is:

Springer Nature Customer Service Center GmbH
Europaplatz 3
69115 Heidelberg, Germany

Batch number: 10756376

Printed by Printforce, the Netherlands